YO-AFI-863

AN ABSTRACT FOR ACTION: APPENDICES

AN ABSTRACT FOR ACTION: APPENDICES

JEROME P. LYSAUGHT, Ed.D.

Director

*National Commission for the Study of
Nursing and Nursing Education*

McGRAW-HILL BOOK COMPANY
New York/St. Louis/San Francisco
Düsseldorf/Johannesburg/Kuala Lumpur
London/Mexico/Montreal
New Delhi/Panama/Rio de Janeiro
Singapore/Sydney/Toronto

AN ABSTRACT FOR ACTION: APPENDICES

Library of Congress Catalog Card Number 73-126176

1234567890 MAMM 7987654321

*This book was set in Med. Theme by Universal Graphics,
and printed on permanent paper and bound by The Maple
Press Company. The editor was Joseph J. Brehm.
Eugene Capriotti and John A. Sabella supervised production.*

This investigation
was supported by the W. K. Kellogg Foundation
and the Avalon Foundation,
and by a private individual.

COMMISSIONERS

President of the Commission

LEROY E. BURNEY, M.D.
President
Milbank Memorial Fund
New York, New York

Vice President of the Commission

BOISFEUILLET JONES, LL.B.
President
Emily and Ernest Woodruff Foundation
Atlanta, Georgia

Secretary of the Commission

*ELEANOR LAMBERTSEN, Ed.D.
Dean, School of Nursing
Cornell University-New York Hospital
New York, New York

DOROTHY A. CORNELIUS
Executive Director
Ohio Nurses' Association
Columbus, Ohio

*Indicates members of Commission during study phase.

CONTENTS

INTRODUCTION

Every investigation necessarily produces a variety of materials and unintended consequences. In order to share these benefits — and likewise the adversities — the commission and staff early determined that there should be a set of Appendices to the final report that would present a documentary of our methods, our interim discoveries and decisions, and specially pertinent data that influenced the outcomes.

When one has spent three years in the company of a staff visiting hundreds of locations and talking with thousands of people, the information generated approaches overload proportions. Therefore, this volume represents a judgment process on the part of the staff. We have attempted to select the materials, analyses, and documents that we thought were most useful to the critical reader. The culling process began with dozens of files and culminated in the eighteen papers included here.

It is emblematic of the relationship between commission and staff that the former read, discussed, criticized, and eventually approved each chapter of the first volume of *An Abstract for Action*. At the same time, the commission unanimously agreed that the Appendices were to be the staff statement — and that absolutely no screening, editing, or intervening clearance would be exercised. As the director of a national inquiry, I don't know any better way of explaining the quality of our commission than by saying they decided this and abided by their decision. I hope they feel in reading these materials for the first time that their virtue has been rewarded. You will find in this volume no dissenting stands, no revelations, and no exceptions engineered by the staff. The *rapport*, from beginning to end, of our investigation built not only confidence, but full, open communications. Thus, there is no surprise between commission decision and staff exposition.

In the first volume, I tried to thank the individuals who contributed so much to the completion of our objectives. In terms of this set of papers, I must particularly single out a few of the staff who were particularly involved. Richard Huse collected, over the course of the study, most of the documentation used in these Appendices, and then turned writer to aid in their transmission. Charles Russell essayed the monumental task of analyzing and reporting the successive reactions to our findings and recommendations. Maryann Powers fitted into her schedule of tours to Ireland the development of descriptions of our regional meetings and other papers. Sydney Sutherland, continuing her Pilgrim's Progress toward the definition of an Assistant's role, found that this included the synthesis and reporting of several documents. Needless to say, all of the aforementioned completed their tasks — and on time. It is their probable regret that the director still maintains certain compulsive features of Marine Corps life, including a belief in deadlines. One can sum up staff performance in two words, "Semper Fidelis." For versatility, one could add with the Coast Guard, "Semper Paratus."

Having ascribed the virtues to commission and staff, and remarking on the outstanding performance of our secretaries, Jill Orioli and Kay Thompson, it remains for the director to accept responsibility for decisions on inclusion plus acts of omission and commission. I do not mind assuming such a role; everyone else worked too patiently, too arduously, and too loyally to be anything but praised. To them go the credits; to the director should be addressed the shortcomings.

With this publication we enter a new phase — that of implementing our report and its recommendations. Here we move from investigator to change agent. And here we hope to find the same support, the same exhilaration, and the same challenge that we encountered in our study. From these experiences will develop a new era for nursing and a new era in health care. It will be our enduring satisfaction that our commission and staff will have hastened the day for both outcomes.

Jerome P. Lysaught
Director

25 June 1970

STUDY STAFF

DR. JEROME P. LYSAUGHT
Director

DR. CHARLES H. RUSSELL
Associate Director

MISS SYDNEY ANNE SUTHERLAND
Assistant to the Director

MR. RAYMOND BURROWS
Research Associate

MR. RICHARD E. HUSE
Research Associate

MISS MARYANN E. POWERS
Research Associate

MR. HERMAN KAUZ
Staff Administrator

MISS GILDA M. ORIOLI
Secretary

MRS. JUDITH D. WHITNEY
Secretary

APPENDIX A

METHODOLOGY OF THE STUDY*

From the inception of our staff work, it was obvious that our inquiry into nursing would assume the dimensions of a classic descriptive study. There had been a succession of studies in American nursing that had contributed sufficient information to constitute the exploratory phase of investigation. At the same time, the requirements of problem parameters, population size, and economic exigency militated against the overall use of experimental designs. Nevertheless, the need to deduce certain kinds of causal inferences from the data meant that certain procedures should be done in experimental fashion and that all precaution had to be taken in the descriptive approaches to protect against bias and invalidity.

While research methods in the social sciences must frequently be non-experimental, this does not mean that they cannot be planned and executed in such ways that accurate and meaningful results are obtained. As Selltiz, *et al.*, admonish, "The procedures to be used in a descriptive study must be carefully planned. Because the aim is to obtain complete and accurate information, the research design must make much more provision for protection than is required in exploratory studies. . . . These considerations of economy and protection against bias enter at every stage."[1]

* Related commentary on this study is included in Chapters 1 and 7 of the final report.

The steps generally associated with a descriptive study are:

a. Formulation of study objectives.
b. Designing the methods of data collection.
c. Selection of samples.
d. Collection and checking of data.
e. Analysis of results.

Because each of these processes involves the possibility of error, it was essential from the beginning that some form of feedback system be regularly induced so that matters of both procedure and substance would be subject to review, criticism, and correction as necessary.

A form of programming was invoked to serve both as a conceptual scheme for succeeding phases of the study and as a safeguard against unintended bias or inaccuracy. The development of a critical decision path automatically divided the study into five phases:

I.   Preliminary Activities — October 1967 to January 1968
II. Intensive Planning — January 1968 to April 1968
III. Execution, Part 1 — April 1968 to March 1969
IV. Execution, Part 2 — March 1969 to August 1969
V.   Synthesis — August 1969 to June 1970

These dates are intended to separate the phases generally, but are not wholly deterministic. That is, they can serve as general guides, but since the activities of one period tended to flow into those of the following phase, not all tasks were completed at the point of interim separation.

Perhaps the clearest means of presenting the methodology of the study is to discuss each of the five phases in terms of its rationale, processes, and outputs. This will then provide both a conceptual scheme and an introduction to the various appendices included in this volume.

PHASE I. PRELIMINARY ACTIVITIES

On October 1, 1967 the Director of the study staff began full-time work on the project. The first efforts were necessarily directed toward acquiring additional staff members (Figure A-1) to serve as a nucleus group, and assessing the task to be attacked. Over a period of a few weeks, three core staff members were appointed: Dr. Charles Russell, Vice President of Bryant College; Raymond Burrows, formerly an opinion research specialist with the Xerox Corporation; and Richard Huse, a staff specialist with the Office of Research Administration of The University of Rochester.

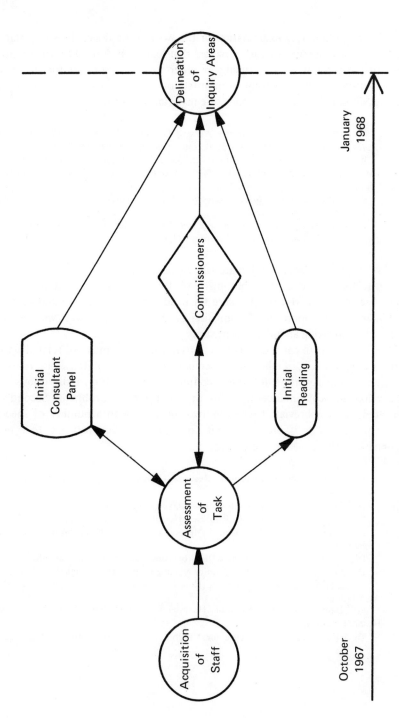

Figure A-1. Phase I. Preliminary Activities

In the preliminary examination of the work to be done, the study staff had the benefit of a number of earlier papers that had been drafted for the purpose of delimiting the problems of nursing in order to obtain support for the national study. Authorized by the joint committee of the American Nurses' Association and the National League for Nursing, the materials included:

a. A prospectus entitled *Better Nursing Education for Improved Patient Care and Health Guidance* prepared for the joint committee by Esther Lucile Brown.

b. A "Proposal to Foundations" prepared by the joint committee, including a statement and supplementary statement on objectives for a Commission on Nursing Education.

c. A paper entitled *Current Issues in Nursing* prepared at the request of the joint committee by Myrtle K. Aydelotte.

d. A report on *Studies in Nursing and Their Impact Upon the Nursing Profession* prepared for the joint committee by Joseph H. Cash.

While these papers and materials represented a valuable overview of the concerns that led to the establishment of the Commission, it is important to emphasize that these documents were the products of the joint committee and had no binding effect upon the Commission or the study staff who were given the charge of establishing an independent study proposal.

For the staff to carry out its functions properly, a number of related activities were planned. Each of the staff members engaged in initial library research, studying current government reports, contemporary literature, and previous studies to develop an acquaintanceship with the field and its problems. Secondly, we consulted in an abbreviated series of two meetings with a number of specialists whom we asked to sketch out and comment on the problems that needed examination. These meetings included:

Dr. Faye Abdellah, Chairman, Research Grants Branch, Division of Nursing, U. S. Public Health Service.

Dr. Blanche Geer, Department of Sociology, Syracuse University.

Dr. Mary Harper, Franklin D. Roosevelt Hospital, Montrose, N. Y.

Dr. George Hlavka, Advanced Systems Laboratory, Thompson-Ramo-Wooldridge Systems, Inc.

Dr. Wanda McDowell, Executive Director, American Nurses' Foundation.

Dr. Doris Roberts, Chief, Community Nursing Branch, U. S. Public Health Service.

Dr. C. H. William Ruhe, Secretary, Council on Medical Education, American Medical Association.

Mr. Daniel Schechter, Director, Hospital Continuing Education Trust, American Hospital Association.

Dr. William Selden, Study Director, Virginia Commonwealth Study of Nursing.

The wide-ranging discussions that took place gave us an opportunity to examine the kinds of problems that had begun to emerge from the literature, and also gave us a first glimpse into the variety of positions that had been taken by health organizations in recent years toward the difficulties of health care delivery.

Over this same general period of time we also contacted the core group of twelve Commissioners individually to keep them acquainted with our developing formulation of inquiry areas and to provide them an opportunity to reflect back their own insights into the field that was to be examined. By January of 1968, the staff was able to prepare for Commission examination a statement of purpose and a general proposal for the initial areas of study. From the prospectus, and from the consensus of the Commissioner's objectives, the staff assumed the following as investigative responsibilities:

1. Delineating reasonable expectations for nursing care and nursing services needed by the community.
2. Assessing the resources required for safe, effective and economical nursing and for the education of nursing personnel.
3. Identifying major obstacles to effective nursing and nursing education.
4. Assessing nursing education and services in terms of leadership and preparation required to provide high quality nursing care.
5. Recommending means for making quality nursing service broadly accessible.

To attain these ends, the staff initially formulated a plan calling for four general study areas:

1. *Economic Factors.* These include salary levels and fringe benefits which affect recruitment, attrition, occupational status, and job satisfaction; the costs of education, and the return on educational investment to the economy.
2. *The Nursing Role in the Various Phases of Health Care.* This must be defined in order to identify the objectives of educational programs. Traditional role expectations are being radically affected by changes in health care, but they still have a major impact on job status and satisfaction. Additionally, role requirements are a central feature of efficient manpower utilization in providing quality health care to all who need it.
3. *Educational Patterns.* The contemporary educational institutions provide a bewildering variety of routes into a complex occupation, differ in quality, produce graduates with varying preparations who must cope with rapid health and educational changes with varying degrees of adequacy.
4. *Organizational and Professional Considerations.* These are the agents and centers of controversy. They influence the establishment of standards, are instrumental in fitting the occupation into society, provide important means to introduce action and change, and are the guiding force in establishing legal requirements.

More specific information was contained in a 19-page draft proposal to the Commission specifying, for each of the four areas, the particular centers of interest, information on the nature of the particular inquiry, questions for investigation, and initial hypotheses. Since this was to be essentially a descriptive study, our concentration was on the formulation of questions to be answered, but since portions of the investigation could be expected to be handled through one or another experimental form, it was considered useful even at this initial phase to suggest hypotheses.

To illustrate the content of this first draft, the following examples are excerpted from the proposal:

Study C NURSING EDUCATION, PRACTICES, TRENDS, AND CHANGES

Centers of Interest

Perhaps the most incongruous feature of nursing is the variety of educational programs that lead to the same title, namely that of Registered Nurse. A nurse may receive this credential after pursuing an educational program in a hospital, or in a junior college, or in a senior college; following a period of 1 1/2, 2, 3, 4 or even 5 years and accompanied by no academic degree, an associate degree, a baccalaureate degree, or even a master's degree.

This variety gives rise to two of the major subjects requiring investigation. First, there is the question of the specific nature, degree, and importance of the variations that result from the different types of preparation. Second, there is the problem of transition from one type of program to another encountered by persons who wish to advance their education in order to rise to positions of leadership and greater responsibility. . . .

Nature of the Study

In making the study a stratified sample of nursing preparatory institutions will be selected. On one dimension, these will vary by academic level: university based programs, college programs, junior college programs, and hospital school programs. On a second dimension, the sample will vary with length of actual preparation. On the third dimension, there will be an effort made to select from varying geographic areas, and size of institution. . . .

Questions for Investigation

Once we have established the "sample group" we shall employ visitations, questionnaires, information from accreditation sources, transcripts, and other instruments to get at such information as this:

1. What kinds of students are enrolled in nursing programs? How do they compare with other students in multiple-purpose institutions? What is their attrition? How does it compare?

2. What kinds of individuals comprise the faculty? What is their preparation? What is their responsibility to the educational program, to nursing service, to their other duties? . . . .

Testable Hypotheses

While a number of hypotheses or research questions will grow out of the examination of data collected for the purposes above, it is still useful to suggest some basic points of view to be subjected to early analysis since they relate so importantly to the kinds of recommendations that the Commission may entertain. For this purpose, the following "null" statements are suggested:

1. There is no difference in practice between the activities of a nurse in a general hospital who has been educated through a diploma school of nursing and a nurse who has been trained in a baccalaureate school of nursing.
2. There is no difference in academic preparation between nurses prepared through a baccalaureate program and those prepared through a junior college or community college program.

As an integral part of this first approximation to study design, we attempted to formulate statements on the results we expected to obtain. At the conclusion of each study section, then, there was a listing of anticipated results. An excerpt from the area on nursing education is shown below:

Results

At the conclusion of this phase of the study, we would expect that recommendations could be generated in the following areas:

1. What institutional changes should be made in terms of nurse-preparatory training? Should some institutions be ended, others enlarged, or new ones created?
2. What should be the institutional roles for each of the institutions currently involved in nursing education? . . . .

The first phase of the investigation was concluded on January 21, 1968 when the proposal, its accompanying documentation, and auxiliary materials were transmitted to the Commission. Following a meeting with that body, and follow-up discussions with individual Commissioners, we were asked to prepare revised drafts of the proposals that would go into even more detail on planning.

One near-parenthetical note might be added. When the joint committee of the ANA-NLN prepared a prospectus for foundations regarding the proposed study, they had used the working title of the National Commission for the Study of Nursing Education. In this preliminary phase of staff work, it seemed obvious to us that the charges to the Commission were necessarily broader than the system for nursing education. For this reason, we proposed, and the Commission adopted, the title of National Commission for the Study of Nursing and Nursing Education. This seemed much more compatible with the total set of objectives — if, also, a bit more cumbersome.

PHASE II.   INTENSIVE PLANNING

Beginning in the latter part of January, 1968 the staff developed in rapid order a second and third draft of the study proposal. The second draft was an effort to capitalize on the suggestions and criticisms of the Commission while the third draft was a total re-working of the document for submission to the Commission for formal approval as a plan for action. Essentially, the second draft of the proposal was for staff notation and discussion while the third draft was the explicit document for Commission study. Perhaps the greatest single change in construction and treatment between the two papers occurred in the decision to modify the number of study areas internal to the proposal. In the first draft, we had spoken of economics, roles, education, and professional considerations. With the recognition that some duplication had been built into this arrangement, and with the benefit of the first feedback opportunities from consultants and Commissioners, we revised this to include only three areas:

1. Area A: The Nursing Role
2. Area B: Nursing Education
3. Area C: Nursing Career Development

In general, the former areas of economics and professional considerations were coalesced into the new Area C (Figure A-2). In addition, however, certain study sections were reapportioned among all the remaining areas and the proposal represented a re-analysis of all investigations.

In March of 1968, the completed redraft was submitted to the Commission. The research proposal now consisted of a 17-page general plan, similar in construction to the first paper, but showing evidence of reformulation. In addition, detailed working papers were developed for each of the three areas extending the discussion of plans and objectives. These comprised a total of 45 additional pages intended to give specific information to guide the Commission in its deliberations. To illustrate the added specificity of this third generation proposal, the following extract is taken from the working paper on the study of nursing education:

> In the remainder of this paper, we shall describe the methodology and instruments that will be employed in the first year, or year and a half, of the study in order to develop baseline data on Area B. This will then be followed by specific and conceptual investigations designed to formulate recommendations to be considered by the Commission. In order to emphasize the initial concerns that are involved in this aspect of the total design, we shall list the particular sub-areas to be included in the first phase of the investigation:
>
> 1. The educational institutions, their needs, problems, plans, and activities; . . .
>
> In order to obtain an appraisal of these various institutions, their current posture, and planned future, we anticipate approaching each institution on the basis first of a mailed questionnaire that would consist of two separate parts. One would go to the dean,

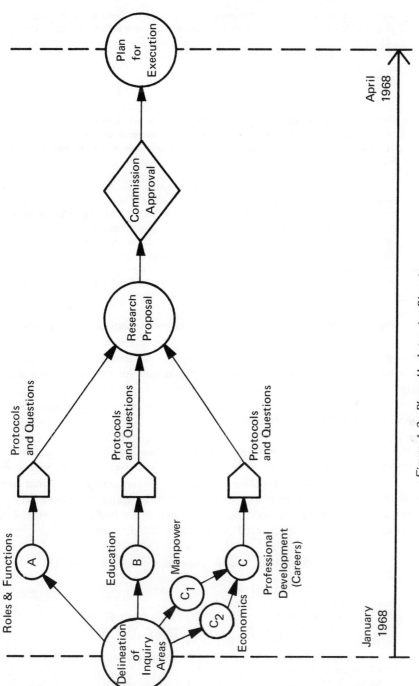

Figure A-2. Phase II. Intensive Planning

director, or head of the nursing program; the second would go to the head of the governing institution, the president of the university, the director of the hospital, the chief officer of the community college. From these instruments, we would seek to obtain these kinds of information:

A. Questionnaire to Heads of Programs

Each dean, director, or head of the nursing education program would be asked to reply initially to an open-ended questionnaire which asks him to list and describe the most serious problems facing nursing education, the most acute need facing his own particular institution, and to suggest the one primary change that he would like to see instituted to improve nursing education in his own situation.

It is anticipated that these replies may be grouped under one of five categories: finance-centered, faculty-centered, curriculum-centered, student-centered, or general problems. By coupling the compelling needs of professional nursing, as specified by the respondents, to the serious problems facing their own institution, we may be able to derive an almost quantitative measure of both need and potency of the several problems. That is, we should be able to distinguish basic, underlying problems that *must* be solved from those acute difficulties that ought to be solved or allayed in the more distant future. In this way, we may be able to develop some rational and temporal sequence of recommendations for the Commission to act upon. . . .

The "working papers" represented the essential plans and protocols for the conduct of the research, and they became the basis for the ensuing discussion with the Commission. By the end of April 1968, the Commission had formally approved the research design and had signified their willingness for the execution phase to begin.

PHASE III. EXECUTION, PART 1

With the formal adoption of the research proposal, the Commission also acted upon a number of other proposals presented by the staff. Two critical suggestions involved the appointment of continuing advisory bodies (Figure A-3) that could fulfill the function of consultants -- and do so over the entire life-span of the staff. With the concurrence of the Commission, two permanent bodies were established. The nursing advisory panel consisted of the following individuals:

Myrtle K. Aydelotte, Ph.D., Director, Department of Nursing Service, The University of Iowa.
Jeanne Berthold, Ph.D., Professor, Frances Payne Bolton School of Nursing, Case Western Reserve University.
Luther Christman, Ph.D., Dean, School of Nursing, Vanderbilt University.
Margaret E. Courtney, Ph.D., Associate Director, The Johns Hopkins School of Nursing.
Ellen Fahy, Ed.D., Dean, School of Nursing, State University of New York at Stony Brook, Health Sciences Center.
Katherine D. Foster, former Director of Nursing, the University of Connecticut Health Center, presently Nurse Coordinator, Boston Maternal and Infant, Children and Youth Program.

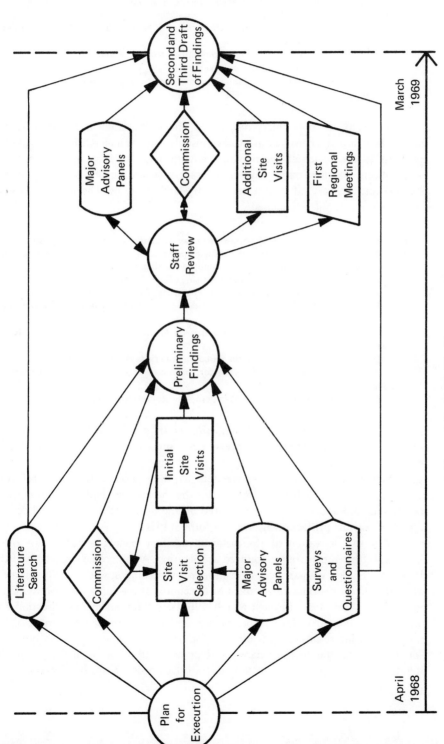

Figure A-3. Phase III. Execution, Part 1

Sister Virginia Kingsbury, former Nursing Education Consultant, Daughters of Charity of St. Vincent DePaul.

Beatrice Perlmutter, Ed.D., Head, Department of Nursing, Bronx Community College of the City of New York.

Doris E. Roberts, Ph.D., Chief, Community Nursing Branch, Division of Nursing, Department of Health, Education, and Welfare.

Kathryn Smith, Ed. D., Dean and Professor, School of Nursing, University of Colorado.

Because of the preliminary discussions, the staff also felt that it was essential that we have a permanent health professions advisory council -- not to provide the antithesis to the advice of the nurses, but to provide a critical input from those organizations that necessarily have to interact with the nursing profession in the planning and delivery of health care in the United States. The individuals who served on this committee included:

Stuart H. Altman, Ph.D., Associate Professor of Economics, Brown University.

Barbara Bates, M.D., Associate Professor of Medicine, The University of Rochester.

Charles E. Berry, Associate Dean, School of Nursing, St. Louis University.

Ivan J. Fahs, Ph.D., Upper Midwest Nursing Study, Minneapolis.

Robert J. Haggerty, M.D., Professor of Pediatrics, The University of Rochester.

Edmund D. Pellegrino, M.D., Vice President for the Health Sciences, State University of New York at Stony Brook.

William Ruhe, M.D., Secretary, Council on Medical Education, American Medical Association.

Daniel Schechter, Assistant to the Director, American Hospital Association.

William K. Selden, Ph.D., Director, Commonwealth of Virginia, Governor's Committee on Nursing.

Peter Terenzio, Executive Vice President, The Roosevelt Hospital.

In addition to the body of Commissioners, these two panels were intended to serve as our primary feedback centers. Each succeeding step of the study, its analysis of data, the specification of findings, and the evolvement of recommendations were to be presented to these bodies for their reflexive commentary and criticism. In this way, the permanent bodies could provide longitudinal aid and critiques — bolstered by the use of other bodies and devices intended to assure protection against any form of bias.

With the activation of the principal advisory panels, a number of other projects shifted into more pronounced acceleration. A comprehensive search of the literature, coupled with an analysis of other relevant studies, was formally initiated. While this effort continued over most of the course of the study, the twelve-month period from April 1968 through March 1969 saw the fundamental direction and execution of the work. (See Appendices F and G for a concise treatment of the more significant results of this effort.). Similarly, in conjunction with both the Commission and the advisory panels — supplemented by our own findings in the literature — we began the construction of a list of possible site visit locations. Our intent, of course, was to verify or refute by actual on-site examination a number of the claims and speculations that we had encountered over the preliminary phases of the study. (A documentary account of the site visit selection and activity is provided in Appendix H.) Finally, we began the construction of a number of surveys and questionnaires that were intended to tease out the information that was called for in the working papers of the third draft proposal for study design. These included, at this stage, a questionnaire for deans and directors of preparatory programs, a survey of the heads of harboring institutions, an inventory of nursing students and faculty, and a special report form for nursing school faculty. (Copies of all these questionnaires may be found in Appendix R. Discussion of the student and faculty questionnaires is provided in Appendices I and J. Information from the deans and institutions' questionnaires is treated in *passim* over the text of the final report.)

Particularly because the Commission was interested in the determination of the site visits — and the processes that were to be used in securing valid information — special efforts were involved in their participation in the screening process and in the development of site visit guides. To this latter end, a ten-page form was developed that contained general questions for each staff interviewer along with checklists for educational institutions and service innovations — all designed to facilitate the recording and analysis of data. A portion of this interviewing guide is reproduced below.

As indicated in the programmatic diagram of Phase III, the collected data from initial surveys, site visits, literature searches, and consultant discussions were collected in early 1969 in a preliminary set of findings. These were first reviewed critically by the staff in a series of day-long conferences, then transmitted to the nursing and health professions advisory panels. With these two groups, we invoked the use of Likert-scale reaction forms asking the individuals to respond to each finding on a five-point attitude scale. The findings, along with advisory panel commentary, were provided to the Commission, along with the same type of response inventories. Our strong feeling was that this kind of feedback device would ensure that each individual had an opportunity to reflect back feelings and criticisms while we would be able to get both a reading of basic agreement-disagreement and a measure of potency (strength) of agreement or disagreement. The Commissioners and advisers individually completed and returned the questionnaires.

In the same general time period, we attempted to expand our efforts at reality testing and validity measurement by invoking the aid of large numbers of individuals outside the compass of our advisors and Commissioners. The first series of regional conferences was held in the spring of 1969 (see Appendix E and Appendix B: the former describes the regional meetings; the latter details reactions to the second draft of findings). Actually, the advisory panels and Commissioners reacted to the first draft of findings; the regional meeting participants responded to

NATIONAL COMMISSION FOR THE STUDY OF NURSING
AND NURSING EDUCATION
208 Westfall Road
Rochester, New York 14620

INTERVIEW RECORD

Interviewer _____ Date _____AM
                                                                      PM

Institution _____

Address _____ City _____

Project or Program Title _____

Type (s) of Program or Project _____

Interviewee(s) _____
                                    Name   Title

_____

_____

_____

_____

Director, or Principal Investigator _____
       (If not interviewed)

Published Material (Collected, or to be sent) _____

_____

a slightly modified document constituting the second draft. From the total
reactions, combined with input from additional site visits and the literature search,
we derived the third draft of findings. This was, in turn, subjected to national
review (see Appendix C).

The development of the third draft of the findings, and their subsequent
presentation to the Commission represented the conclusion of the third phase of
the study. At that point in time, our findings, sources, and investigative questions
had been shared with over 600 individuals and organizations, including nurses,
physicians, health administrators, and consumers of health service so that we had

the benefit of their reaction and criticism as we analyzed the validity and generalizability of our work to that point.

PHASE IV. EXECUTION, PART 2

Between March and August of 1969 (Figure A-4), the major remaining portion of the investigation was completed preparatory to the drafting of the final report and summary. With the acknowledgement by the Commission of the third draft of findings, the staff began the transitional efforts toward the construction of recommendations.

The literature search was pressed toward a conclusion (although scanning and annotation was continued through June of 1970 for the 20 weekly, monthly, and quarterly journals that comprised our basic "current" sources). Appendix G provides further details and an annotated listing of some of the sources utilized.

Likewise, the site visits were completed with a very few exceptions, and these last were picked up in the early fall of 1969. The processing and analyses of surveys and questionnaires were accomplished, including the computerized analysis of the Nursing Schools Environments Inventory (Appendix I).

The first draft of the proposed recommendations was an admittedly rough document intended essentially for quick reaction by our advisory panels and our Commissioners. In addition to these groups, only a small local *ad hoc* panel was asked to react to this preliminary draft. This group included:

> Virginia Brantl, R.N., then enrolled as a graduate student at The University of Chicago, but serving as a faculty member at The University of Rochester.
> Mary Ann Eeells, R.N., then enrolled as a graduate student at The University of Rochester.
> Edith Olson, R.N., Coordinator of Nursing Programs, Rochester Regional Medical Program.
> Sister Victoria Nolan, then Director, School of Nursing, St. Mary's Hospital, Rochester, New York.

Their reactions provided us with useful information from student and practitioner points of view that aided us in editing statements for the second draft.

More extensive, and certainly more crucial to the entire scheme of the investigation, were the comments and reactions of the Commissioners and the two national advisory panels. As with the successive drafts of the findings, the individual participating in the reaction survey was asked to complete a Likert-type scale for each sub-portion of each recommendation. This actually meant, for example, that each Commissioner and advisor had to make over 250 decisions concerning the draft of proposals. Each decision was recorded in terms ranging from "strongly agree" to "strongly disagree" through a five point scale. To illustrate the transitional process involved in one area of the recommendations, we shall show

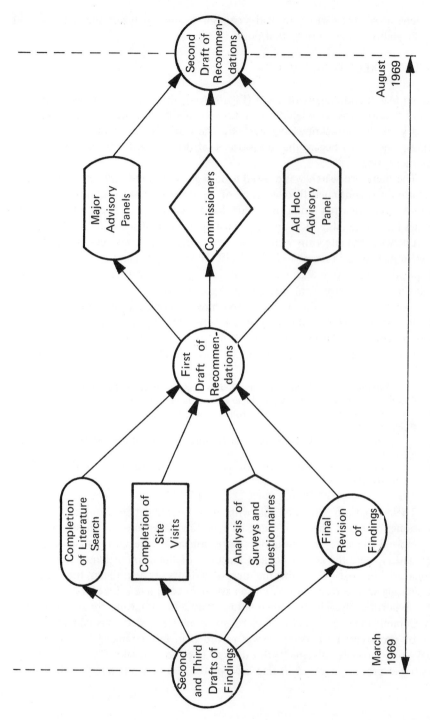

Figure A-4. Phase IV. Execution, Part 2.

excerpts from the same set of recommendations at succeeding stages of the feedback process. For example, the first portion of recommendations in the area of nursing education at the point of the second draft read as follows:

INDICATED RECOMMENDATIONS

Study Area B
Question Number 1

Trends in the institutional patterns for nursing education.

1. For a variety of reasons including cost, societal expectations and educational advantages, diploma schools of nursing should be redirected in their efforts. We recommend that:

(#92)   a. Those diploma schools that are strong and vital, endowed with a qualified faculty, suitable educational facilities, and motivated for excellence should be encouraged to become associate degree granting institutions;

(#93)   b. An *ad hoc* advisory commission be set up in each of the six regional accrediting associations to investigate and recommend requirements and conditions for the extension of degree granting powers to qualified diploma schools in their region;

(#94)   c. All other diploma schools, those that do not wish to apply for degree granting powers and those that fail to achieve the requirements of the regional accrediting bodies, be consolidated into a smaller number of programs involving a larger number of students in order to reduce the per unit costs of education and in order to make better allocation of qualified faculty;

Reactions from each of these groups were recorded and subjected to analysis and discussion. As indicated in Appendix D, succeeding drafts of the recommendations enjoyed a great deal of consensual agreement, but we were anxious to explore every indication of unsureness or disagreement to determine whether we had data to support the points in question. Moreover, we were extremely interested in the appended commentaries of our readers who suggested additional areas to consider, or bits of information to explore.

From this preliminary work, which seems brief in the description, but which was quite timetaking in the performance, we completed the revision and editing of the second draft of the recommendations, and eventually moved on to the final phase of the investigation.

PHASE V. SYNTHESIS

The second draft of recommendations was again transmitted to the advisory panels and the Commissioners. Two additional major evaluation groups were included in our feedback design at this point as well. The first consisted of small groups selected from the four major organizational units that had been involved in our data collection -- and ultimately would be among the most affected by our recommendations. These groups were:

1. The American Nurses' Association
2. The National League for Nursing
3. The American Medical Association
4. The American Hospital Association

Each of these bodies was asked to name a small group of representatives to meet with our staff people in work sessions to review the second draft of the recommendations (Figure A-5), and to complete reactionnaires for each of the points of each recommendation. The discussions allowed the participants to explore not only any and all of the proposed recommendations, but the background data and processes. The response inventories were carefully collated and analyzed, and the data was provided to the Commission.

Following these meetings, the staff prepared a third draft of the recommendations that took into account the responses of the Commissioners, the advisory panels, and the professional body representatives. To indicate the kind of shaping process that had been accomplished, the following excerpt shows the beginning recommendations for nursing education from that third draft:

NURSING EDUCATION

Study Area B
Question Number 1

Trends in the Institutional Patterns for Nursing Education

1. For a variety of reasons including cost, societal expectations, and educational advantages, the future pattern of nursing education should be developed within the framework of our institutions for higher education. We recommend that:
a. Each state have, or create, a master planning committee that will take nursing education under its purview, such committees to include representatives of nursing, education, other health professions, and the public, to recommend specific guidelines, means for implementation, and deadlines to ensure that nursing education is positioned in the mainstream of American educational patterns.
b. Those hospital schools that are strong and vital, endowed with a qualified faculty, suitable educational facilities, and motivated for excellence be encouraged to seek and obtain regional accreditation and become degree granting institutions in their own right.
c. All other hospital schools of nursing, those that do not wish to apply for degree granting powers and those that fail to achieve the requirements of the regional accrediting bodies, move systematically and with dispatch (under the guidance of the state master planning committee), to effect inter-institutional arrangements with junior collegiate or collegiate institutions so that. . . .

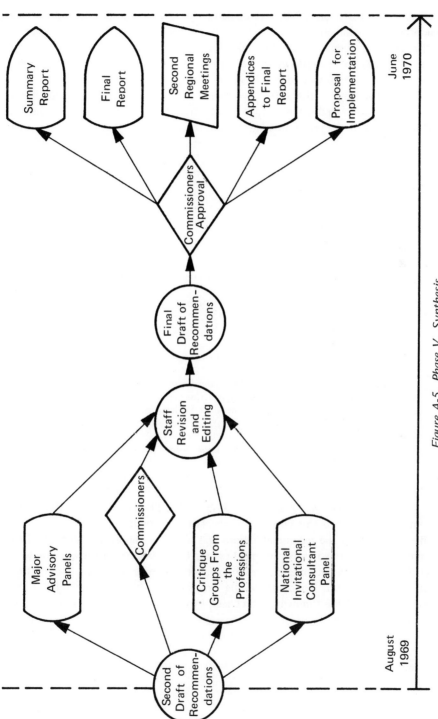

Figure A-5. Phase V. Synthesis

Upon completion of this document, the staff essayed one last outside feedback and commentary. Over the course of the investigation, a number of individuals had demonstrated their particular competence in areas that we were involved in studying, and had indicated their great personal interest in the outcomes of the work. In no way did this mean that they were endorsing — or even necessarily favoring — the effort we were making. With the approval of the Commission, we invited a panel of these individuals to come to Rochester, to study this third draft of the recommendations and react to them. Members of the group were:

ROBERT ABRAMS, M.D., *Director*, Clinical Research Center, Downstate Medical Center, Brooklyn, New York.

ALLAN C. ANDERSON, *Executive Director*, Strong Memorial Hospital, Rochester, New York.

VIRGINIA BARHAM, Ph. D., *Nursing Education Consultant*, State Board of Nurse Registration, San Francisco, California.

JOHN DANIELSON, Council of Teaching Hospitals, Association of American Medical Colleges, Washington, D.C.

WILLIAM DEMARIA, M.D., *Associate Professor of Pediatrics*, Duke University, Durham, North Carolina.

LOUIS DREXLER, *Administrator*, Worcester Hahnemann Hospital, Worcester, Massachusetts.

MARTHA PITEL, Ph.D., *Chairman*, Department of Nursing, University of Kansas Medical Center, Kansas City, Kansas.

JOHN SBARBARO, M.D., *Medical Coordinator*, Neighborhood Health Programs, Department of Health and Hospitals, Denver, Colorado.

EUGENE J. SMITH, The American Society of Hospital Nursing Service Administrators, AHA, and *Director of Nursing*, Charlotte Memorial Hospital, Charlotte, North Carolina.

MAMIE WANG, Outpatient Nursing Department, The New York Hospital—Cornell Medical Center, New York, New York.

A final effort was made to polish and edit the fourth draft of the recommendations, and this constituted the last staff input to this portion of the study. The draft of the recommendations was now transmitted to the body of the Commission, and in two successive meetings the Commissioners went word by word over each recommendation and altered, expanded, or re-arranged the draft to their unanimous agreement. To continue the example from the recommendations on nursing education, the following is an excerpt from the fourth draft as modified by Commissioner action:

NURSING EDUCATION

Study Area B
Question Number 1

Trends in the Institutional Patterns for Nursing Education

1. For a variety of reasons including cost, societal expectations, and educational advantages, the future pattern of nursing education should be developed within the framework of our institutions for higher education. We recommend that:

a. Each state have, or create, a master planning committee that will take nursing education under its purview, such committees to include representatives of nursing, education, other health professions, and the public, to recommend specific guidelines, means for implementation, and deadlines to ensure that nursing education is positioned in the mainstream of American educational patterns.

b. Those hospital schools that are strong and vital, endowed with a qualified faculty, suitable educational facilities, and motivated for excellence be encouraged to seek and obtain regional accreditation and degree granting powers.

c. Other hospital schools of nursing, move systematically and with dispatch (under the guidance of the state master planning committee), to effect inter-institutional arrangements with junior collegiate or collegiate institutions so that. . . .

With formal action by the Commission adopting the fourth draft of the recommendations (as modified in the Commission discussions), the staff was able to proceed with the final steps of synthesis. These actions included:

1. Preparation of the Summary Report that was published in the February, 1970 issue of the *American Journal of Nursing.*

2. Writing of the complete final report published in 1970 by the McGraw-Hill Book Company under the title of *An Abstract for Action.*

3. Writing of the present volume of appendices to amplify the content of the final report and provide a description of methods and materials.

4. Planning and conducting the series of 1970 Regional Conferences to inform the professions and the public of the report and recommendations of the Commission.

5. Developing a proposal for implementing the recommendations through a continuing staff and commission that would serve as change agents in cooperation with the professions and the public.

A summary report of the purposes and participation in the 1970 regional meetings is provided in Appendix Q.

CONCLUSION

Throughout the current investigation a determined effort was made to utilize not only a wide variety of sources, but to involve a broad distribution of individuals, organizations, and points of view in order to ensure that validity and reliability would obtain. This effort largely centered about the built-in provision of feedback throughout each phase of the inquiry as indicated on the several programmatic phase charts. While no investigation is fool-proof or absolute, the inclusion of frequent and sustained interactions between knowledgable and vocal bodies ensured that no opportunity was lost for correction, challenge, and criticism.

Essentially, while the Commission held final authority and responsibility for the report and recommendations, and while the staff had primary accountability for the conduct and development of the investigation, it must also be recognized that both these groups were the beneficiaries of the time and talents of literally thousands of individuals and organizations throughout the country. Figure A-6 is a simplified indication of the variety of inputs that came to the staff—and in no way accounts for the many individuals and groups that had access to the Commission over the course of the more than two and one half years of its existence. The staff accepts its responsibility for the development and conduct of the investigation—and for the methodology employed—but it also acknowledges its debt to the various constituencies that helped in the accumulation and analysis of data. Without their aid, it would have been an impossible task. With their help, the recommendations embody a wide consensus of viewpoints toward enhancing both nursing care and the nursing profession. Through such involvement, feedback, and critical examination, the report represents *An Abstract for Action.*

FOOTNOTE

1. Claire Selltiz et al., *Research Methods in Social Relations*, Holt, Rinehart, and Winston, New York, 1962 (Revised One-Volume Edition) p. 67.

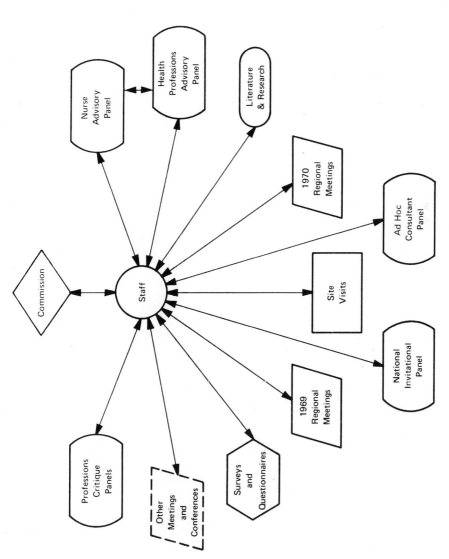

Figure A-6. Staff Interface

APPENDIX B

TABULATION OF REACTIONS TO THE SECOND DRAFT OF THE PRELIMINARY FINDINGS

A major interest during the preparation of the report of this Commission was to test the validity of the emerging findings against the thinking of other persons interested in the outcomes of the study. Such a process was necessary to acquire the accuracy of understanding required to make relevant and useful recommendations.

It was recognized that the test should involve persons representing the full spectrum of interests in health care, including the lay consumer, health planners, and insuring agencies as well as representatives of the various health professions. These persons would make a valuable contribution to eventual content of the report through exposure to the study findings at the formative stage. Their reactions would help to single out issues of particular importance or concern that would require special attention. Moreover, their participation would help to promote an exchange of ideas among those who would be directly affected by the Commission report, inform them of the progress of the study, and very possibly begin to build a climate of understanding that could help to secure acceptance and implementation of the Commission recommendations.

The method used was to adapt one of the procedures employed by the study staff to keep the Commission informed of the results of the inquiries in progress. The staff had prepared a set of questions and probable findings in each of the areas under consideration (roles, education, and careers) and submitted these to the

Commission and the advisory panels. Both the Commissioners and panelists were asked to record their reactions by two means: first, suggesting additional questions for investigation; and second, rating each of the individual findings on a five point reaction scale of agreement, uncertainty or disagreement. Each question and related set of findings was accompanied by citations to sources, such as books, reports, survey questionnaires, and interviews, that provided basic documentation. The respondents were also asked to record any comments if they so desired.

An initial draft of questions and probable findings was circulated internally to the study staff, Commission, and advisory panels. The second draft that was used in the wider survey and is reported in this Appendix incorporated modifications suggested by the initial review. There was a total of 30 questions and 99 findings in this draft. Area by area the figures were: roles, 10 questions, 30 findings; education, 8 questions, 36 findings; careers, 12 questions, 33 findings.

This draft was also circulated internally, but it was reviewed more widely at regional conferences held by the staff and at a program sponsored by the Upper Midwest Study Group on Nursing. Each of these various groups included representatives of the several parties and professions who would be directly affected by the Commission recommendations. The total number of persons who eventually returned reaction forms was 156. The numbers by group were as follows: Commissioners, 8; Health Advisory Panel, 6; Nurse Advisory Panel, 6; Conference Participants—Washington, D. C., 24; St. Louis, 30; San Francisco, 17; other conference invitees unable to attend, 36; Upper Midwest Study Group, 29.

OVERALL RESPONSE TO THE SURVEY

Perhaps the most striking result of the survey was the high rate of agreement with the statement of both questions and preliminary findings. *There were no suggestions for investigation of additional questions,* indicating that the study had addressed the main issues concerning nursing and nursing education as seen by a well informed group of persons.

A similar picture of general support appeared with respect to the findings. The respondents had the options of recording agreement, uncertainty, and disagreement with respect to each.* The overall rate of agreement (Figure B-1) was more than 74 percent, with only 19 percent uncertainty, and less than 7 percent disagreement. Only 6 of the 99 findings aroused 15 percent or more of the respondents to disagreement and 80 percent attracted 10 percent or less disagreement (see detailed reports by study area).

---

* Actually a Likert scale response instrument was used allowing for a 5 point scale: strongly agree, agree, uncertain, disagree, strongly disagree. This allowed us to consider potency as well as direction.

OVERALL REACTIONS

	Agree 74.3 percent			Uncertain 19 percent	Disagree 6.7 percent

	Agree (percent)	Uncertain (percent)	Disagree (percent)
Study Area A: Nursing Roles	79.0	15.7	5.3
Study Area B: Nursing Education	72.4	20.9	6.7
Study Area C: Nursing Careers	72.0	20.1	7.9

Figure B-1.   Synthesis of Reactions to Questions and Preliminary Findings in Survey 1.

Positive agreement was markedly high, especially when considered in light of the opportunity to register uncertainty as well as disagreement. Seventy per cent or more of the survey group reacted affirmatively to nearly three quarters of the findings. Only one quarter of the findings produced a combined response of uncertainty and disagreement greater than 30 percent.

Two major objections can be raised to counter this landslide of evidence of favorable response. One is that differences of point of view might have been eliminated through the involvement of some of the persons polled in prior discussions of the study. Those individuals who had had an opportunity to discuss the working papers with the study staff could have dropped their objections owing to their knowledge of the background thinking.

There is reason to believe, however, that this did not occur. More than a third (65) of the respondents did not take part in any discussions of the questions and findings with the study staff. These included the Upper Midwest Study Group and those invited but unable to attend the regional conferences. The patterns of response for these groups did not differ markedly from those of others.

A second objection takes in the general proposition that the investigation was so conducted that it would unintentionally tend to produce agreement. Thus the respondents might have all shared similar views before they ever saw the survey forms, or the statements were too general, too vague, or too innocuous to elicit any contrary reactions.

The evidence also appears unfavorable to such an interpretation. First, a substantial number of the findings did run counter both to established positions of major health professional organizations, which were represented among the respondents, and to what many persons think is the conventional wisdom regarding the issues under study. These controversial findings did in fact elicit disagreement, though not from a majority. Second, the rate of agreement for most of the findings was too high to support the view that they were vague, general, or innocuous.

Third, the respondents were encouraged to make written comments or express objections in face-to-face discussions with the study staff. Both types of exchanges resulted in genuine participant involvement that would not have occurred had the material under consideration been bland. Disagreement was forcefully expressed when it did occur.

Finally, the persons involved were chosen to represent a wide range of points of view regarding nursing and nursing education, and some were selected to represent different ideas than those expressed in the findings. Most, if not all the respondents were distinguished for their independence of mind.

Consensus Among the Fields Surveyed

Despite the above factors, a genuine consensus was evident that leads to the second major finding of the survey. It appears that there was a relatively high convergence of points of view among the respondents, irrespective of background or professional affiliation. This finding suggested the possibility that there is enough unanimity of opinion among persons concerned with health care to build agreement regarding the means for resolving the problems in nursing. The prospect held out for agreement and possibly concerted action among the major segments in health care led the study staff to make a broader survey. This second survey, reported in Appendix C, tended to confirm the original finding of consensus.

While the analysis of the over-all results of the first survey indicated agreement in general, it was necessary to examine the results in each of the study areas. This analysis was made to discover if individual findings required further study and revision. It was also made to identify issues or sets of findings that were particularly controversial and would require special consideration in the development of recommendations.

SURVEY RESULTS ON STUDY AREA A: NURSING ROLES

The most notable feature of the survey in this area (Study Area A) was the high rate of agreement (Table B-1). The average rate was 79 percent, with five of the findings exceeding 90 percent. This area also aroused little over-all disagreement, and a low level in those instances that did occur. The average was 5.3 percent disagreement, with a rate in excess of 10 percent in only three instances.

A strong consensus emerged with regard to the findings on trends and changes in health care and their impact on some aspects of the nurse's role. Thus, statements to the effect that the public will require more comprehensive and economical care, that technology will replace routine work, and that government activity in health care will increase, obtained 93 percent, 89 percent, and 86 percent agreement respectively. It was also agreed that nurses in the future will function as team members (89 percent) and share skills with other team members (94 percent), although it was felt that they will acquire additional unique skills (85 percent). The further belief was that they will take increased responsibility in care of the critically ill (95 percent), improve the integration of psychological factors with physical care (87 percent), and take more leadership in health promotion and long-term care (81 percent).

Two notable instances of particularly high agreement arose in regard to administrative aspects of the present role of nurses. One was the statement that nurses are currently expected to perform many functions apart from direct care of individuals, which attained 91 percent agreement, only 3 percent disagreement, and 6 percent uncertainty. The other, proposing that improved patient care will require departure from the utilization of nursing talent for non-nursing functions, drew virtually unanimous consent, with 96 percent agreement, 1 percent disagreement, and 3 percent uncertainty.

TABLE B-1. RANGES AND MEANS—STUDY AREA A: NURSING ROLES

	Mean (percent)	Range (percent)
Agree	79.0	44 to 96
Uncertain	15.7	2 to 55
Disagree	5.3	1 to 12

Another notable instance was the reaction to the statement that nursing should be defined into levels according to the scope of responsibility in various positions rather than divided into "professional" and "technical" classes. This statement might have elicited strong disagreement from the nursing group because it differed from the official position of the American Nurses' Association, which had endorsed the concept of professional and technical categories. Despite this difference, there was 76 percent agreement, 17 percent uncertainty, and only 7 percent disagreement.

Uncertainty arose both in regard to certain specific changes in the role of the nurse and to the effects of technology. Thus the proposition that communication technology will increase personal contact and quality of treatment drew 69 percent agreement but 23 percent uncertainty and 8 percent disagreement. That technological advance will cause nurses to have more responsibility for observation and assessment of illness, only secured 66 percent agreement but 30 percent uncertainty. A rate of 26 percent uncertainty and 12 percent disagreement—the high disagreement figure for this study area—was accorded to the statement that nurses will increasingly be concerned with cost control. Comparatively great uncertainty occurred over the prediction that the nurse would function in a role of patient advocate, with 24 percent uncertainty but 71 percent agreement.

One of the higher instances of disagreement (11 percent) accompanied by uncertainty (24 percent) was registered to the statement that men will serve equally as well as women in most health care situations. Despite 74 percent support, one of the higher rates of disagreement (12 percent) occurred also in regard to the finding that nurses will develop working familiarity with computers. The highest rate of uncertainty in the area, 55 percent, arose in regard to perception of innovations, and apparently occurred as a result of indecision about how to interpret the findings stated.

A series of questions and findings pertaining to innovations in health care earned somewhat lower support and greater uncertainty than many of the others. Seventy-eight percent accord was granted to the proposition that public support in the future would tend to foster mass health care approaches and non-profit organizations. Less agreement was registered to two statements concerning organizational response to innovations. These were, that conflict between established and new community organizations would in some instances foster and in others inhibit experimentation (75 percent agreement), and that recently established health power structures might be more receptive to initiating new services than older existing services would be (74 percent agreement).

In summary, the highest degree of agreement in this study area concerned the larger trends in health care and their impact on the role of the nurse. Change in the health system was anticipated, particularly with regard to the need to modify practices to permit nurses to concentrate their efforts on care activities. The consensus was that nurses in the future would enter into a more significant role on the health team, and assume rising levels of responsibility. Acknowledgement of these changes reflected a general concern with meeting the public needs for health care.

SURVEY RESULTS ON STUDY AREA B: NURSING EDUCATION

The issues regarding nursing education (Study Area B) were generally acknowledged to be the most controversial in the entire study. Here the likelihood of sharp disagreement and a low level of agreement seemed great. Yet, the reactions to the findings (Table B-2) in this area were highly affirmative, with an average of 72.4 percent agreement and only 6.7 percent disagreement. A slight shift toward greater uncertainty, much of it due to lack of information on the part of some respondents, was the only difference between the response to this study area and to the area of the nurse's role (20.9 percent compared to 15.7 percent).

The first question concerned trends and major issues in nursing education. Here the findings on the future of the diploma school were expected to produce strongly divergent opinions. Three key findings dealt with the subject. All drew overwhelming support, with at least 90 percent agreement and no more than 3 percent disagreement in any case. The statements were: the number of diploma schools will continue to fall for a combination of social, economic, and educational

TABLE B-2. RANGES AND MEANS—STUDY AREA B: NURSING EDUCATION

	Mean *(percent)*	*Range* *(percent)*
Agree	72.4	44 to 94
Uncertain	20.9	3 to 48
Disagree	6.7	2 to 20

reasons; stronger hospital schools will work out cooperative arrangements with institutions of higher education; community junior colleges will show the greatest rate of growth in establishing nursing education programs. The only question seems to have been over the pace of change, for to the statement, "little in the way of 'revolutionary' institutional change seems likely," there was 60 percent agreement, 23 percent uncertainty, and 17 percent disagreement.

Markedly strong support also appeared for the assertion that health care facilities must assume greater responsibility for extended orientation and on-the-job training for new nurses (93 percent agreement). However, the proposition that junior college programs lack satisfactory clinical preparation for their students encountered an unusually low level of agreement (53 percent) and a comparatively strong demurrer (20 percent) along with relatively great uncertainty (27 percent). There was fairly high concurrence (74 percent) that nursing education programs cannot meet the numerical demand for graduates.

The findings about the major problems in nursing education also rated a high level of agreement. These included statements establishing an order of importance for the problems, with a strong consensus that lack of qualified faculty precedes inadequate financial support.

The statements regarding nurse faculty members did secure support, but were also subject to high rates of uncertainty. Written comments on the reaction forms indicated that the uncertainty was due primarily to lack of information on the part of some respondents. The highest levels of agreement occurred in response to the statements that nurse faculty members lack research competence (65 percent) and that graduate study opportunities are restricted and limited chiefly to content in education and administration (60 percent).

Other findings related to those regarding nursing faculty appeared in two sets of questions, one on graduate programs and the other on continuing education for nurses in practice. These responses showed strong endorsement for the need for advanced education (75 percent) but also above average disagreement (12 percent). Support of the need for continuing education was nearly unanimous (93 percent). Very little disagreement was registered to the propositions that nurses must assume more personal responsibility for maintaining pace with advancing knowledge and that colleges will develop centers for continuing education of nurses (2 percent, 3 percent disagreement).

Two questions dealt with the matters of curriculum and development of allied health programs. In regard to curriculum, the respondents endorsed and expressed virtually no disagreement to the finding that there is growing emphasis on preparing nurses as clinical practitioners rather than educators or administrators (83 percent and 1 percent). Above average agreement and little disagreement also arose concerning the finding that few institutions are making large scale and systematically evaluated curriculum changes (75 percent and 4 percent). The high rates of uncertainty in the latter instance and in the findings on recent growth of research courses and honors programs were again due to lack of information on the part of some respondents.

The probability that some allied health schools will subsume preparation of nurses gained 67 percent agreement but 9 percent opposition and 24 percent uncertainty. However, the finding that efforts to develop a core curriculum in health sciences have not succeeded secured only 41 percent agreement, 12 percent disagreement, and 47 percent uncertainty. A statement noting increasing independence of junior and community colleges in organizing health curricula earned 64 percent support, 4 percent disagreement, and 32 percent uncertainty.

Students in nursing were the subject of one series of findings. Strong support arose for the proposition that there will be greater differentiation in the social and economic backgrounds in the recruits for nursing, with increased representation of the disadvantaged and upper middle class (87 percent agreement). Growing student discontent with traditional forms of nursing education was also anticipated by the respondents (85 percent agreement). The prediction that retention and completion rates for nursing students will improve drew 62 percent assent but a fairly high rate of uncertainty at 35 percent. Lowest support was registered for the statement that there would continue to be sharp differentiation in job placement among graduates of the various nursing programs (56 percent agreement, 20 percent disagreement).

Taken as a whole, the response to the findings on nursing education portend replacement of diploma school programs by college programs. Agreement peaked on the statements relevant to this issue. The importance of inservice and continuing education was also strongly endorsed, perhaps reflecting not just the rapidity of change in health sciences but anticipation of an expanded nurse role as indicated in the first study area. Stress on growth of the clinical component in nursing education was evident. The belief that students would be a significant factor in the press for new approaches was recorded. The probability that change in nursing education is imminent emerged as a distinct view held by the respondents.

SURVEY RESULTS ON STUDY AREA C: NURSING CAREERS

Study Area C dealt with the subject of nursing careers. The emphasis was on factors involved in the professional status of nursing that influence manpower, including the perception of nursing as a field of employment, salary levels, interprofessional relations, and the like. These subjects, particularly the issue of manpower, were also potentially controversial, but the current of response (Table B-3) was strongly affirmative with 72 percent agreement, 20.1 percent uncertainty, and 7.9 percent disagreement overall.

TABLE B-3. RANGES AND MEANS—STUDY AREA C: NURSING CAREERS

	Mean (percent)	Range (percent)
Agree	72	44 to 88
Uncertain	20.1	6 to 42
Disagree	7.9	1 to 22

In spite of the potential for controversy, two of the points regarding manpower elicited a high rate of agreement, both at the 85 percent level. These were that economic influences are combining with increasing complexity of health service to build a more sophisticated role for nurses, and that manpower planning must provide for both highly educated nurses and quantitatively large numbers of less well educated nursing personnel. In contrast, the statement that the need for large numbers of nurses might be reduced in the future through labor saving technology, better utilization, and related innovations, met a fairly high degree of disagreement, 11 percent, and a high degree of uncertainty, 35 percent.

Some statements relating the future of diploma schools to manpower and economic issues also secured a favorable response. These included the point that diploma schools will continue to play an important part in meeting nurse manpower requirements over the next five to ten years (88 percent agreement), and that in remote geographic regions they may do so for the foreseeable future (86 percent agreement). Statements to the effect that public allocation of funds for nursing education will grow as shortages reach a critical level and that inadequate endowment had deterred private colleges from entering the field of nursing education produced quite high agreement and practically no disagreement (85 percent and 81 percent agreement to 3 percent and 1 percent disagreement).

Two findings regarding manpower and education produced above average rates of disagreement and uncertainty. The first asserted the desirability of organizing programs in nursing patterned after the Master of Arts in Teaching or the Master of Business Administration in order to attract graduates of liberal arts colleges and mature women. Though 53 percent of the respondents agreed to this proposal, 11 percent disagreed and 36 percent were uncertain. The other asserted that since diploma school educational resources were substantial they needed to be considered in future planning, resulting in 9 percent dissent, 22 percent uncertainty, and 69 percent agreement.

The statement regarding men as a factor in meeting future manpower needs, though gaining agreement from a 72 percent majority, was subject to 18 percent uncertainty and 10 percent dissent. There was 10 percent disagreement and 19 percent uncertainty over the finding that more men will enter nursing as the rewards of the career improve. To the point that men will enter nursing if career information is properly presented there was 15 percent disagreement and 25 percent uncertainty.

The topic of career advancement elicited a high rate of agreement in part, but also some disagreement and uncertainty. The need for advancement was strongly affirmed, with 87 percent agreement. The proposition that the presence of levels of practice in nursing is conducive to career opportunity and that means for granting recognition to introductory levels of nursing have been inadequate both stirred 12 percent dissent though they did gain 74 percent and 76 percent support. The finding that a core curriculum could contribute to career mobility was subject to 27 percent uncertainty.

It is interesting to observe that although they did not attain the highest levels of support, statements favorable to constructive interprofessional relations did attract an affirmative response. Correspondingly, the highest level of disagreement in the entire study was registered on a statement contrary to constructive interprofessional relations. Thus 81 percent of the respondents agreed that hospital administrators recognize the value of a sophisticated role for nurses and will play an important part in the future of nursing, and only 4 percent and 7 percent disagreed. With respect to medicine, 71 percent agreed with the statement that physicians will favor a sophisticated role for nurses, whereas 22 percent disagreed and 34 percent were uncertain regarding a statement which implied that physicians were attempting to and would succeed in efforts to control nursing.

Another area of strong agreement concerned the consumer, where the finding that consumer influence over health affairs is increasing secured 85 percent support. A related statement, that the consumer is not now but soon may become a significant force achieved 77 percent agreement but 13 percent disagreement.

As with the other areas, some of the higher rates of uncertainty accompanied high disagreement or were caused by the fact that there were respondents who felt that they lacked the factual knowledge required to make a judgment. In other cases, genuine uncertainty prevailed. An instance of this type was the statement that shifts in control of health services (such as the rise of community boards) will hasten expansion of the nurse's role (25 percent uncertainty). Others concerned two findings on the influence of the National League for Nursing in educational accreditation and one on developments in the area of licensure, which had uncertainty rates of 34 percent, 26 percent, and 27 percent.

The general pattern of reactions to this study area included acknowledgement of the consumer as a growing force in health care. The tendency of economic factors to raise the level of the nurse's role was recognized, accompanying the support accorded in the first survey section to the influence of change in health care toward growing responsibility for nurses. Comparatively little hope, however, was registered for resolving nurse manpower problems through automation and technology. The need for career advancement in nursing was expressed. The respondents endorsed the importance of good interprofessional relations, suggesting an overall synthesis of the findings in this area around the point that the needs of health care in the future will only be met to the extent that the respective professions join in a common endeavor.

SUMMARY

In summary, our purpose in conducting this survey was to test the ideas being developed in the study, identify controversial issues, and share the thinking of the Commission with those who would be affected by its recommendations. We sought to fulfill this purpose by presenting the initial questions and findings prepared by the study staff to 156 persons representing the full range of the parties involved. We secured their judgments through written comments, reactions recorded on a scale of agreement and disagreement, and through face-to-face discussions.

This procedure revealed that the respondents were generally in agreement with the preliminary questions and findings of the study staff. No additional questions were suggested. Agreement with the great majority of the findings was strong; disagreement was low; uncertainty was greatest where the respondents lacked information on specific details. Variation in the responses to the individual areas of the study—nursing roles, education, and careers—represented a modest shift toward greater uncertainty rather than increased disagreement. No area of the study was found to contain a greatly different response pattern from the other areas of inquiry.

The major area of agreement concerned the prospective changes in the health care system. These included a growing demand for health care, enlarged health promotion service, increased use of a team approach, and greater application of technology. Consensus was also indicated regarding the related subjects of greater consumer activity in decisions affecting health care and a growing need for continuing education.

Findings regarding the potentially controversial issue of the future of the diploma school secured strong support. Thus there was almost universal agreement with the proposition that the number of diploma schools will continue to fall in the years ahead. The finding that there is an acute shortage of nurse faculty members was also accorded a high rate of support, indicating that the preparation of nurses by well qualified persons will remain a priority need despite any future decline in numbers of programs.

Findings regarding the quantity and quality of nurses which might have produced controversy also obtained support. There was general acknowledgement that preparation of clinical leaders in nursing along with substantial numbers of other persons are required to meet the needs for numbers of nurses to perform the various kinds of roles. The importance of good interprofessional relations to develop the role of nurses to meet future health care needs was also indicated.

While support for the study findings was strong throughout, the largest degree of uncertainty and disagreement appeared to concern the pace of change and the specific details of change. Generally speaking, however, the respondents seemed to anticipate steady development rather than a sudden or radical departure from present practice.

The results of this survey also indicated how certain of the findings could be restated to increase the relevance of the eventual recommendations to the future of health care. More importantly, they revealed the possibility that a consensus might be developed among the major professional groups involved. The further analysis of the findings, therefore, was projected through a survey of national organizations reported in the next section of these appendices. If the evidence of consensus continued to show in this survey, a critical aspect of the Commission's recommendations would concern identifying processes whereby the various parties might work out problems together to meet the health care needs of the American public.

On the following pages, an itemized list of questions, preliminary findings, and respondent reaction is displayed. For the sake of brevity and simplicity, the questions and findings have been somewhat shortened. A copy of the complete questionnaire constructed for the Third Draft of the Findings is provided in Appendix R and the reader can quickly relate the material provided there with the abbreviated version of this, the Second Draft.

TABLE B-4. DATA FROM SECOND DRAFT

Questions, Preliminary Findings, and Respondent
Reaction to the Second Draft of the
Staff Findings

Study Area A: Nursing Roles	Agree (percent)	Uncertain (percent)	Disagree (percent)
1. How will trends in health care and progress in health sciences affect the role of the nurse			
a. Technological innovation will replace most routine work	89	5	6
b. Nurses will work as team members	89	7	4
c. Public demand will require comprehensive, economical care	93	5	2
d. Nurses will specialize more	79	12	9
e. Communication technology will increase personal contact and quality of treatment	69	23	8
f. Government will be more active in employment, planning, and standard setting	86	10	4
2. How will the responsibilities of nurses change in the future			
a. Nurse responsibility in care of critically ill will grow	95	5	3
b. Nurses will give more attention to health promotion, disease prevention	82	12	6
c. Nurses will be more active in leadership of team in health promotion, long-term care	81	15	4
d. Nurses will become increasingly concerned with methods of cost control	62	26	12
e. Through use of technology, nurses will have more responsibility for observation and assessment of degree of illness	66	30	4
3. How will the future performance of nurses change? Nurses will demonstrate			
a. Improved integration of physical care and psychological assurance	87	10	3

TABLE B-4. DATA FROM SECOND DRAFT

	Agree (percent)	Uncertain (percent)	Disagree (percent)
b. Increased willingness to deal with personal factors in health care, such as fear of death	76	18	6
c. Working familiarity with computers, and uses of other technology	74	14	12
d. Greater responsibility for serving as the patient advocate	71	24	5
e. Capacity to adapt care to patient environments with same standards of quality	79	17	4

4. How will change affect the unique skills of nurses and involvement of men in nursing care

a. Nurses will share some capabilities with other personnel	94	5	1
b. Nurses will acquire additional unique skills	85	9	6
c. Men will serve equally as well as women in most situations	65	24	11

5. Will future patient care be improved by delineating nursing into "professional" and "technical?" Will nurses have an expanded role in psychological aspects of care

a. It is preferable to define nursing by levels of competence required by the scope or responsibilities of a position rather than by "technical" or "professional"	76	17	7
b. Nurses will increase their human relations skills as they assume responsibility for increasingly complex problems	85	11	4

6. Observations of nursing practice in innovative settings indicate that

a. Care for the seriously ill, deprived, aged, and young will be emphasized, but nursing may also need to give special attention to the "not-so-ill" to assure adequate care for this group	71	20	9

TABLE B-4. DATA FROM SECOND DRAFT

	Agree (percent)	Uncertain (percent)	Disagree (percent)
7. Can health care innovations be evaluated in terms of increased quality of care as perceived by patients and professionals			
a. Factors other than perceived improvement in quality of care, such as patient involvement in care regimens, easier access, must be considered in assessing innovations	44	55	1
8. Will development of health care require new levels of nursing skills and capabilities			
a. New settings will require skill levels and specialization that differ from current practice, but greater uniformity among similar settings. Some may require fewer skill levels, others more	84	12	4
9. Do differences exist between present institutional expectations of nurses and expectations in innovations; how can these be resolved			
a. Currently nurses are expected to perform many institutional functions in addition to direct care	91	6	3
b. Improved patient care will require changes in these expectations and related institutional operations	96	3	1
c. The relevant changes must be initiated by health professionals and institutions or the public will intervene	79	17	4
10. What factors affect introduction and acceptance of innovations, and how will these influence the future role of nurses			
a. Public agency personnel through control of allocation of resources for innovation will foster mass health care and non-profit organizations	78	19	3

TABLE B-4. DATA FROM SECOND DRAFT

	Agree (percent)	Uncertain (percent)	Disagree (percent)
b. Conflict between established and emerging community parties will in some cases create an environment inimical to innovation and foster it in others	75	18	7
c. Established health power structures, acceding to community wishes, will attempt to provide new services that may be more receptive to innovation than existing services	74	21	5

Study Area B: Nursing Education

1. What are the discernible trends in the institutional patterns for the preparation of nurses? Which educational institutions, or groupings of institutions, will be changing? What will be the nature of those changes

	Agree (percent)	Uncertain (percent)	Disagree (percent)
a. The number of hospital schools of nursing will continue to be reduced for a combination of economic, social, and educational reasons	94	3	3
b. The larger and stronger hospital schools will work out cooperative programs with institutions of higher education	92	6	2
c. The greatest growth among institutions will be that of the community junior college with more of them becoming engaged in the health field	90	7	3
d. The community and junior college programs characteristically lack satisfactory clinical training for their students	53	27	20
e. In all likelihood, the combined output of all institutions (based on current and projected figures) will be inadequate to provide needed supply	75	19	6
f. Little in the way of "revolutionary" institutional change seems likely	60	23	17

TABLE B-4. DATA FROM SECOND DRAFT

	Agree (percent)	Uncertain (percent)	Disagree (percent)
g. Some hospital schools of nursing will reduce the length of their program from three to two and one-half years	54	38	8
h. Hospitals and other health care facilities must assume responsibility for extended orientation and on-the-job training programs for first-time nurse employees	93	4	3

2. What are the most pressing problems and needs currently of nursing preparatory institutions? What are short-term and long-term answers to these needs

a. Probably the single most pressing need is for qualified faculty—with no quick or easy solution in sight	87	7	6
b. Finances rate a close second. Nursing schools are distinguished by lack of endowment, high costs in comparison to many other institutions (arts and science, for example)	87	10	3
c. Other problems include: lack (and geographic maldistribution) of qualified student applicants; hospital schools untilled; some other schools having to turn away qualified students	75	17	8

3. What are the strengths, weaknesses and trends among nursing faculty?

a. Over one out of five faculty members do not have a college degree	44	48	8
b. Over three out of five have no better than baccalaureate preparation	54	42	4
c. Graduate opportunities are restricted and most frequently aimed at limited educational objectives	60	28	12

TABLE B-4. DATA FROM SECOND DRAFT

	Agree (percent)	Uncertain (percent)	Disagree (percent)
d. Nurse faculty members do not have research competence	65	25	10
e. There is little experimentation in applying innovative changes in teaching methodology	58	25	17

4. What changes are taking place among the body of nursing students in terms of academic excellence, differing socio-economic-racial background, etc.? What effects will this have on future institutions educating nurses

a. Wider range of socio-economic groups being drawn into nursing with upper middle class entering collegiate programs and disadvantaged students being more actively recruited at all levels	87	9	4
b. Slightly higher completion and retention rates for nursing students will be projected	62	35	3
c. Student unrest and discontent with many of the traditional institutions and programs will become manifest	85	10	5
d. Continued sharp differentiation in job placement among graduates of different preparatory programs	56	24	20

5. What changes are taking place in, or are being recommended for, the nursing curriculum

a. Few institutions are really involved in large-scale changes, and many of these are relatively uncontrolled for purposes of measurement and evaluation	75	21	4

TABLE B-4. DATA FROM SECOND DRAFT

	Agree (percent)	Uncertain (percent)	Disagree (percent)
b. One rather clear trend, however, lies in the direction of more and better preparation toward the role of the nurse clinician. This will include different and higher skills than are now being "trained for" in some instances, but will be more patient centered than some programs that seem designed for education or administration	83	16	1
c. A few schools are beginning to introduce research methods and basic statistics in curriculum	60	39	1
d. A few schools are developing "honors" programs for students	49	49	2

6. What changes are taking place in other "health schools" that will affect the future of nursing education

	Agree (percent)	Uncertain (percent)	Disagree (percent)
a. The probability is increasing that there will be a number of allied health schools that will attempt to subsume the preparation of nurse practitioners	67	24	9
b. That most attempts at the development of a core curriculum in the health sciences have been unsuccessful and that less and less of the core is being taught to all students	41	47	12
c. That junior and community colleges are becoming more independent and self-directed in their development of health curricula	64	32	4

TABLE B-4. DATA FROM SECOND DRAFT

	Agree (percent)	Uncertain (percent)	Disagree (percent)
7. What are the needs for advanced (either graduate or specialized) education in nursing			
a. Advanced education is among the most critical needs in all nursing	78	10	12
b. Qualified faculty are well-nigh unobtainable	71	21	8
c. Imperative need for advanced clinical education	83	14	3
d. Inadequate funds, finances, student aid, etc.	78	14	8
8. What are the needs for continuing and in-service education in nursing in order to provide for up-dating and up-grading			
a. New aspects of health care and delivery are going to increase the variety and rapidity of in-service education	93	4	3
b. Social change will place increased emphasis on continuing education and the development of better articulated career ladder types of opportunity	93	4	3
c. The need for increased numbers of qualified "faculty" for in-service education will likely be greater than the current number of faculty engaged in hospital schools of nursing. Qualifications will be higher. Shortages will be even more exaggerated	76	21	3
d. Colleges and universities will expand and/or establish continuing education centers for professional nurses	83	14	3
e. The individual professional nurse must assume greater responsibility for her own development of expertise than that which is presently expected of the employer	83	15	2

TABLE B-4. DATA FROM SECOND DRAFT	Agree (percent)	Uncertain (percent)	Disagree (percent)
Study Area C: Nursing Careers			
1. What general economic factors are influencing the development of the nurse's functions, and what is the significance of these combined forces for manpower planning			
a. Persistent manpower shortages, a rising level of nurse's salaries are compelling nurses into leadership roles, and creating a demand by employers for higher standards of education	71	20	9
b. These factors combined with increasing sophistication of health service are creating a more demanding role for nurses	85	12	3
c. Manpower planning should acknowledge the need to prepare two groups of nursing personnel: 1) highly educated person prepared at baccalaureate or higher levels to provide leadership; 2) large numbers of persons to provide routine personal care (associate degree of diploma school, vocational and other nurse training programs)	85	7	8
d. The number of nurses is below the need, but improved technology, concentration of nursing services in care activities, and related trends may improve the manpower situation	54	35	11
2. Are there enough spaces in colleges and universities to prepare the number of highly educated nurses needed in the future? Would the establishment of a post-baccalaureate program for nursing (similar to the MAT or MBA), attract liberal arts graduates into nursing			
a. The number of spaces in colleges is well below the number required to meet the need for personnel trained at this level	72	26	2

TABLE B-4. DATA FROM SECOND DRAFT

	Agree (percent)	Uncertain (percent)	Disagree (percent)
b. Women college graduates in the liberal arts, including mature women able to enter the labor force, would respond favorably to master's level programs in nursing similar to the MAT in teaching or the MBA in business	53	36	11
c. Accreditation standards of the National League for Nursing would permit approval of such programs	48	48	4
3. Do the manpower requirements for nursing personnel dictate that the diploma schools be retained and continue to provide graduates to fill nursing positions			
a. The diploma school will continue to play a significant part in the preparation of nurses over the next 5 to 10 years	88	6	6
b. In some geographic regions remote from educational institutions, the diploma school will continue to serve a function for the foreseeable future	86	9	5
4. What is the comparative magnitude of all financial expenditures for nursing education? Do the resources of diploma schools need to be taken into consideration in planning for nursing education in the future?			
a. The allocation of public and private funds to nursing education will grow in magnitude as the shortage of nurses reaches a critical level	85	12	3
b. Compared to medicine, dentistry, teaching, and social work the investment in nursing education is very modest. It is also low in relation to the importance of the contribution of nursing to sound health care	75	23	2

TABLE B-4. DATA FROM SECOND DRAFT

	Agree (percent)	Uncertain (percent)	Disagree (percent)
c. The endowment of schools of nursing is comparatively low; foundation support is also low. These factors are serious deterrents to the entry of private colleges into the field of nursing education	81	18	1
d. Diploma school resources probably represent the major part of the investment in nursing education, and need to be taken into account in future planning	69	22	9
5. Does the need to provide upward mobility in American society require the organization of a career ladder for advancement within nursing? Is it necessary to view nursing education as such a ladder to permit advancement from one level to another			
a. In a full employment economy upward mobility is essential to retain personnel	87	9	4
b. The structure of nursing into levels provides an excellent setting for implementing current public policy respecting career advancement	74	14	12
c. Lack of adequate means for the recognition of lower levels of education by higher levels has created excessively long periods of education and has discouraged upward mobility	76	12	12
d. Development of a core curriculum in all health fields leading into various careers could materially improve the possibilities for mobility	66	27	7
6. Do the facts regarding career patterns of women and nurses in particular indicate that more men need to enter the field			

TABLE B-4. DATA FROM SECOND DRAFT

	Agree (percent)	Uncertain (percent)	Disagree (percent)
a. In spite of increasing participation by women in the work force and career persistence by women college graduates, insufficient numbers can make the long-term commitments to supply an adequate pool of highly trained nurses	72	18	10
b. Men will enter nursing more willingly as the career improves	71	19	10
c. Men can be attracted to the field if career information is properly presented	57	28	15

7. Should the role of the advanced levels of nursing practice be expressed in state licensing laws by means of developing a license above the RN; or is the Academy of Nursing the proper agency to recognize this level of practice?

Should licensing laws be so designed as to require persons who hold the RN to complete the bachelor's degree? Should such laws also call for periodic demonstration of competence as a requirement for renewal of licensure

	Agree	Uncertain	Disagree
a. The Academy of Nursing will develop as one avenue of recognition of the advanced levels of nursing practice. The possibility also exists that special licensing or certification, as is now the case for public health nurses in some states, will grow, especially for practice in particular settings	67	26	7
b. Other professions, notably teaching, have brought about phased improvement of practitioners over a period of years through raising educational requirements. A similar pattern might have broad appeal in nursing	67	27	6

TABLE B-4. DATA FROM SECOND DRAFT

	Agree (percent)	Uncertain (percent)	Disagree (percent)
c. There is no requirement for demonstration of competence as a condition for renewal of licensure, but the issue is before all health professions and can be viewed as an important factor in improving the quality of nursing care	81	14	5

8. Does the national concern over the physician shortage and the effort within medicine to maintain and expand control over "auxiliaries" suggest that nurses will be converted to medical auxiliaries? In any case, are there indications that medicine will recognize the role of the nurse in terms of an increasingly scientific content and rising level of specialization

	Agree	Uncertain	Disagree
a. The evidence suggests that organized medicine is moving to establish and increase its authority over the standards of practice and accreditation of education programs for patient care personnel, and that this could extend to nursing. The possibility of such a development appears to appeal to some nursing groups functioning in special areas of practice	44	34	22
b. There is some support in medicine for a significantly more sophisticated role for the nurse which suggests that medicine will accept such a role if the case for it is properly made	71	24	5

9. Will the recent change in federal legislation enlarging the number of agencies recognized for accreditation purposes in qualifying for federal funds for nursing education weaken the standing of the National League for Nursing? Will it weaken efforts to prepare nurses for an increasingly scientific and specialized practice

TABLE B-4. DATA FROM SECOND DRAFT

	Agree (percent)	Uncertain (percent)	Disagree (percent)
a. Current opinion in nursing and hospital groups is that the change in legislation enlarging the number of agencies recognized for accreditation in nursing education will not materially affect the standing and influence of the National League for Nursing	46	34	20
b. Standards for the accreditation of educational programs will reflect the rising standard of nursing practice no matter what agency is responsible for accreditation	72	14	14

10. Is there an arena for resolving issues of preparation and utilization between consumers and providers of health service

	Agree (percent)	Uncertain (percent)	Disagree (percent)
a. The consumer is in the process of building representation through health insurance plans, third party contractors, federal departments and agencies, and Congress, but the arena for resolving issues of preparation and utilization does not yet exist	85	10	5
b. Under these circumstances, consumers are probably a neutral, although potentially significant, force in delineating the nurse role	77	10	13

11. What are the implications of current struggles (among community groups, levels of government) over control within the health field for development of the nurse role? What is the posture of Congress and other sources of support in health care (primarily foundations) regarding the emergence of an advanced level of nursing practice

TABLE B-4. DATA FROM SECOND DRAFT

	Agree (percent)	Uncertain (percent)	Disagree (percent)
a. Since hospitals have been the dominant agency in defining the nurse role, it is possible that a shift in control of the setting in which health service is delivered (such as to community clinics supervised by community boards) will hasten the development of the nurse role	68	25	7
b. Recent Congressional and foundation programs have provided funds for programs that would tend to develop levels of the nurse role	82	16	2
12. What part do hospital administrators play in defining and implementing the role of the nurse; and what arguments will convince them of the value of viewing a role for nurses as being at a complex level			
a. Hospital administrators have had and will continue to have very considerable influence over the role of the nurse	81	12	7
b. Hospital administrators will recognize the value of a sophisticated role for the nurse when they can observe, as in the case of highly qualified nursing personnel in coronary and intensive care units, it as contributing to the effective operation of the institution	81	15	4

APPENDIX C

TABULATION OF REACTIONS TO THE THIRD DRAFT OF THE PRELIMINARY FINDINGS

Following an initial survey of reactions to the issues and preliminary findings placed before the Commission by the study staff, the decision was to conduct a much wider poll of groups in the health field. The purposes were, as in the first instance to: test the thinking of the staff and Commission; identify points subject to particular controversy; and prepare the way for presentation and possible acceptance of the Commission recommendations. One new dimension was added to these purposes, that of testing the unexpectedly high degree of consensus shown among the different health care groups reacting to the original survey.

The results of this second survey (hereafter referred to as Survey II) strongly supported the results of the first survey. The response to the issues and findings before the Commission was overwhelmingly affirmative. There was marked evidence of an unexpectedly high degree of consensus among the fields represented. These significant results strongly suggested the possibility that major advances in health care delivery and strengthened relationships among the health professions might be at hand.

In view of these findings the reasons for the choice of the groups included in the survey are of more than usual importance. The decision was to poll state level organizations in the health field, supplemented by the addition of health insurers, planners, heads of nursing education programs, and directors of nursing service departments.

The state organizations were selected for two reasons. First, the persons responding could be assumed to have a wide acquaintance with the issues in the survey, but at the same time they could be expected as organizational representatives to reflect the thinking in their respective regions and fields: nursing, medicine, and health service administration. Second, individuals serving in state-level posts could be expected eventually to play an important part in implementing the recommendations of the Commission. Obtaining the views of such persons and providing them with foreknowledge of the Commission's work was essential.

The health insurers and planners were included both because they would be likely to approach the survey from the point of view of the delivery of health care and their importance as segments of the health care industry. The addition of the nursing educators and the service directors was made to gain the perspective of those who have day-to-day decision making responsibilities in many of the areas covered in the study.

The question of which persons to include in the sample, and the adequacy of the number of respondents needed to represent thinking in the health field, were, of course, considered. These will be discussed in some detail later. However, over and above the quality of the sample, no previous survey is known to have included all these groups in responding to issues as broad in scope as those represented in this study. The responses, therefore, embody a significant body of opinion in the health field. The numbers of respondents in each group were: nursing—26 state associations, 17 state leagues, 29 state boards, 143 educational program directors, 135 nursing service directors; state medical societies, 13; state hospital associations, 7; state health departments, 28; health insurers, 13; health planners, 20.

These groups were surveyed in the same way as was reported in Appendix B. An edited set of the questions and probable findings was prepared. For the most part, this was closely related to the original version; there were some changes in language and some added questions, findings, and sources, but none of the original points was eliminated.

These sets were printed and bound in booklet form and mailed with a response sheet to record agreement, uncertainty, and disagreement. The booklets also provided substantial space for individual comment. The instructions asked that individuals list only the names of their organizations, with no information that could lead to personal identification. As desirable as it might have been to have more detailed information on the respondents, it was considered important to assure anonymity so that each respondent would have maximum freedom of expression.

OVERALL RESPONSE TO THE SURVEY

The survey produced a very high rate of agreement. The contrast with the overall response in Survey I provides particularly clear evidence on this point. Whereas a majority of the Survey I groups had discussed the questions and findings with the study staff, the Survey II groups had not. Yet the rate of agreement of the first group was lower (74.3 percent) than was that of the second group (77.8 percent) (see Table C-1).

TABLE C-1. OVERALL AND GROUP REACTIONS TO QUESTIONS AND PRELIMINARY FINDINGS DRAFT III

	Agree *(Percent)*	*Uncertain* *(Percent)*	*Disagree* *(Percent)*
Overall Reaction	77.83	12.44	9.70
Nurses (350)	84.43	8.66	6.90
State Health Department (28)	84.48	7.78	7.73
State Medical Society (13)	74.75	13.78	11.46
State Hospital Association (7)	75.24	8.72	16.04
Health Insurance (13)	78.20	15.19	6.61
Health Planners (20)	69.91	20.56	9.52

Note: The overall average was secured by averaging the percentages for each group independently and then averaging the sum of these averages. The nurse groups were combined into a single figure because the groups were generally consistent with one another in their responses.

The evidence of affirmative response may also be observed by examining the rate of agreement for each Survey II group independently and contrasting these with the overall response to Survey I. With only one exception each Survey II group produced a higher rate of agreement than was registered overall in Survey I. The exception was the health planning group, where the high degree of uncertainty was an off-setting factor.

The overall rate of disagreement was low in this study, with an average of less than 10 percent, but somewhat higher than the overall rate of disagreement (6.7 percent) in Survey I. The group by group rates of disagreement were also higher. In this case, no group was an exception.

Corresponding to the large proportions of the groups recording agreement or disagreement, there was a general low level of uncertainty. The nurses, health departments, and health service administrators rated less than 10 percent uncertainty. The medical societies, though somewhat higher at 13.78 percent, had a lower degree of uncertainty than the overall average for Survey I, and lower than the figure recorded for any single study area (roles, education, careers) in that investigation. Owing to unfamiliarity with some of the factual details contained in the survey, the health insurers and planners necessarily responded with higher rates of uncertainty.

In view of the strong tide of agreement, a number of issues arise concerning the validity of this survey. These questions are generally the same as in the case of Survey I. The findings might have been innocuous and would not have provoked much disagreement under any circumstances. The respondents could have been persons who were interested in the survey to begin with and as such would have been favorably disposed to the findings. The groups selected might not really represent their fields, and, in any case, the number of respondents may have been too low to provide a meaningful sample.

There is reason to believe that none of these contentions has major substance. In regard to innocuousness, many of the findings were clearly controversial, dealing with topics on which professional sensitivities are well known. Others stated views that were contrary to formally adopted organizational positions. Reactions in a number of cases were strong and supported by elaborate commentaries. The rate of disagreement was, in fact, higher than in Survey I.

It is reasonable to believe that the respondents may have been more interested in the survey than non-respondents. It is reasonable, too, to assume that they would represent the full range of opinion of persons in their kinds of organizations and quite probably in their field. That is, persons who were interested in the survey would have been quite as likely to be in disagreement as to have been in agreement. Strong feelings in either direction would be equally likely to provoke a response.

Perhaps the most compelling point is the nature of the response from the health insurers and planners. These clearly showed less familiarity with the issues. At the same time, and partly because of the record of their unfamiliarity, they can be considered to represent an independent body of opinion. This group of respondents had no profound commitment to any profession's point of view, and undoubtedly represented a primary concern with health service and costs. As independents, these groups can be viewed as casting an objective vote, with distinct majorities confirming the reactions of their profession-related colleagues.

In light of these considerations it is probable that this survey accurately reflects both the thinking of the groups involved and the opinions of the health field practitioners in general. From a statistical point of view, it might be desirable to replicate the poll to assure a more randomized sample. It is likely, however, that the results would differ little from the present data. We believe, therefore, that significant segments of opinion in the health care field agreed to the relevance of the issues under study by the Commission and to the key findings in the three areas of investigation.

Consensus Among the Fields Surveyed

The results of the survey suggest strongly that a high rate of consensus exists among the groups in the health field. Table C-1 shows that the percentage differences among the groups are small. With the exception of the health planning group where the factor of uncertainty had a strong influence, the differences in overall agreement among the groups are less than 10 percent. The same generalization applies to disagreement.

Certain of the groups in the survey show nearly identical levels of response. The nursing and state health departments both had an 84 percent affirmative rate. The physicians and health service administrators were together in the percentage of favorable reactions. The insurers and planners both had a fairly high rate of uncertainty.

Despite these and other affinities, inspection of the results on individual findings (see detailed responses at the close of this appendix) shows that the groups tended to rise and fall together in their rates of response. When a finding was approved, it was often approved by large majorities of every group. When disapproval occurred, it was also generalized. Then, too, there were instances where groups, such as nursing and administration, which showed fairly consistent patterns of difference, came together on key points. This was part of a trend toward strong common responses on major issues.

REACTIONS TO FINDINGS ON STUDY AREA A: NURSING ROLES

The evidence of consensus becomes more specific as one examines the reactions to detailed findings in each of the study areas. The first area included findings concerning the development of health sciences and the health care system relevant to identifying emerging features of the role of the nurse. It aroused the highest level of agreement in the study (Table C-2).

The most affirmative reactions were accorded to broad statements on trends in health care and the emergence of a team approach. Thus, strong majorities acknowledged that computers and other technological innovations would replace much routine work, and that consumers will demand more comprehensive, less wasteful, and greater specialization in care. Almost 100 percent of all groups concurred that nurses will share capabilities with other personnel and gave high approval to related statements predicting team membership and skill in team work for nurses.

TABLE C-2. OVERALL AND GROUP REACTIONS-STUDY AREA A: NURSING ROLES

	Agree (Percent)	Uncertain (Percent)	Disagree (Percent)
Overall Reactions	82.90	7.28	9.80
Nurses (350)	88.86	5.55	5.59
State Health Department (28)	90.33	4.42	5.52
State Medical Society (13)	78.69	8.56	12.75
State Hospital Association (7)	78.72	5.20	16.08
Health Insurance (13)	83.58	7.75	8.67
Health Planners (20)	77.23	12.22	10.55

While there was general support for most of the findings on changes in the health care system, deviations among the groups occurred in some instances. The nurses, health department respondents, administrative and medical groups, and insurers were quite sure that government will employ more health personnel in the future, but 20 percent of the planners did not think so. The view that innovations in care practice can occur in any setting gained support, but the proposition that these are most likely to occur in new kinds of settings, such as the Kaiser plan and O. E. O. clinics, earned a high rate of disagreement from medicine (62 percent), with 35 percent of the planners and 25 percent of the nursing service directors also opposed. There was an affirmative reaction to the point that the public will initiate change through its own agencies if existing institutions do not, but hospital administration split evenly on the issue (43 percent agree, 43 percent disagree, 14 percent uncertain).

The future role of the nurse was subject to some highly interesting evidence of support as well as opposition and divergent views. Considering a general consequence of technology, there was strong agreement that use of improved instruments for communication would make treatment more personal, with only a mild demurrer registered by medicine and administration. When specifically applied to the nurse's role in the view that nurses will use computers and other technology in giving care, there was a rise to above average disagreement for all groups excepting administration.

There was very strong endorsement for a statement that cast nursing in its traditional chief role of service in the hospital. The statement was that nurses will increase their capabilities for dealing with the critically ill, which earned a 100 percent agreement from medicine, health departments, and insurers, 96 percent from nurses, 86 percent (one disagreement) from the administrative group, and 80 percent (with 15 percent uncertainty) from the planners.

However, statements that cast nurses in a different role involving community-based practice and related attributes of professional responsibility and skill were subject to some dissent. Thus the statement that nurses will devote more resources to "total family" mental and physical health maintenance, gained nearly 100 percent agreement from the nurses, health departments, and planners, 85 percent accord from insurers, but only 46 percent from medicine (23 percent disagreement, 31 percent uncertainty), and 42 percent from administrators (29 percent each for uncertainty and disagreement).

More than 90 percent of the nurses agreed, too, with the finding that practitioners in their field would increase their competence for dealing with psychological aspects of death, dismemberment, and disfigurement, with unanimous support from health departments and 84 percent insurers, but only 75 percent planners, 70 percent medicine, and 57 percent administration. There was surprisingly high agreement with the statement that nurses in the future would intercede more frequently on behalf of the patient if doctors are remiss. Medicine gave 54 percent assent and only 38 percent disagreement, but 86 percent of the hospital administration and health departments groups concurred, and over 80 percent from nursing thought so. Both insurers and planners were rather in disagreement and uncertain (31 percent and 30 percent disagreement; 38 percent and 25 percent uncertain) although 45 percent of the planners did approve the findings.

Somewhat higher accord was granted to two statements that forecast nurses in special roles in the care of ambulatory patients, the aged, and persons in rural areas. These were received with high rates of agreement and no instance of major disagreement.

The findings that nurses are now too much engaged in and also chiefly rewarded for, administrative and institutional operating functions rather than patient care secured general endorsement except from administrators and planners. The figures were: nursing over 90 percent agreement, health departments 92 percent, insurers 84 percent, medicine 77 percent agreement to 15 percent disagreement, planners 65 percent agreement to 25 percent disagreement, administration 57 percent agreement to 43 percent disagreement.

Finally, the view that men can perform nursing roles as well as women had a favorable response. A large majority (93 percent) of the nurses thought so, and few disagreed. One hundred percent of the administrative group, 96 percent of the health departments and 84 percent and 90 percent of the insurers and planners respectively also agreed. Only medicine failed to show as strongly in the consensus, with 23 percent disagreement against 77 percent agreement.

Two questions dealt with the kinds of capabilities nurses need for patient care, considering the quality of judgment and the technical skill involved. It is worth distinguishing the reaction of the nurses to these statements because it illustrates the generalization that there was agreement from all groups even on findings that were controversial.

The statements involved used the terms "technical" and "professional", and the findings were that: a) the capabilities required by an individual nurse in meeting patient care needs often range from "technical" (skill) to "professional" (judgment); b) the use of the terms "technical" and "professional" are unsuitable designations because the process of care usually requires both. The second of these two statements was contrary to an official position adopted by the American Nurses' Association, which had explicitly endorsed the suitability of the terms "technical" and "professional" for classifying nurses in a position statement adopted in 1965. It is certain that most if not all of the nurses were familiar with the position statement.

The groups supported the first statement by a large majority with 97 percent of the nurses in agreement. A substantial majority also supported the second statement, including 75 percent of the nurses. Despite this approval, the sentiment in favor of "technical-professional" designations came out in the response of the hospital administration representatives (29 percent disagreement) and some nurses, who recorded the following rates of disagreement and uncertainty: state associations, 12 percent disagreement, 12 percent uncertainty; state leagues, 24 percent uncertainty; state boards, 24 percent disagreement, 7 percent uncertainty; educators, 18 percent disagreement, 5 percent uncertainty; service directors, 10 percent disagreement, 9 percent uncertainty.

A pair of findings illustrates that consensus did exist among the groups in the respect that they moved together toward agreement, disagreement, or uncertainty. The first statement suggested that, in the future, a gap will exist between actual nursing care and institutional goals for quality of care. This rated a below average level of agreement with corresponding above average disagreement and uncertainty for all groups excepting medicine. The second statement asserted that future pronouncements on goals may more accurately relate to practice than they now do owing to the effect of research by nurses. This statement rated lower levels of agreement and correspondingly higher uncertainty and disagreement from all groups excepting those in the administration field.

A summary of the responses to the findings on the role of nurses showed that there was a high level of agreement on the broad future trends of health care. Specific trends, such as the impact of technology, and a shift of the role of the nurse to greater involvement in community oriented care, secured somewhat less agreement but were nevertheless supported by the majority. A favorable response even in cases of controversial findings appeared in the medical response to the nurse acting as a patient advocate, and the nurse disapproval of the "technical-professional" designations. Consensus appeared in the tendency of the groups to move in concert throughout the various categories.

REACTIONS TO FINDINGS ON STUDY AREA B: NURSING EDUCATION

Nowhere in this study was consensus among the groups of greater importance. In no other area of study was the fact of consensus more clearly in evidence.

This generalization at first sight may appear unwarranted. The rate of overall agreement, 71 percent, was the lowest for the three study areas; uncertainty, at more than 18 percent, the largest; disagreement, at over 10 percent, the highest (Table C-3).

TABLE C-3. OVERALL AND GROUP REACTIONS-STUDY AREA B: NURSING EDUCATION

	Agree (Percent)	*Uncertain (Percent)*	*Disagree (Percent)*
Overall Reactions	71.05	18.68	10.25
Nurses (350)	79.48	9.51	11.01
State Health Department (28)	78.09	11.95	9.96
State Medical Society (13)	68.81	20.92	10.27
State Hospital Association (7)	73.03	11.70	15.27
Health Insurance (13)	69.90	25.94	5.16
Health Planners (20)	58.02	32.10	9.88

Yet, three general facts suggest that this comparison with the other study areas does not reflect the true tone of the response to this set of findings. The first analysis is that the hospital administration and the nurse groups were closer together in this area than any other. The second finding is that a rise in uncertainty rather than heightened disagreement tends to account for reduced agreement. Finally, analysis of the detailed responses to the individual findings shows disagreement, in many instances, was of a positive rather than negative nature.

Perhaps the most significant record of major agreement and general consensus in the entire study appeared in the response to the findings on the future of diploma schools. This topic was the most controversial issue dealt with by the Commission. Yet, the response to the statement that diploma schools will continue to decline for social, economic, and educational reasons was overwhelmingly affirmative, with nearly 100 percent acceptance from nursing and health departments, 92 percent from medicine, 86 percent from administration, 92 percent from insurers, and 80 percent from planners. A related finding on the assimilation of diploma schools by colleges gained a similarly high rate of support, and the prediction of major growth of junior college nursing programs received even stronger acknowledgement.

Other statements on general aspects of nursing education were also approved. Nearly 100 percent of all groups agreed that service institutions must establish extended orientation and in-service training programs. Most thought that many community college programs now lack adequate clinical preparation. With some uncertainty from all groups, and mild disagreement from the nurses, there was acceptance of the finding that the numbers of nurse graduates will be insufficient to meet demand.

An example of the generalization that much of the disagreement was in a positive direction occurred in a statement on the pace of change in nursing education. This was subject to far greater disagreement and uncertainty than other points on trends. All groups either disagreed quite strongly (20 percent or more) or were uncertain (20 percent or more) in regard to the statement that "little in the way of 'revolutionary' institutional change seems likely," excepting administration where 71 percent agreement was offset by 29 percent disagreement. Another statement, that many hospital schools will reduce the length of their programs, produced a common reaction toward uncertainty and disagreement.

Findings on two other topics rated very strong approval. One was that the chief problem in nursing education is shortage of faculty, with finances standing second. The other concerned the area of continuing education. In this latter case, the consensus was almost 100 percent on the two general findings relating to the issue, and also highly affirmative for most groups on the specific point that colleges will establish centers for continuing education of nurses. The only disagreement to a finding on continuing education really affirmed the importance of such study. This was the view that employers do not expect nurses to take responsibility for their own development, which aroused over 50 percent objection from all groups, with insurers, administrators, and nurses standing together at over 70 percent. Clearly, too, this common response illustrates the consensus among the groups.

We have previously observed that the high rate of uncertainty recorded in this study area was a result of lack of information on the part of many of the respondents. This was especially true in regard to findings about nurse faculty members. For example, the stated fact that over one out of five faculty members do not hold a college degree aroused over 50 percent uncertainty from most of the respondents, excepting the nursing and health department groups which generally agreed.

Despite the high uncertainty common to the statements on faculty, there was increased agreement on three important points. The proposition that graduate programs in nursing have emphasized teaching and administration (rather than clinical studies) secured majority approval from all groups but administration. The expectation that clinical studies would rise to greater prominence in graduate programs gained about 90 percent approval from nurses and health departments, 71 percent from administration, 69 percent from medicine, 62 percent from insurance and 45 percent from planning. The view that most nurse faculty members lack research competence rated acceptance from three quarters of each group, excepting insurers, and planners where majorities did concur.

Findings concerning students in nursing had a somewhat mixed reception though a majority of most groups agreed in every case. There was strong affirmation of the view that more upper-middle class and disadvantaged students would enter nursing education, but a statement that the retention of students would improve had weak endorsement across the board. Nursing, administration, insurance, and health departments gave better than 70 percent majorities to the finding that student unrest would foster change in the nursing curriculum, but medicine and planning mustered only slightly more than 50 percent. The proposition that there would be sharp differentiation in job placement among graduates of different types of programs gained a slight majority from most of the groups, but failed with administration and planning.

In the area of the nursing curriculum there was some interesting evidence of agreement in spite of the presence of uncertainty. All the groups in nursing agreed that few institutions were engaged in large-scale curriculum change. Nearly a majority of each of the other groups concurred. Better than half of all the groups, excepting insurance and planning, saw more emphasis in the nursing curriculum on preparation of clinicians and more attention to differences in student ability, though administration also dropped from the majority here. With the exception of medicine and planning, the highest rates of agreement regarding graduate programs were recorded on a statement distinguishing a shift toward an emphasis on research.

A set of statements also related to curriculum, concerned development of programs in other fields. There was some concurrence, fairly high uncertainty, but little disagreement that the emerging allied health schools might attempt to subsume nursing preparation. An even division, excepting administration, arose on the point that core curriculum experiments had not succeeded. The nurses, and health departments agreed that junior colleges were defining their health programs with increasing independence, with support from planning and administration.

The important subject of financing of nursing education showed results that were not necessarily negative for the study but somewhat negative on the issue involved. Through the evidence of financing of junior colleges, some of the groups were quite sanguine in their appraisal of the willingness of the public to support nursing education. Nursing, administration, and planning, with about 40 percent disagreement each, were only lukewarm. A somewhat higher percentage of all groups felt that the public in the future may give better support, and a clear majority agreed that private colleges have avoided the field owing to poor foundation backing. There was very high agreement that increased support for institutions and individuals was essential to meeting the demands that will be placed on nursing education.

One of the rare instances of a sharp difference among the groups appeared in the set of findings on the need for advanced education for nurses. The findings indicated that advanced education is among the most critical needs in nursing. Administration excepted, more than half of each group did agree. However, nursing supported by the health departments stood practically alone in very strong endorsement of the statement. The rates were: nurses over 95 percent agreement; health departments 93 percent agreement; insurers 69 percent agreement, 23 percent disagreement; planners 55 percent agreement, 30 percent disagreement, 15 percent uncertainty; medicine 54 percent agreement, 46 percent disagreement; administration 43 percent agreement, 43 percent disagreement, 14 percent uncertainty.

Contrasted with these results is a turnabout toward strong agreement in favor of advanced clinical education, with the respondents presumably visualizing in-service programs and a stronger clinical component in graduate studies. Agreement among nurses was nearly 99 percent, supported by 93 percent, health departments; 85 percent, medicine; 72 percent, administration; 70 percent, planning; and 69 percent insurance. There was also very substantial agreement that faculty to staff graduate programs are practically unobtainable, and, excepting administration, majority acknowledgement that the financial resources available for graduate education are inadequate.

Taken as a group, the responses to the findings on nursing education show a markedly positive endorsement. There was concurrence on the future of diploma education. The key place of a faculty shortage in nursing education was affirmed, and the critical need for more public support approved. The groups strongly favored continuing education with a marked emphasis on clinical content and a slim majority for formal graduate study. The existence of a consensus among the fields seemed quite conclusive in the general upward and downward swell of the responses.

REACTIONS TO FINDINGS ON STUDY AREA C: NURSING CAREERS

One characteristic of the response in the area of nursing careers was that some of the findings tended to set the nursing group apart (Table C-4). Overall agreement was strong at nearly 80 percent. It was accompanied by the lowest rate of disagreement—slightly more than 9 percent—for all three areas, and moderate uncertainty at 11.38 percent. The tendency of nursing to separate away appeared in the disagreement percentage for this field, where the figure of 4 percent was the lowest for any group in any of the studies.

TABLE C-4. OVERALL AND GROUP REACTIONS-STUDY AREA C: NURSING CAREERS

	Agree (Percent)	*Uncertain (Percent)*	*Disagree (Percent)*
Overall Reactions	79.55	11.38	9.06
Nurses (350)	84.96	10.94	4.01
State Health Department (28)	85.02	6.98	8.00
State Medical Society (13)	76.77	11.86	11.37
State Hospital Association (7)	73.97	9.26	16.77
Health Insurers (13)	82.82	11.18	6.00
Health Planners (20)	74.50	17.37	8.13

The first two sets of questions dealt with manpower issues in nursing. There was very high agreement that manpower planning needs to provide both for a leadership group, including clinicians as well as teachers, researchers, and administrators; and for a numerically large group to perform the bulk of nursing services. There was also agreement that recurrent shortages and rising salaries were thrusting registered nurses into leadership positions.

A substantial majority of most groups felt that effective utilization and technology could contribute to the solution of nurse manpower problems. In this they differed from the Survey I respondents, though the shift may have been due to modified statement of the finding. Even stronger agreement arose for the statement that proportionately fewer nurses may be available to deliver an increased volume of service, requiring improved quality of nursing practice, management, leadership, and preparation of substitute personnel.

Expansion of nursing manpower resources was the concern of several findings. Most groups agreed very strongly that successful recruitment and retention programs required a complex of approaches rather than any single solution. However, the non-nursing groups disagreed with the finding that turnover in the field is due to an inadequate role rather than to the female composition of the profession and low wages. Here the nurses and health departments differed from their colleagues.

Also related to manpower was the point on the capacity of nursing education to prepare the numbers of nurses needed. There was strong agreement that diploma schools would be important for the next five to ten years, and even greater support for the view that diploma school resources should be utilized for clinical education and in-service programs over the long term. Excepting for the planning and administration groups, fairly substantial majorities felt that baccalaureate education programs need expansion. A slightly less favorable response was accorded to the statement that nursing could attract liberal arts graduates and mature women by offering masters level clinical programs for such persons. The final point, that programs of this type would gain accreditation, earned a high rate of uncertainty owing to lack of respondent information.

The potential for increasing the number of men in nursing was explored. Strong agreement attached to the statement that more men should enter the field, with 100 percent of the administration group and nearly 90 percent of the nurses in favor. It was quite strongly agreed that men would enter the field as the salary and career improves, with highs again recorded by administration and nursing. Less approval was given to the statement that recruitment programs are not now aimed at men, though substantial majorities did agree and administration once more was unanimous in support.

The concept of upward career mobility secured a generally positive reception, though some findings showed lower rates among certain groups. Interestingly, only the hospital administration respondents recorded substantial opposition (43 percent) to the finding that nurses have had opportunity to move upward into administration and teaching and not in clinical practice. This group, too, scored 29 percent disagreement whereas the others chiefly concurred with the finding that upward mobility has been discouraged by lack of recognition for nursing education below the baccalaureate level. Consistent with the positive attitude toward the core curriculum apparent in the findings in nursing education, there was wide-spread concurrence that such a program could improve career mobility.

The favorable reaction of medicine to one of the findings on career advancement—that medicine ought to be open as a career avenue for nurses—was pertinent to two later questions on interprofessional relations. The latter dealt specifically with the attitudes of physicians and administrators toward the role and contributions of nurses in health care. Most of the groups felt that physicians should and did have good consociate relations with nurses.

The nurses, however, differed from the others on two of the findings, and the hospital administration group joined them in one case. The nurses expressed much lower than customary agreement and some dissent to the statement that medicine was seeking to establish collaborative relationships with other professions in defining roles and education. Most agreed firmly that such relations might be possible if based on consociate association, but agreement again fell to a comparatively low level and disagreement rose on the point that physicians are willing to enter into such a relationship. The administration representatives joined the nurses in sharing an impression of medical attitudes that differed from that of other respondents.

Generally speaking the view of relationships between nurses and administrators seemed to be more positive. All groups believed that administrators now have and will continue to have a major influence in defining the role of the nurse, though a mild demurrer was registered by the nursing field itself. The belief that administrators are willing to recognize a sophisticated clinical role for nurses received practically universal support with minimal objection from nurses.

A further test of interprofessional attitudes occurred in the case of findings about the effects and future of accreditation of nursing education. The nurses were practically unanimous that accreditation has improved the quality of education programs, but the other groups were not nearly so sure even though majorities agreed in every case. A similar pattern appeared regarding the point that accreditation had not negatively affected the supply of nurses. There was somewhat higher support for the proposition that accreditation standards would rise in the future as a reflection of growing complexity of health services.

Consumer influence, policies of health care, and costs were the subject of the closing series of findings. Widespread agreement appeared for the view that consumers are growing more vocal and influential both in their demand for health care and in defining the role of the nurse. Similar responses were registered in regard to the tendency of new community health services to create a more responsible role for nurses, and for public authorities to react by supporting growth of more sophisticated types of nursing functions.

The relationship of nursing to costs in health care had not appeared in Survey I, so the responses here are new. Substantial majorities of every group but the planners acknowledge that excellence in nursing practice can act as a control on costs. Even larger majorities, taking in all groups, thought that better management practices by nurses, especially in utilization of personnel, could control costs. Slightly less approval appeared for the view that nurses could contribute to savings in health care by assuming some roles previously performed by physicians, with a notable 90 percent from planners somewhat offset by the 29 percent dissent of administration. The nurses generally felt quite strongly that their profession in the past has contributed to cost savings through improved procedures, with 62 percent concurrence from medicine, 57 percent from administration, 54 percent from insurance, and 40 percent uncertainty against 45 percent agreement among planners.

A comprehensive interpretation of the response to this section of the survey suggests that though nurse manpower problems will persist, they are not beyond solution. Better utilization and salaries, technological advance, imaginative recruitment and retention programs, sound approaches to education, and career advancement can offset the persistent manpower shortage in this critical field. A belief in the importance of effective interprofessional relations was apparent, with some evidence that there is room for improvement. A rise in consumer activity was projected, and a resulting tendency to thrust nurses into more sophisticated roles was generally anticipated. The importance of controlling costs in health care emerged in the favorable response to nursing's contribution in this area.

SUMMARY

Two major conclusions stand out from this review of the response of different groups to this survey. It seems inescapable that major professional and related group segments concerned with health care agreed with the analysis and findings of the Commission. It is equally evident that a broad consensus exists on solutions to the problems of nursing, and that this was particularly the case in regard to the most controversial issue in the study, namely the future development of nursing education in a collegiate and university context.

In view of these circumstances, the possibilities for interprofessional cooperation are great. Through such a common approach, the detailed issues in the role of the nurse, the means for meeting consumer demands without unduly raising costs, the application of technology, and organization of an efficient system for care delivery can be resolved. This Commission is in a position to make a major contribution, through forceful endorsement of interprofessional cooperation, toward reaching the ultimate goal of sound health care for the American public.

Notes to Table C-5:

SNA	— State Nurses' Associations (26)	SMS	— State Medical Societies (13)
SLN	— State Leagues for Nursing (17)	SHA	— State Hospital Associations (7)
SBN	— State Boards of Nursing (29)	SHD	— State Health Departments (28)
NED	— Nursing Education Directors (143)	HI	— Health Insurers (13)
NSD	— Nursing Service Directors (135)	HP	— Health Planners (20)

A copy of the instrument appears in Appendix R. Numbered findings can be correlated with the response data shown in Table C-5.

Table C-5. Itemized Response Data from the Third Draft of Preliminary Findings

STUDY AREA A: NURSING ROLES	SNA (26)	SLN (17)	SBN (29)	NED (143)	NSD (135)	SMS (13)	SHA (7)	SHD (28)	HI (13)	HP (20)
					Percent					
Probable Finding No. 1										
Agreement	100	100	100	95	95	85	86	100	92	90
No Opinion	0	0	0	1	2	0	0	0	0	5
Disagreement	0	0	0	4	3	15	14	0	8	5
Probable Finding No. 2										
Agreement	100	100	100	97	98	85	100	96	100	90
No Opinion	0	0	0	1	1	0	0	0	0	0
Disagreement	0	0	0	2	1	15	0	4	0	10
Probable Finding No. 3										
Agreement	96	100	97	99	98	92	86	92	100	90
No Opinion	0	0	0	1	0	0	14	4	0	5
Disagreement	4	0	3	0	2	8	0	4	0	5
Probable Finding No. 4										
Agreement	96	94	90	90	96	92	100	89	100	70
No Opinion	0	0	3	5	2	8	0	4	0	15
Disagreement	4	6	7	5	2	0	0	7	0	15
Probable Finding No. 5										
Agreement	96	100	97	88	88	62	71	92	84	90
No Opinion	4	0	3	6	4	15	0	4	8	5
Disagreement	0	0	0	6	8	23	29	4	8	5
Probable Finding No. 6										
Agreement	88	76	83	78	86	77	100	86	84	75
No Opinion	8	18	10	9	4	8	0	7	8	5
Disagreement	4	6	7	13	10	15	0	7	8	20

Table C-5. Itemized Response Data from the Third Draft of Preliminary Findings

	SNA	SLN	SBN	NED	NSD	SMS	SHA	SHD	HI	HP
Probable Finding No. 7										
Agreement	100	94	97	96	97	100	86	100	100	80
No Opinion	0	6	3	2	2	0	0	0	0	15
Disagreement	0	0	0	2	1	0	14	0	0	5
Probable Finding No. 8										
Agreement	100	94	100	94	94	46	42	96	85	95
No Opinion	0	6	0	4	2	31	29	4	0	0
Disagreement	0	0	0	2	4	23	29	0	15	5
Probable Finding No. 9										
Agreement	84	100	97	92	94	84	86	93	77	60
No Opinion	12	0	3	6	2	8	0	7	23	15
Disagreement	4	0	0	2	4	8	14	0	0	25
Probable Finding No. 10										
Agreement	100	100	94	92	92	85	86	100	92	90
No Opinion	0	0	3	3	3	15	0	0	0	0
Disagreement	0	0	3	5	5	0	14	0	8	10
Probable Finding No. 11										
Agreement	100	94	97	93	94	85	72	92	92	75
No Opinion	0	0	0	5	3	0	14	4	0	20
Disagreement	0	6	3	2	3	15	14	4	8	5
Probable Finding No. 12										
Agreement	96	94	100	89	90	84	71	93	77	70
No Opinion	4	6	0	9	8	8	0	7	8	10
Disagreement	0	0	0	2	2	8	29	0	15	20

Table C-5. Itemized Response Data from the Third Draft of Preliminary Findings

	SNA	SLN	SBN	NED	NSD	SMS	SHA	SHD	HI	HP
Probable Finding No. 13										
Agreement	100	94	94	96	97	85	71	100	92	80
No Opinion	0	6	3	2	3	0	0	0	0	15
Disagreement	0	0	3	2	0	15	29	0	8	5
Probable Finding No. 14										
Agreement	96	94	90	95	93	70	57	100	84	75
No Opinion	4	6	7	2	2	15	14	0	8	20
Disagreement	0	0	3	3	5	15	29	0	8	5
Probable Finding No. 15										
Agreement	88	76	79	80	82	62	86	82	69	65
No Opinion	4	6	14	10	6	15	0	7	8	20
Disagreement	8	18	7	10	12	23	14	11	23	15
Probable Finding No. 16										
Agreement	88	88	79	81	76	54	86	86	31	45
No Opinion	12	12	4	11	10	8	0	7	38	25
Disagreement	0	0	7	8	14	38	14	7	31	30
Probable Finding No. 17										
Agreement	100	94	93	92	82	62	71	96	84	90
No Opinion	0	6	7	6	13	23	0	4	8	5
Disagreement	0	0	0	2	15	15	29	0	8	5
Probable Finding No. 18										
Agreement	96	100	94	99	96	100	100	100	92	95
No Opinion	0	0	3	1	2	0	0	0	0	5
Disagreement	4	0	3	0	2	0	0	0	8	0

Table C-5. Itemized Response Data from the Third Draft of Preliminary Findings

	SNA	SLN	SBN	NED	NSD	SMS	SHA	SHD	HI	HP
Probable Finding No. 19										
Agreement	96	100	97	98	93	100	72	100	69	90
No Opinion	0	0	0	0	4	0	14	0	0	10
Disagreement	4	0	3	2	3	0	14	0	31	0
Probable Finding No. 20										
Agreement	92	100	94	96	86	77	100	96	84	90
No Opinion	0	0	3	2	5	0	0	0	8	10
Disagreement	8	0	3	2	9	23	0	4	8	0
Probable Finding No. 21										
Agreement	96	100	97	96	97	84	86	100	77	85
No Opinion	4	0	0	1	1	8	0	0	8	15
Disagreement	0	0	3	3	2	8	14	0	15	0
Probable Finding No. 22										
Agreement	76	76	69	77	81	84	71	82	85	80
No Opinion	12	0	7	5	9	8	0	11	15	20
Disagreement	12	24	24	18	10	8	29	7	0	0
Probable Finding No. 23										
Agreement	100	88	94	93	86	85	72	100	77	85
No Opinion	0	12	3	5	6	0	14	0	8	5
Disagreement	0	0	3	2	8	15	14	0	15	10
Probable Finding No. 24										
Agreement	96	88	97	90	88	92	72	100	77	80
No Opinion	4	6	3	8	5	0	14	0	8	10
Disagreement	0	6	0	2	7	8	14	0	15	10

Table C-5. Itemized Response Data from the Third Draft of Preliminary Findings

	SNA	SLN	SBN	NED	NSD	SMS	SHA	SHD	HI	HP
Probable Finding No. 25										
Agreement	80	82	90	80	78	77	72	86	92	75
No Opinion	8	18	7	7	5	8	14	7	8	5
Disagreement	12	0	3	13	17	15	14	7	0	20
Probable Finding No. 26										
Agreement	84	82	83	86	94	92	100	85	92	80
No Opinion	12	18	3	12	5	8	0	4	0	20
Disagreement	4	0	14	2	1	0	0	11	8	0
Probable Finding No. 27										
Agreement	92	94	94	92	89	84	86	96	92	90
No Opinion	4	6	3	2	3	8	0	0	8	0
Disagreement	4	0	3	6	8	8	14	4	0	10
Probable Finding No. 28										
Agreement	31	65	76	78	65	30	43	82	100	65
No Opinion	0	29	17	10	12	8	43	11	0	0
Disagreement	19	6	7	12	23	62	14	7	0	35
Probable Finding No. 29										
Agreement	92	82	90	84	85	70	100	85	100	90
No Opinion	8	12	7	11	13	15	0	4	0	10
Disagreement	0	6	3	5	2	15	0	11	0	0
Probable Finding No. 30										
Agreement	69	47	66	57	56	62	57	43	77	50
No Opinion	19	24	24	25	28	15	14	11	15	25
Disagreement	12	29	10	18	16	23	29	46	8	25

Table C-5. Itemized Response Data from the Third Draft of Preliminary Findings

	SNA	SLN	SBN	NED	NSD	SMS	SHA	SHD	HI	HP
Probable Finding No. 31										
Agreement	84	82	90	85	86	85	71	86	77	65
No Opinion	12	6	7	7	2	15	0	7	15	30
Disagreement	4	12	3	8	12	0	29	7	8	5
Probable Finding No. 32										
Agreement	84	65	80	70	72	85	71	78	69	65
No Opinion	8	0	10	12	7	15	0	4	23	25
Disagreement	8	35	10	18	21	0	29	18	8	10
Probable Finding No. 33										
Agreement	76	82	69	67	77	54	86	64	54	45
No Opinion	12	6	10	16	8	23	0	29	38	45
Disagreement	12	12	21	17	15	23	14	7	8	10
Probable Finding No. 34										
Agreement	92	100	100	88	82	77	57	92	84	65
No Opinion	4	0	0	2	3	8	0	4	8	10
Disagreement	4	0	0	10	15	15	43	4	8	25
Probable Finding No. 35										
Agreement	92	88	90	89	93	85	43	92	84	90
No Opinion	8	6	7	5	2	15	14	4	8	0
Disagreement	0	6	3	6	5	0	43	4	8	10
Probable Finding No. 36										
Agreement	61	94	72	77	85	100	86	92	84	65
No Opinion	12	6	7	8	5	0	0	4	8	15
Disagreement	27	0	21	15	10	0	14	4	8	20

STUDY AREA B:
NURSING EDUCATION

	SNA	SLN	SBN	NED	NSD	SMS	SHA	SHD	HI	HP
Probable Finding No. 37										
Agreement	100	100	100	98	92	92	86	96	92	80
No Opinion	0	0	0	0	2	0	0	0	0	20
Disagreement	0	0	0	2	6	8	14	4	8	0
Probable Finding No. 38										
Agreement	81	88	76	86	93	92	100	89	100	85
No Opinion	4	6	14	4	5	8	0	7	0	15
Disagreement	15	6	10	10	2	0	0	4	0	0
Probable Finding No. 39										
Agreement	88	94	100	97	89	92	100	93	100	95
No Opinion	8	0	0	1	7	0	0	7	0	5
Disagreement	4	6	0	2	4	8	0	0	0	0
Probable Finding No. 40										
Agreement	80	94	83	75	87	92	100	85	92	75
No Opinion	8	0	10	11	8	8	0	11	8	25
Disagreement	12	6	7	14	5	0	0	4	0	0
Probable Finding No. 41										
Agreement	96	88	90	96	93	77	86	92	92	65
No Opinion	0	0	0	2	2	23	14	4	8	20
Disagreement	4	12	10	2	5	0	0	4	0	15
Probable Finding No. 42										
Agreement	50	64	48	56	61	54	71	50	62	60
No Opinion	12	18	14	14	10	31	0	14	23	20
Disagreement	38	18	38	30	29	15	29	36	15	20

Table C-5. Itemized Response Data from the Third Draft of Preliminary Findings

	SNA	SLN	SBN	NED	NSD	SMS	SHA	SHD	HI	HP
Probable Finding No. 43										
Agreement	69	82	83	83	76	54	71	61	54	50
No Opinion	19	12	7	5	10	15	0	25	23	30
Disagreement	12	6	10	12	14	31	29	14	23	20
Probable Finding No. 44										
Agreement	100	94	97	98	92	100	100	100	100	85
No Opinion	0	0	0	0	2	0	0	0	0	10
Disagreement	0	6	3	2	6	0	0	0	0	5
Probable Finding No. 45										
Agreement	100	100	100	99	93	100	100	100	77	65
No Opinion	0	0	0	0	3	0	0	0	15	25
Disagreement	0	0	0	1	4	0	0	0	8	10
Probable Finding No. 46										
Agreement	96	100	97	90	92	92	71	92	77	70
No Opinion	0	0	3	5	5	8	0	4	23	20
Disagreement	4	0	0	5	3	0	29	4	0	10
Probable Finding No. 47										
Agreement	84	100	87	73	77	85	86	82	62	60
No Opinion	4	0	3	14	16	15	0	18	23	30
Disagreement	12	0	10	13	7	0	14	0	15	10
Probable Finding No. 48										
Agreement	73	64	55	48	53	38	29	39	23	30
No Opinion	8	24	24	27	29	54	57	39	62	55
Disagreement	19	12	21	25	18	8	14	22	15	15

Table C-5. Itemized Response Data from the Third Draft of Preliminary Findings

	SNA	SLN	SBN	NED	NSD	SMS	SHA	SHD	HI	HP
Probable Finding No. 49										
Agreement	92	82	76	76	70	46	43	67	46	46
No Opinion	4	18	21	15	25	46	43	29	54	50
Disagreement	4	0	3	9	5	8	14	4	0	5
Probable Finding No. 50										
Agreement	69	94	69	78	80	69	42	75	77	55
No Opinion	8	6	7	5	5	23	29	11	23	45
Disagreement	23	0	24	14	15	8	29	14	0	0
Probable Finding No. 51										
Agreement	96	88	94	89	91	69	71	89	62	45
No Opinion	4	6	3	7	6	31	29	11	38	50
Disagreement	0	6	3	4	3	0	0	0	0	5
Probable Finding No. 52										
Agreement	92	94	97	84	83	77	71	79	54	55
No Opinion	4	0	0	8	12	23	29	14	46	45
Disagreement	4	6	3	8	5	0	0	7	0	0
Probable Finding No. 53										
Agreement	69	65	56	62	68	54	72	43	31	40
No Opinion	4	0	10	6	17	38	14	18	69	55
Disagreement	27	35	34	32	15	8	14	39	0	5
Probable Finding No. 54										
Agreement	96	94	90	90	82	100	71	86	85	80
No Opinion	4	6	3	4	9	0	29	14	15	20
Disagreement	0	0	7	6	9	0	0	0	0	0

Table C-5. Itemized Response Data from the Third Draft of Preliminary Findings

	SNA	SLN	SBN	NED	NSD	SMS	SHA	SHD	HI	HP
Probable Finding No. 55										
Agreement	58	65	66	45	48	54	42	57	39	30
No Opinion	23	29	17	30	30	15	29	25	46	65
Disagreement	19	6	17	25	22	31	29	18	15	5
Probable Finding No. 56										
Agreement	84	82	90	77	81	54	71	75	77	55
No Opinion	8	6	3	11	14	31	0	14	23	40
Disagreement	8	12	7	12	5	15	29	11	0	5
Probable Finding No. 57										
Agreement	57	59	59	64	51	54	43	57	61	30
No Opinion	8	12	0	12	13	8	0	11	31	40
Disagreement	35	29	41	42	36	38	57	32	8	30
Probable Finding No. 58										
Agreement	50	88	69	51	62	46	42	65	38	45
No Opinion	15	6	10	15	23	46	29	21	54	45
Disagreement	35	6	21	34	15	8	29	14	8	10
Probable Finding No. 59										
Agreement	77	88	90	81	77	54	57	82	47	40
No Opinion	19	0	3	12	15	31	29	4	38	55
Disagreement	4	12	7	7	8	15	14	14	15	5
Probable Finding No. 60										
Agreement	92	94	94	86	74	31	86	89	69	45
No Opinion	8	0	3	9	23	46	14	4	31	55
Disagreement	0	6	3	5	3	23	0	7	0	0

Table C-5.　Itemized Response Data from the Third Draft of Preliminary Findings

	SNA	SLN	SBN	NED	NSD	SMS	SHA	SHD	HI	HP
Probable Finding No. 61										
Agreement	54	71	94	76	55	54	43	60	62	40
No Opinion	38	29	3	19	40	38	57	36	38	60
Disagreement	8	0	3	5	5	8	0	4	0	0
Probable Finding No. 62										
Agreement	50	71	55	55	49	84	57	79	77	40
No Opinion	12	0	0	6	8	8	0	0	0	20
Disagreement	38	29	45	39	43	8	43	21	23	40
Probable Finding No. 63										
Agreement	54	70	45	51	46	62	42	71	70	40
No Opinion	15	12	21	23	20	30	29	11	15	25
Disagreement	31	18	34	26	34	8	29	18	15	35
Probable Finding No. 64										
Agreement	84	76	76	76	74	69	86	96	100	60
No Opinion	12	12	17	10	12	31	0	0	0	35
Disagreement	4	12	7	14	14	0	14	4	0	5
Probable Finding No. 65										
Agreement	92	88	93	90	78	62	86	79	77	55
No Opinion	8	12	7	7	16	30	14	21	23	35
Disagreement	0	0	0	3	6	8	0	0	0	10
Probable Finding No. 66										
Agreement	100	100	100	99	96	84	100	96	92	80
No Opinion	0	0	0	0	2	8	0	4	8	10
Disagreement	0	0	0	1	2	8	0	0	0	10

Table C-5. Itemized Response Data from the Third Draft of Preliminary Findings

	SNA	SLN	SBN	NED	NSD	SMS	SHA	SHD	HI	HP
Probable Finding No. 67										
Agreement	69	59	72	63	53	54	72	64	46	50
No Opinion	23	35	21	22	32	38	14	29	54	50
Disagreement	8	6	7	15	15	8	14	7	0	0
Probable Finding No. 68										
Agreement	38	53	45	49	53	38	86	61	15	45
No Opinion	58	35	52	36	35	31	0	25	77	45
Disagreement	4	12	3	15	12	31	14	14	8	10
Probable Finding No. 69										
Agreement	77	70	69	68	66	38	57	75	23	55
No Opinion	15	24	28	21	23	54	29	21	77	40
Disagreement	8	6	3	11	11	8	14	4	0	5
Probable Finding No. 70										
Agreement	96	100	100	95	84	54	43	93	69	55
No Opinion	4	0	0	0	2	0	14	0	8	15
Disagreement	0	0	0	5	14	46	43	7	23	30
Probable Finding No. 71										
Agreement	92	88	100	95	89	92	72	93	77	65
No Opinion	8	6	0	3	9	8	14	7	23	30
Disagreement	0	6	0	2	2	0	14	0	0	5
Probable Finding No. 72										
Agreement	100	100	100	96	92	85	72	93	69	70
No Opinion	0	0	0	2	1	0	14	0	23	25
Disagreement	0	0	0	2	7	15	14	7	8	5

Table C-5. Itemized Response Data from the Third Draft of Preliminary Findings

	SNA	SLN	SBN	NED	NSD	SMS	SHA	SHD	Hi	HP
Probable Finding No. 73										
Agreement	76	88	97	79	77	54	43	75	62	55
No Opinion	12	12	3	16	17	38	43	14	38	40
Disagreement	12	0	0	5	6	8	14	11	0	5
Probable Finding No. 74										
Agreement	100	88	97	93	98	92	100	92	100	85
No Opinion	0	6	0	5	1	8	0	4	0	10
Disagreement	0	6	3	2	1	0	0	4	0	5
Probable Finding No. 75										
Agreement	100	100	100	98	100	92	100	100	100	95
No Opinion	0	0	0	2	0	8	0	0	0	0
Disagreement	0	0	0	0	0	0	0	0	0	5
Probable Finding No. 76										
Agreement	81	76	76	80	81	62	71	75	92	60
No Opinion	15	18	14	12	8	30	29	18	8	30
Disagreement	4	6	10	8	11	8	0	7	0	10
Probable Finding No. 77										
Agreement	96	100	100	88	83	100	86	96	77	55
No Opinion	4	0	0	5	11	0	14	4	23	35
Disagreement	0	0	0	7	6	0	0	0	0	10
Probable Finding No. 78										
Agreement	31	29	14	19	25	38	29	25	54	25
No Opinion	4	6	3	6	3	8	0	11	31	20
Disagreement	65	65	83	75	72	54	71	64	15	55

STUDY AREA C:
NURSING CAREERS

	SNA	SLN	SBN	NED	NSD	SMS	SHA	SHD	HI	HP
Probable Finding No. 79										
Agreement	92	94	97	94	88	69	100	92	85	80
No Opinion	8	0	0	4	7	31	0	4	15	15
Disagreement	0	6	3	2	5	0	0	4	0	5
Probable Finding No. 80										
Agreement	96	88	97	92	96	92	86	93	100	90
No Opinion	0	6	0	4	2	0	14	0	0	5
Disagreement	4	6	3	4	2	8	0	7	0	5
Probable Finding No. 81										
Agreement	96	82	93	94	95	85	86	96	100	80
No Opinion	0	6	0	2	0	15	0	0	0	5
Disagreement	4	12	7	4	5	0	14	4	0	15
Probable Finding No. 82										
Agreement	84	100	90	89	89	100	100	92	100	85
No Opinion	8	0	0	4	5	0	0	4	0	5
Disagreement	8	0	10	7	6	0	0	4	0	10
Probable Finding No. 83										
Agreement	96	94	97	90	93	85	71	92	92	85
No Opinion	0	6	3	2	4	0	0	4	0	0
Disagreement	4	0	0	8	3	15	29	4	8	15
Probable Finding No. 84										
Agreement	100	94	97	94	96	84	86	100	92	90
No Opinion	0	6	3	1	2	8	0	0	8	5
Disagreement	0	0	0	5	2	8	14	0	0	5

Table C-5. Itemized Response Data from the Third Draft of Preliminary Findings

	SNA	SLN	SBN	NED	NSD	SMS	SHA	SHD	HI	HP
Probable Finding No. 85										
Agreement	96	100	94	95	93	77	86	100	100	95
No Opinion	4	0	3	2	5	0	0	0	0	0
Disagreement	0	0	3	3	2	23	14	0	0	5
Probable Finding No. 86										
Agreement	62	65	59	68	53	23	29	67	30	25
No Opinion	15	0	3	5	5	0	14	4	8	5
Disagreement	23	35	38	27	42	77	57	29	62	70
Probable Finding No. 87										
Agreement	88	100	97	91	84	77	57	85	69	45
No Opinion	8	0	3	6	11	8	0	4	23	45
Disagreement	4	0	0	3	5	15	43	11	8	10
Probable Finding No. 88										
Agreement	65	64	72	66	60	54	57	64	47	45
No Opinion	23	18	7	22	20	15	0	29	38	40
Disagreement	12	18	21	12	20	31	43	7	15	15
Probable Finding No. 89										
Agreement	46	41	48	44	36	23	14	32	38	20
No Opinion	54	53	52	49	57	62	72	68	62	70
Disagreement	0	6	0	7	7	15	14	0	0	10
Probable Finding No. 90										
Agreement	92	94	97	92	95	92	86	93	85	100
No Opinion	8	0	0	2	2	0	0	0	0	0
Disagreement	0	6	3	6	3	8	14	7	15	0

Table C-5. Itemized Response Data from the Third Draft of Preliminary Findings

	SNA	SLN	SBN	NED	NSD	SMS	SHA	SHD	HI	HP
Probable Finding No. 91										
Agreement	96	94	100	94	96	92	100	100	100	100
No Opinion	4	6	0	4	2	0	0	0	0	0
Disagreement	0	0	0	2	2	8	0	0	0	0
Probable Finding No. 92										
Agreement	100	88	100	93	96	92	86	96	100	100
No Opinion	0	12	0	4	1	0	0	0	0	0
Disagreement	0	0	0	3	3	8	14	4	0	0
Probable Finding No. 93										
Agreement	80	82	90	71	78	77	72	85	100	95
No Opinion	8	12	3	14	6	15	14	4	0	5
Disagreement	12	6	7	15	16	8	14	11	0	0
Probable Finding No. 94										
Agreement	81	94	94	83	78	85	57	85	92	85
No Opinion	4	0	3	2	2	0	0	4	8	10
Disagreement	15	6	3	15	20	15	43	11	0	5
Probable Finding No. 95										
Agreement	96	82	93	91	95	85	57	89	77	85
No Opinion	0	12	0	2	1	15	14	7	15	15
Disagreement	4	6	7	7	4	0	29	4	8	0
Probable Finding No. 96										
Agreement	92	88	87	81	89	77	86	96	85	95
No Opinion	4	0	10	12	7	15	0	4	15	5
Disagreement	4	12	3	7	4	8	14	0	0	0

Table C-5. Itemized Response Data from the Third Draft of Preliminary Findings

	SNA	SLN	SBN	NED	NSD	SMS	SHA	SHD	HI	HP
Probable Finding No. 97										
Agreement	77	64	83	61	70	77	57	75	77	65
No Opinion	15	18	3	11	12	8	14	0	0	30
Disagreement	8	18	14	28	18	15	29	25	23	5
Probable Finding No. 98										
Agreement	81	94	93	93	88	85	100	96	77	85
No Opinion	4	6	7	5	6	15	0	4	15	15
Disagreement	15	0	0	2	6	0	0	0	8	0
Probable Finding No. 99										
Agreement	100	94	94	84	86	77	100	85	77	75
No Opinion	0	0	3	8	4	8	0	11	15	25
Disagreement	0	6	3	8	10	15	0	4	8	0
Probable Finding No. 100										
Agreement	69	76	79	84	87	77	100	75	77	85
No Opinion	4	0	7	4	5	23	0	11	23	0
Disagreement	27	24	14	12	8	0	0	14	0	15
Probable Finding No. 101										
Agreement	80	94	94	72	74	54	72	93	62	40
No Opinion	12	0	3	20	15	38	14	7	23	45
Disagreement	8	6	3	8	11	8	14	0	15	15
Probable Finding No. 102										
Agreement	77	76	83	79	73	54	57	92	100	55
No Opinion	8	6	3	11	12	38	14	4	0	40
Disagreement	15	18	14	10	15	8	29	4	0	5

Table C-5. Itemized Response Data from the Third Draft of Preliminary Findings

	SNA	SLN	SBN	NED	NSD	SMS	SHA	SHD	HI	HP
Probable Finding No. 103										
Agreement	81	82	90	80	81	69	57	86	84	70
No Opinion	15	12	3	8	6	23	29	0	8	30
Disagreement	4	6	7	12	13	8	14	14	8	0
Probable Finding No. 104										
Agreement	62	58	58	57	69	84	86	53	77	45
No Opinion	23	24	21	24	18	8	0	18	23	45
Disagreement	15	18	21	19	13	8	14	29	0	10
Probable Finding No. 105										
Agreement	96	88	93	90	92	85	100	100	100	85
No Opinion	0	6	7	8	3	0	0	0	0	15
Disagreement	4	6	0	2	5	15	0	0	0	0
Probable Finding No. 106										
Agreement	58	64	69	56	66	85	57	68	92	85
No Opinion	15	12	3	9	5	0	14	11	8	10
Disagreement	27	24	28	35	29	15	29	21	0	5
Probable Finding No. 107										
Agreement	100	100	100	98	94	62	57	93	61	55
No Opinion	0	0	0	0	1	15	29	7	31	35
Disagreement	0	0	0	2	5	23	14	0	8	10
Probable Finding No. 108										
Agreement	100	82	97	92	86	77	57	85	69	60
No Opinion	0	6	0	5	7	15	29	11	23	35
Disagreement	0	12	3	3	7	8	14	4	8	5

Table C-5. Itemized Response Data from the Third Draft of Preliminary Findings

	SNA	SLN	SBN	NED	NSD	SMS	SHA	SHD	HI	HP
Probable Finding No. 109										
Agreement	54	64	83	65	71	69	29	53	70	75
No Opinion	15	12	0	8	8	23	57	11	15	15
Disagreement	31	24	17	27	21	8	14	36	15	10
Probable Finding No. 110										
Agreement	100	94	100	86	89	69	100	89	92	90
No Opinion	0	0	0	13	9	31	0	11	0	5
Disagreement	0	6	0	1	2	0	0	0	8	5
Probable Finding No. 111										
Agreement	88	88	97	87	86	77	71	96	92	75
No Opinion	8	0	0	10	8	8	0	0	8	15
Disagreement	4	12	3	3	6	15	29	4	0	10
Probable Finding No. 112										
Agreement	100	100	100	92	90	70	86	96	92	95
No Opinion	0	0	0	6	9	15	0	0	8	5
Disagreement	0	0	0	2	1	15	14	4	0	0
Probable Finding No. 113										
Agreement	84	88	94	88	89	77	86	85	77	75
No Opinion	12	12	3	11	11	15	14	11	23	25
Disagreement	4	0	3	1	0	8	0	4	0	0
Probable Finding No. 114										
Agreement	77	82	93	90	91	100	100	82	92	85
No Opinion	4	6	0	2	1	0	0	0	8	15
Disagreement	19	12	7	8	8	0	0	18	0	0

Table C-5. Itemized Response Data from the Third Draft of Preliminary Findings

	SNA	SLN	SBN	NED	NSD	SMS	SHA	SHD	HI	HP
Probable Finding No. 115										
Agreement	88	88	86	84	89	100	100	92	100	85
No Opinion	4	0	7	5	5	0	0	4	0	10
Disagreement	8	12	7	11	6	0	0	4	0	5
Probable Finding No. 116										
Agreement	88	100	94	94	89	84	71	89	92	60
No Opinion	8	0	3	4	7	8	0	4	0	15
Disagreement	4	0	3	2	4	8	29	7	8	25
Probable Finding No. 117										
Agreement	100	94	100	97	97	92	86	100	100	80
No Opinion	0	6	0	2	2	0	0	0	0	10
Disagreement	0	0	0	1	1	8	14	0	0	10
Probable Finding No. 118										
Agreement	88	82	86	75	79	85	57	82	92	90
No Opinion	8	6	7	15	6	0	14	4	8	0
Disagreement	4	12	7	10	15	15	29	14	0	10
Probable Finding No. 119										
Agreement	88	82	87	69	80	62	57	71	54	45
No Opinion	4	0	3	11	8	30	14	18	31	40
Disagreement	8	18	10	20	12	8	29	11	15	15

APPENDIX D
REACTIONS TO PRELIMINARY RECOMMENDATIONS

I n May 1969 the study staff made a strategic decision that was to prove critical for the successful completion of the Commission report by the target date of January 1970. This decision was to prepare a preliminary draft of recommendations for review by various groups in the health field (as well as the Commission). The results of this review were to be used to formulate a set of recommendations for final action.

The initial step in this process was to discuss a first draft with the nurse and health professions advisory panels at two separate meetings in June. The draft was an extensive document which was greatly modified over time, but contained all the major recommendations that were later subjected to intensive examination by representatives from nursing, medicine, and health services administration meeting separately, and as interdisciplinary groups.

The fundamental features of the review procedure had to be developed for this series of meetings. This included mailing in advance to each of the participants a set of the recommendations on the three study areas — roles, education and careers. These and all later documents were written in short, numbered paragraphs for each section of each recommendation. The participants were provided with answer sheets, numbered to correspond to each sub-paragraph, for recording agreement, disagreement, or uncertainty. This arrangement permitted individuals to react either to any whole concept underlying a set of recommendations or to specific points expressed in given paragraphs. The Commissioners and the major advisory panels participated at this stage through returning similar forms of the instrument.

Following the initial exchange with the advisory panels, and a study of the Commissioners' reactions, the staff drew up a second draft of the recommendations. This was discussed at a meeting with the Commission in late August and became the focal point of the second phase of the review that took place from September through early December. It contained 213 numbered paragraphs, 41 in the area of roles, 93 in education, and 79 in careers. Table D-1 illustrates the progress of selected recommendations of the second draft.

This second phase of the review consisted of a series of meetings with well-informed persons representing the main groups concerned with the outcomes of the report — nursing, medicine, and health service administrators. These groups, coupled with the majority of lay persons on the Commission and study staff, were considered to represent both professional and consumer points of view.

Invitations to take part in a discussion of the recommendations were sent to the presidents and executive directors of the American Nurses' Association, the National League for Nursing, and the American Hospital Association. The staff had earlier accepted an offer made by Dr. William Ruhe, member of the health advisory panel and executive director of the Council on Medical Education of the American Medical Association, to arrange a September meeting with representatives of his Council and the AMA Committee on Nursing. It was explicitly made clear that these discussions were informal and, in no sense, indicated support by any organization for the recommendations, or any part thereof. Plans were also made for separate meetings with an inter-disciplinary group of panelists who had previously met individual staff members during site visits, and a joint meeting of the two advisory panels.

The selection of persons to act as representatives and choice of dates for the meetings were decided by the organizations, with the staff offering to be available at their convenience. The nursing groups had the closing word of commentary, with the order of meetings as follows:

September 20, Chicago — American Medical Association. Council on Education and Committee on Nursing Representatives.

October 10, Chicago — American Hospital Association. Type VIII Membership and Society of Nursing Service Directors Representatives.

October 31, New York — American Nurses' Association. Staff Representatives.

November 1, New York — American Nurses' Association. Representatives of ANA Commissions.

November 6, Cleveland — National League for Nursing. Board Representatives.

November 10, Rochester — Joint Meeting Nurse and Health Professions Advisory Panels.

November 18, Rochester — Interdisciplinary Panel.

December 5, New York — National League for Nursing. Staff Representatives.

Based on these meetings, the staff prepared a third draft of the recommendations, which it submitted for discussion at a December 10 meeting of the Commission. This had the essential features of the text submitted for final approval in early January 1970 and incorporated into the Commission report.

The reactions to the second draft were on the whole very favorable. The views of the Commissioners parallelled those of the review groups. Yet, in its initial response the Commission did tend toward a somewhat more generous approval than the other reviewers, perhaps reflecting a sense of confidence established between it and the study staff.

The first area to be reviewed, at most of the discussion sessions, was that of roles. In this area there was ready acceptance of the recommendations that nursing concentrate on clinical functions; keep pace with advances in health science; adapt technology to humane, individualized care; secure funding for research and work on the evolution of roles jointly with medicine. Less agreement was registered for the proposition that nursing consider two areas of practice, the one pertaining to the traditional field of care of the acutely ill, hospitalized patient (episodic care); the other, an emerging area of practice directed primarily to families and community, and chiefly concerned with health promotion and disease prevention (distributive care).

Also subject to some uncertainty and dissent and later modified were specific recommendations on defining the roles of assistants to nurses, joint appointments of persons in clinical practice and education, the agency responsible for research on standards of health care, and nurse leadership of the health team. Much of the underlying thought for these recommendations was retained by rewording and incorporating relevant discussion in the full report of the Commission.

The Commissioners differed from the others chiefly in responding somewhat more critically to several points in this area. One was the proposal that the American Nurses' Association should define the role of personnel in the nurse's assistant category. Another was a recommendation stating that the nurse specialist should "organize" other health care personnel. The third was that third party payers should investigate profit allowances to reduce health care costs.

The reacting groups were in slightly more disagreement than the Commission on the proposition that the American Nurses' Association should formulate plans for career advancement of aides and assistants. They expressed more doubt and disagreement over the recommendation that there should be joint appointments of persons to posts involving both nursing practice and education.

In the area of education, there was immediate strong endorsement of recommendations favoring expansion of nurse faculty resources; opportunity for educational advancement; the use of technology in education; greater financial support for educational research and wide adoption of innovations; cooperation among the health fields in development of curriculums; and continuing education.

The draft recommendations on diploma schools were expected to be controversial and proved to be so. Much dissent was accorded to all of them and to the proposal for establishing study committees that could incorporate the concepts of episodic and distributive nursing into the curriculum, providing some specialization at the baccalaureate level.

Half of the Commissioners concurred with the other respondents in a negative reaction to the initial proposal that strong diploma schools should become colleges. Most, however, concurred on the point that the regional accrediting associations should set up *ad hoc* committees to recommend the terms under which such schools could become degree granting, and that states should provide financial assistance to diploma school students for enrolling in college courses. Beyond this the Commission, with few exceptions, was quite consistently in agreement. There was, however, slightly more Commission reaction against recommendations on specific figures and the wording of the proposal that states set up planning committees for nursing education, which many interpreted to mean that the state would make all decisions on authority to establish nursing education programs.

The third area of the study on the nursing career secured favorable responses on recommendations favoring career advancement, nurse involvement in planning and decision making in health affairs and institutions, and attention in manpower planning to utilization of nurses in distributive as well as episodic capacities, and mandatory licensure. Increased uncertainty or disapproval were registered on recommendations for a blue ribbon commission to study nurses' salaries (though salary improvement was favored), and the study of respective functions of the National League for Nursing and American Nurses' Association.

There was also some uncertainty and opposition to the point that registered nurses remain a single licensed group and refrain from adding another license for advanced levels of practice. Similar response was accorded to a related proposal in favor of reexamination of the individual's qualifications for practice that was interpreted literally to mean written testing rather than regular review. Proposals for specific action by medical and hospital organizations to support nursing were subject to doubt or disagreement although the essential principles were approved.

Very little difference arose between the Commission and other groups in this section. What little there was occurred primarily in the form of more frequent expression of uncertainty by the group reviewers than the Commissioners. This extended to the idea that the Commission should recommend salary structures, peer groups should take part in the promotion of nurses who lack academic qualifications, the license renewal proposals, medical organization action to support nurses, and specific recommendations for study and promotion of the nurse's role in cost saving.

Viewed in the overall, the exposure of the draft recommendations to a large number of persons and groups made a vital contribution to the work of the Commission. On the purely practical level, it resulted in a tighter document, with much material eliminated, pared down, and clearly sharpened.

The staff was able to test thoroughly the recommendations it considered most fundamental, such as: the establishment of state committees to plan for the development of nursing education; the orientation of nursing to clinical practice and development of the clinical role through joint practice commissions with medicine; and the measures to assure an adequate supply of nurse manpower through improvement of the nursing career. Moreover, it was able to sustain the case for those aspects of the recommendations that were most controversial, particularly the movement of preparation for nursing into the mainstream of higher education.

The ultimate concern of the Commission was with action. It was conscious of the many excellent reports on nursing that had preceded its own work. Nevertheless, it perceived a timeliness to the present report in the forward thrust of the health field. In accepting the preliminary critique of informed segments of the health professions in its own four meetings to discuss the recommendations, it was able to formulate unanimously its own major concepts — research to build a scientific practice of nursing, relevant education, and a rewarding career. The Commission sought to create a platform that could bring unified action from nursing in concert with other health professions — anticipating improved health care for the American public.

TABLE D-1. PROGRESS OF SELECTED RECOMMENDATIONS

Reaction to Recommendations* (2nd Draft)			Recommendation (2nd Draft)	Recommendation in Final Report
Agree (Percent)	Uncertain (Percent)	Disagree (Percent)		
53	29	18	A special committee be created in each state, to work with existing state agencies and departments, consisting of representatives of the State Nursing Association, State League for Nursing, State Board of Nursing, State Medical Society, State Hospital Association, State Nursing Home Association, consumers, and insurers to recommend specific guidelines, means for implementation, and deadlines for inter-institutional agreements between diploma schools and institutions of higher education.	Each state have, or create, a master planning committee that will take nursing education under its purview, such committees to include representatives of nursing, education, other health professions, and the public, to recommend specific guidelines, means for implementation, and deadlines to ensure that nursing education is positioned in the mainstream of American educational patterns.
88	12	0	A national Joint Practice Commission be established between medicine and nursing to discuss and make recommendations concerning the congruent roles of the physician and nurse in providing quality patient care, with particular attention to: the rise of the nurse clinical specialist; the introduction of the physician's assistant; the increased activity of other professions and para-professions in areas long assumed to be the concern solely of the physician and/or the nurse.	A national Joint Practice Commission, with state counterpart committees, be established between medicine and nursing to discuss and make recommendations concerning the congruent roles of the physician and the nurse in providing quality health care, with particular attention to: the rise of the nurse clinician; the introduction of the physician's assistant; the increased activity of other professions and para-professions in areas long assumed to be the concern solely of the physician and/or the nurse.

*Based on reaction forms returned by participating groups.

TABLE D-1. PROGRESS OF SELECTED RECOMMENDATIONS

79	18	3	State counterpart Joint Practice Commissions be established between medicine and nursing to discuss and make recommendations for the congruent roles of physicians and nurses and to recommend both to their legislatures and to the national commission such changes or alterations in basic health practice acts, licensure, and regulation as they deem necessary to ensure the provision of quality health care.	
61	24	15	In order to meet the growing demands for health care, and to hasten the development of an emphasis on health maintenance and disease prevention that will supplement our current system for cure and restoration, we recommend that: a. The education and training of nurses begin at the generalist level to lead to a concentration in episodic or distributive types of health settings. 1. Episodic settings, like our current hospitals, would be primarily devoted to cure and restoration; 2. Distributive settings, like well-baby clinics or school nursing, would be devoted to health maintenance and disease prevention.	Two essentially related, but differing, career patterns be developed for nursing practice: a. One career pattern (episodic) would emphasize nursing practice that is essentially curative and restorative, generally acute or chronic in nature, and most frequently provided in the setting of the hospital and in-patient facility. b. The second career pattern (distributive) would emphasize the nursing practice that is designed essentially for health maintenance and disease prevention, generally continuous in nature, seldom acute, and most frequently operative in the community or in newly developed institutional settings.

TABLE D-1. PROGRESS OF SELECTED RECOMMENDATIONS

91	9	0	All clerical, technical, and managerial functions which do not involve direct patient care be performed by non-nursing personnel. This would include the provision of supplies, the keeping of non-clinical records, and the performance and supervision of housekeeping services;	Continued study be given to the use of technology, organizational practices, and specialized personnel (e.g., ward clerks and unit managers) that can release nurses from non-nursing functions while maintaining nursing control over the delivery of nursing care.
			Demonstratedly effective innovations be adopted by health care facilities to provide:	
97	0	3	1. Middle management (non-nursing) personnel to function as unit or ward managers in hospitals and other facilities to handle the administrative functions that are necessary to effective and efficient patient care;	
88	12	0	2. Increased use of technology, mechanical, electrical, and data processing systems to automate an increasing amount of the work that is necessary, but is presently done inefficiently and ineffectively by health personnel;	
100	0	0	3. That each innovation be accompanied with educational and planning programs, and with evaluative measures, to ensure that organizational change is accompanied by an actual increase in nursing service and by qualitative improvements in patient care.	

TABLE D-1. PROGRESS OF SELECTED RECOMMENDATIONS

| 61 | 24 | 15 | A national committee for the study and development of the nursing curriculum be established as was previously done in the biological, physical, and social sciences in order to develop objectives, universal goals, alternatives, and sequences for nursing instruction. | No less than three regional or inter-institutional committees be funded for the study and development of the nursing curriculum (similar to previous national studies in the biological, physical, and social sciences) in order to develop objectives, universals, alternatives, and sequences for nursing instruction. These committees should specify appropriate levels of general and specialized learning for the different types of educational institutions, and should be particularly concerned with the articulation of programs between the two collegiate levels. |
| 88 | 12 | 0 | With almost twenty percent of the faculty of nursing schools not having completed a baccalaureate program, and an additional forty percent lacking advanced preparation, it is obvious that there is an acute need to develop a greater number of qualified faculty to teach clinical and advanced nursing subjects. We recommend that:

a. The Congress establish a national Nurse-Specialist Training Act that would contain these provisions:

1. Non-interest bearing loans that would be repaid by five years of subsequent teaching or clinical specialist practice combined with tutorial teaching, said loans to be available for nurse faculty or nurse clinicians pursuing graduate degrees at either the Masters or Doctoral level; | The Congress continue and expand such programs as the Health Manpower Act to provide educational loans to nurses pursuing graduate programs with provision for part or whole forgiveness based on subsequent years of teaching. |

TABLE D-1. PROGRESS OF SELECTED RECOMMENDATIONS

97	3	0	2. Post-graduate fellowships for nursing faculty and clinical specialists, available for one or two semesters, to permit added professional development and re-orientation to changed nursing practice and health care delivery systems;
38	56	6	3. A distribution of openings as follows: Masters 80 percent — Doctorate 20 percent; Nursing Faculty 40 percent — Clinical Specialists 50 percent — Research Specialists 10 percent,
76	21	3	4. Earmarked funds for faculty members currently serving hospital schools of nursing to enable them to obtain additional formal academic preparation required for appointment to faculty posts in community, or other colleges. These funds should have the same forgiveness features based on years of continuing service.
76	21	3	Legislation be enacted in each state to provide institutional grants to all schools of nursing proportional to the number of students enrolled, such grants to be used to defray expenses of operation and expansion, and to provide salary increments for qualified faculty.
			Federal and state funds should be provided to institutions for nursing education: a. For financial support proportional to the number of students enrolled, such moneys to be used to defray expenses of operation and expansion, and to provide salary increments for qualified faculty;

TABLE D-1. PROGRESS OF SELECTED RECOMMENDATIONS

b. For the building and construction of facilities including laboratories and classrooms.

Federal, state and private funds be utilized to implement continuing education programs on either a state-wide or broader basis (as suggested by the current inter-state compacts for higher education) in order to develop short courses, seminars, or other educational experiences. In the face of changing health roles and functions, a greater measure of continuing education programs should be planned and conducted by inter-disciplinary teams.

There is almost universal agreement on the need for more frequent and more effective opportunities for both continuing and in-service education. In view of the needs of the personnel and the demands of the evolving health care system for frequent and continuing up-dating, we recommend that:	85	15	0
a. The U. S. Department of Health, Education, and Welfare establish one set of regions for health planning that will include responsibility for comprehensive and co-operative planning for continuing education for the health related professions, thus eliminating the present multiplicity and over-lap of districts like regional medical programs, mental health, comprehensive health planning regions, etc.,			
b. Within each region established under Recommendation "a" above, there be	82	18	0
1. At least one medical school and clinical treatment complex that could provide facility and faculty for excellent continuing education;			
2. An inter-disciplinary committee including nursing representatives to investigate needs for continuing education, determine needs and resources, and enlist the institutional and individual aid required;	94	3	3

TABLE D-1. PROGRESS OF SELECTED RECOMMENDATIONS

| 94 | 3 | 3 | 3. Establish one institutional or a joint institutional program for continuing education in nursing that would develop short courses, seminars, case presentations, individualized learning materials, and other learning aids for continuing education. This institution should work cooperatively on training developments where nursing and the other health professions could team up for continuing education. Also, this institution should receive funds and financial aid from the health planning region to support this activity. | In addition to increasing the supply of nurses by graduating more students from schools of nursing, the retention of registered nurses in the profession must be vigorously fostered. We recommend that:
a. Health service administrators move to reduce turnover, retain nurses in practice and provide incentives for nurses with families to return to practice by |
| 97 | 3 | 0 | 1. Establishing conditions for nurses to obtain job satisfaction by providing care of a high quality, including such elements as sufficient staff to provide opportunity for adequate patient surveillance and rehabilitation as well as performance of treatments and procedures, planning, teaching and counseling; | Health management and nursing administration seek to reduce turnover, increase retention, and induce a return to practice by nurses through:
a. Building on current improvements in starting salaries to create a strong reward system by developing schedules of substantially increasing salary levels for nurses who remain in clinical practice.
b. Establishing conditions, through organizational and staffing practices, that will give nurses an opportunity to provide optimum care to their patients, including individual planning and implementation of the care plan. |

TABLE D-1. PROGRESS OF SELECTED RECOMMENDATIONS

			Recommendation
97	3	0	2. Paying salaries that are competitive with other health occupations and the service industries; 3. Introducing retraining programs for inactive nurses, flexible employment policies respecting part-time work, maternity leaves, and arrangements for care of families during working hours. c. Adopting personnel policies that provide for planned orientation and in-service education courses, flexible employment policies, respecting part-time work, scheduling, maternity leaves, assistance for continuing and graduate education to qualify for advancement, and leaves for educational purposes.
100	0	0	b. Personnel policies encourage the creation of a career in nursing by providing for continuing education (in-service and attendance at short courses), assistance for formal education to qualify for advancement, and leaves for education.
79	18	3	More programs be established to bring liberal arts and science graduates into nursing preparatory programs, such programs to offer a Master of Science in Nursing and include the general nursing core, an introduction to either distributive or episodic nursing care, and orientation and preliminary training in one of the specialties related to the chosen field. As a model for such a program, educators should examine the Master of Arts in Teaching programs for arts and science graduates. Both professional organizations and educational institutions in nursing increase counseling services and recruitment efforts directed at mature females seeking initial entries into nursing programs. These efforts should include overtures to both high school graduates and college graduates from the liberal arts and sciences. Recruitment into nursing must be fostered by changing the public image and status of the nurse, by publicizing the changing character of the nurse role, the changing functions of the nurse, and the growing capacity of the nurse to

TABLE D-1. PROGRESS OF SELECTED RECOMMENDATIONS

			Recommendation
			perform as a full member of a health team. We recommend that:
85	15	0	a. Nursing, medicine and health administration committees, individually and collectively, take responsibility for a public image campaign and
			1. Direct their appropriate committees to undertake the task of public relations;
79	18	3	2. Organize an inter-association committee for such a purpose (Area C: Q-5; 2).
			Nursing practice, over the years, has become increasingly sophisticated. In order to protect the public and to keep pace with the times, we recommend that:
97	3	0	a. The remaining states which do not have mandatory licensure laws for registered nurses immediately adopt such appropriate legislation;
76	15	9	b. There be only one license in nursing -- the Registered Nurse License. Advanced levels of nursing should be recognized in ways other than a special license;
			c. Nurse licensure laws be revised;
58	21	21	1. Licensure laws should provide for periodic examination of the individual's qualifications for practice as a condition for license renewal;

A single license be retained for registered nurses. Differences in levels of nursing should be recognized through: a) designation of master clinicians by approved bodies for such purposes, presumably the Academy of Nursing; b) state licensing standards for health service units; c) qualifications regarding personnel specified in accreditation standards for health service units, d) institutional personnel policies respecting appointments, grades or ranks, and qualifications for promotion.

TABLE D-1. PROGRESS OF SELECTED RECOMMENDATIONS

| 70 | 24 | 6 | 2. The standards adopted for such re-evaluation should be conventional, namely, presentation of evidence of continuing study and assessment by employers and peers. |
| 76 | 21 | 3 | d. The language of licensing laws in nursing and other health related fields be couched in flexible terms as to permit role evolution in accord with emerging features of health service. Questions of scope of practice and the capacity to perform specific treatments and procedures should be determined in the states by joint committees of medicine and nursing either formally designated, or appointed by the attorney general, and used by him as a resource. |

Institutional personnel policies and standards should reflect the changes taking place in patient care and the health care field. We recommend that:

| 91 | 6 | 3 | a. Differences in levels of nursing personnel be recognized in: 1) institutional personnel policies respecting grades or ranks and qualifications for promotion; 2) qualifications regarding personnel set down in accreditation standards for health service units; 3) state licensing standards for health service units; 4) designation of specialists by approved bodies for such purposes (See Area B: Q-7). |

TABLE D-1. PROGRESS OF SELECTED RECOMMENDATIONS

67	12	21	b. Over a period of time, institutional personnel policies and standards for approval for health service units be altered to require that the bachelor's degree serve as the minimum qualification for a person to function at a level above that of the nurse-generalist.
85	15	0	1. Persons now at these levels who do not hold the degree should be provided with opportunity and assistance to complete the necessary program of study;
76	18	6	2. Review by peers, including administrative personnel, should be provided to approve persons who are exceptions to this standard.
			In order to determine the optimum arrangement of resources, functions, and personnel for nursing and for patient care in the coming decades, we recommend that:
70	24	6	a. The American Nurses' Association and the National League for Nursing join together to retain a management consulting firm to study the functions and structures of both organizations, and such related bodies as the American Nurses' Foundation and the American Journal of Nursing, for the purpose of determining
79	15	6	1. Any areas of duplication or over-lap that could fruitfully be eliminated or reduced;

The national nursing organizations, particularly the American Nurses' Association and the National League for Nursing, press forward in their current study of functions, structures, methods for representation, and inter-relationships in order to determine: a) areas of overlap or duplication; b) areas of unmet needs; and c) areas or functions that could be transferred from one organization to another in the light of changing conditions.

TABLE D-1. PROGRESS OF SELECTED RECOMMENDATIONS

76	18	6	2. Any areas of need that are currently remaining unmet;
70	24	6	3. Any areas or functions that should be transferred from one organization to another in light of changing professional needs or altered systems and practice.

Since there is evidence to indicate that one little-used source of recruitment into nursing is from the ranks of aides and auxiliaries, particularly those from the socio-economic disadvantaged, we recommend that:

88	11	0	1. Federal and state government explore the possibility of offering scholarships and stipends for such recommended candidates to nursing and health education courses, the scholarships to cover tuition and books, the stipend to compensate for lost earnings, to permit them to acquire junior college preparation as an entry into the professional fields of health care;
94	6	0	2. Hospitals, nursing homes, and other health care facilities maintain an observant eye for those individuals in lower job classifications who, despite probable shortcomings in formal education, display outstanding motivation, intelligence, and work habits in the performance of their tasks related to health care in order to inform them of career opportunities and to recommend them to educational institutions that can provide proper remedial work and the opportunity for advancement.

In view of the growing shortage of labor in all areas of the American economy nursing must tap new sources of supply in the manpower pool. We recommend that:

a. Nursing assess the feasibility and potential of attracting larger numbers of talented disadvantaged persons who are capable of contributing to quality care.

b. Public and private agencies and health facilities: a) seek to identify individuals in lower job classifications who, despite probable shortcomings in formal education, display outstanding motivation, competence, and intelligence and encourage them to obtain the necessary preparation to enter nursing education programs; b) provide scholarships and stipends to such individuals in amounts proportional to their demonstrated achievement.

APPENDIX E

REPORT ON THE 1969 REGIONAL CONFERENCES

The timetable for the progress of the study indicated that the preliminary findings, based on the first site visits, the initiation of the literature search, consultation with the two major advisory panels and meetings and discussions of the Commissioners and staff, would be completed by late 1968.

It was decided, at that point, that a survey of the opinions and reactions of a more varied sample of individuals who would be directly concerned with the outcomes of the study would contribute valuable information for the modification of findings and subsequent formulation of the first draft of recommendations.

Rather than a mailed questionnaire, the staff felt a direct discussion would help to draw out questions and opinions. Therefore, a series of three regional meetings of nurses, physicians, educators, consumers, insurers, investigators of health service delivery, and health administrators was planned for the spring of 1969. Consideration of appropriate geographic distribution of sites that would offer easy transportation access from a wide area and where conference facilities were available led to the selection of St. Louis, San Francisco, and Washington, D. C., for meetings on March 3 and 4, March 6 and 7, and March 19 and 20.

To insure that each conference would provide maximum opportunity for discussion and comment, attendance was limited to 45 persons. The lists of individuals to be invited was compiled from a variety of sources. The Commissioners and members of the nurse advisory panel and the health professions advisory panel provided suggestions. The Department of Health, Education, and Welfare, the Insurance Association of America, the AFL-CIO, The Social Security Administration and the National Health Council were among the organizations surveyed for additional advice. Published lists of various committee memberships and conference participants were reviewed for further options. These included, for example, the reports of the AMA-ANA National Conferences for Professional Nurses and Physicians; and the lists of members, panelists, and staff of the National Advisory Commission on Health Manpower.

Finally, 181 invitations were issued in January 1969, with an effort being made to balance representation of nurses, physicians, administrators, insurers, consumers, health service specialists and educators for each conference. The numbers of invitations in each category that were issued for each conference are shown in Table E-1.

TABLE E-1. CONFERENCE INVITATIONS

	St. Louis	*San Francisco*	*Washington, D.C.*
Administrators	9	8	7
Consumers	11	9	12
Educators	6	7	7
Health Service Specialists	5	4	8
Insurers	9	8	8
Nurses	13	12	11
Physicians	8	8	11

A combination of mail and telephone contacts resulted in a final attendance of 33 people in St. Louis, 32 in San Francisco, and 39 in Washington, D. C. The names of attendees for each meeting are shown in Table E-2.

TABLE E-2. REGIONAL CONFERENCE ATTENDEES

St. Louis, Missouri — March 3-4, 1969; Persons in Attendance 33

Wright Adams, M.D., Executive Director, Illinois Regional Medical Program, Chicago, Illinois.

Odin Anderson, Professor and Associate Director, Center for Health Administration Studies, University of Chicago, Chicago, Illinois.

Richard Barr, Assistant Director, University of Kansas Medical Center, Kansas City, Kansas.

Karl Bartscht, Director, Planning, Research and Development, Community Systems Foundation, Ann Arbor, Michigan.

E. H. Borman, Manager, Medical Relations Department, General American Life Insurance Company, St. Louis, Missouri.

Mary A. Brambilla, Nurse Clinician, University of Minnesota Hospital, Minneapolis, Minnesota.

Emily B. Campbell, Associate Professor, School of Nursing, University of Wisconsin, Madison, Wisconsin.

Thelma C. Cobb, Director of Employee's Health and Volunteer Service, Provident Hospital, Chicago, Illinois.

Morton Creditor, M.D., Michael Reese Hospital, Chicago, Illinois.

Harry Davis, Bi-State Regional Medical Program, St. Louis, Missouri.

Margery Drake, The Catholic Hospital Association, St. Louis, Missouri.

David A. Gee, Executive Director, Jewish Hospital of St. Louis, St. Louis, Missouri.

Joe S. Greathouse, Jr., Director, Vanderbilt University Hospital, Nashville, Tennessee.

Fannie Harris, Consumer Representative, Detroit, Michigan.

Emily Holmquist, School of Nursing, Indianapolis Medical Center Campus, Indianapolis, Indiana.

Mrs. John T. Jones, Jr., Consumer Representative, Houston, Texas.

Robert Laur, Coordinator for Professional Education, University of Missouri, Columbia, Missouri.

Lucille Petry Leone, Associate Dean, College of Nursing, Texas Women's University, Dallas, Texas.

Joseph S. Lichty, M.D., Executive Director, Akron General Hospital, Akron, Ohio.

Henrynne A. Louden, Consumer Representative, New Orleans, Louisiana.

Charles E. Morgan, Consumer Representative, Detroit, Michigan.

Mary Ann Muranko, Hospital-Community Liaison Nurse, Children's Psychiatric Hospital, University of Michigan Medical Center, Ann Arbor, Michigan.

Richardson Noback, M.D., Executive Director, Kansas City General Hospital and Medical Center, Kansas City, Missouri.

Robert Owens, Assistant Dean of Instruction, Parkland College, Champaign, Illinois.

Naomi R. Patchin, Assistant Director, Division of Hospital Schools of Nursing, American Hospital Association, Chicago, Illinois.

Albert Pisani, M.D., Presbyterian-St. Luke's Hospital, Chicago, Illinois.

Martha Pitel, Chairman, Department of Nursing Education, University of Kansas Medical Center, Kansas City, Kansas.

Sam Pollock, Consumer Representative, Cleveland, Ohio.

Lucien Pyle, M.D., Medical Arts Building, Topeka, Kansas.

Harold L. Tremain, M.D., Director, Medical Division, Michigan Hospital Service, Detroit, Michigan.

Robert Tupper, M.D., Pontiac General Hospital, Pontiac, Michigan.

William R. Willard, M.D., Vice President for the Medical Center, University of Kentucky, Lexington, Kentucky.

Marie J. Zimmer, Director of Nursing Service, University of Wisconsin Hospitals, Madison, Wisconsin.

San Francisco, California — March 6-7, 1969; Persons in Attendance 32

Curtis Aller, Health Manpower Specialist, Berkeley, California.

Virginia Barham, Nursing Education Consultant, State Board of Nurse Registration, San Francisco, California.

John Bigelow, Washington State Hospital Association, Seattle, Washington.

Mark Blumberg, M.D., Director of Health Planning, University of California, Berkeley, California.

Orville Booth, Executive Vice President, St. Francis Memorial Hospital, San Francisco, California.

Mike Chavoya, Jr., Consumer Representative, Vista, California.

Fred Davis, Professor, School of Nursing, University of California, San Francisco, California.

Marjorie Dunlap, Dean, School of Nursing, University of California, San Francisco, California.

Mrs. Stuart Durkheimer, Board Member, Visiting Nurses Association, Portland, Oregon.

Leon Fox, M.D., San Jose, California.

Rosamond Gabrielson, Executive Director, Department of Nursing, Good Samaritan Hospital, Phoenix, Arizona.

Alfred L. Gunther, Manager, Group Insurance Administration, Metropolitan Life Insurance Company, San Francisco, California.

A. B. Halverson, Executive Vice President, Occidental Life Insurance Company of California, Los Angeles, California.

James Haviland, M.D., Member, Council on Education, American Medical Association, Seattle, Washington.

Algo D. Henderson, Center for Research and Development in Higher Education, University of California, Berkeley, California.

Fred R. Higginbotham, Vice President, Public Relations, Blue Cross and Blue Shield of Texas, Dallas, Texas.

Betty Highley, School of Nursing, University of California Medical Center, San Francisco, California.

Harold Hixon, Administrator, University of California Hospitals, San Francisco, California.

Arnold Hurtado, M.D., Chairman, Department of Medicine, Kaiser Foundation Hospitals, Portland, Oregon.

Hilliard J. Katz, M.D., San Francisco, California.

Clifford Keene, M.D., President, Kaiser Foundation Health Planning, Inc., Oakland, California.

Barbara Kerr, M.D., Intermountain Regional Medical Program, University of Utah Medical Center, Salt Lake City, Utah.

Marie Kurihara, Nursing Care Specialist in Cardiopulmonary Disease, Veteran's Administration Hospital, Long Beach, California.

Ruth Ludemann, Assistant Professor, College of Nursing, University of Arizona, Tucson, Arizona.

Al McNabney, Southern Pacific Hospital, San Francisco, California.

Maryann Powers, Head Nurse, Cardiac Recovery Room, University of Oregon Medical School Hospital, Portland, Oregon.

William Price, Vice President, Kaiser Foundation School of Nursing, Oakland, California.

Jean Quint, School of Nursing, University of California, San Francisco, California.

Mrs. William Smith, Consumer Representative, San Marino, California.

Faustina Solis, Farm Workers Health Service, California State Department of Public Health, Berkeley, California.

Mrs. August J. Turchi, Immediate Past President, Visiting Nurse Association, Portland, Oregon.

Fay Wilson, Chairman, Nursing Department, Los Angeles City College, Los Angeles, California.

Washington, D.C. — March 19-20, 1969; Persons in Attendance 39

Mattie Ansley, Consumer Representative, Atlanta, Georgia.

Jack D. Arnold, Executive Director, Association of Schools of Allied Health Professions, Washington, D. C.

Howard J. Baker, M.D., Vice President, Blue Cross of Greater Philadelphia, Philadelphia, Pennsylvania.

Edwin C. Brown, Secretary-Treasurer, Rhode Island Group Health Association, Providence, Rhode Island.

Penelope Buschman, Clinical Nurse Specialist, Babies Hospital, Columbia Presbyterian Medical Center, New York, New York.

Ione G. Carey, Director, Education, Visiting Nurse Service of New York, New York, New York.

Edward J. Connors, Consultant, Health Services and Mental Health Administration, National Institutes of Health, Bethesda, Maryland.

John Darlson, Assistant to Representative Paul G. Rogers, U. S. House of Representatives, Washington, D. C.

Barbara J. Doody, Advisor to Home Health Agencies, Massachusetts Blue Cross, Inc., Boston, Massachusetts.

John Elliott, Manpower Administration, U.S. Department of Labor, Washington, D.C.

Geraldine Ellis, Assistant Chief, Nursing Department, Clinical Centers, National Institutes of Health, Bethesda, Maryland.

Howard Ennes, Second Vice President, The Equitable Life Assurance Society, New York, New York.

Alfred S. Ercolano, Executive Director, American Nursing Home Association, Washington, D. C.

John Forsythe, Assistant to Senator Ralph W. Yarborough, U. S. Senate, Washington, D. C.

W. Todd Furniss, Director, Commission on Academic Affairs, American Council on Education, Washington, D. C.

William S. Hall, M.D., Director, South Carolina Department of Mental Health, Columbia, South Carolina.

Susan S. Jenkins, Professional Relations Advisor, Bureau of Health Insurance, Social Security Administration, Baltimore, Maryland.

Elizabeth A. Katona, Nurse Clinician, State University Hospital, Downstate Medical Center, Brooklyn, New York.

Robert Kevan, Associate Study Director, Board of Medicine, National Academy of Sciences, Washington, D. C.

Dr. Cynthia Kinsella, Director of Nursing, Mount Sinai Hospital, New York, New York.

Cleo Leggett, Harlem Psychiatric Rehabilitation Center, New York, New York.

Mary Liston, Dean, School of Nursing, The Catholic University of America, Washington, D. C.

Mary MacDonald, Director, Department of Nursing, Massachusetts General Hospital, Boston, Massachusetts.

John C. McMeekin, Administrative Assistant, Pennsylvania Hospital, Philadelphia, Pennsylvania.

Harold Margulies, M.D., Secretary, Council on Health Manpower, American Medical Association, Washington, D. C.

Lawrence E. Meltzer, M.D., Director, Coronary Care Unit, Presbyterian—University of Pennsylvania Medical Center, Philadelphia, Pennsylvania.

Marion Metcalf, Director, Nursing Department, Peter Bent Brigham Hospital, Boston, Massachusetts.

Mabel Morris, Director of Nursing Service, Temple Community Mental Health Center, Philadelphia, Pennsylvania.

Rose Pinneo, Assistant Professor, Department of Nursing, University of Rochester, Rochester, New York.

Marsha G. Poindexter, Consumer Representative, Roxbury, Massachusetts.

Frances Reiter, Dean, Graduate School of Nursing, New York Medical College, New York, New York.

June Remillet, Head, Public Health Nursing, College of Nursing, University of Florida, Gainesville, Florida.

Jessie M. Scott, Director, Division of Nursing, Bureau of Health Professions, Education and Manpower Training, National Institutes of Health, Arlington, Virginia.

William Shannon, Associate Director, American Association of Junior Colleges, Washington, D. C.

Mrs. Peter Soyster, Consumer Representative, McLean, Virginia.

John H. Touhy, M.D., Medical Director, St. Agnes Hospital, Baltimore, Maryland.

Bennetta B. Washington, Director, Women's Centers Job Corps, Office of Economic Opportunity, Washington, D. C.

William Wilson, Administrator, Mary Hitchcock Memorial Hospital, Hanover, New Hampshire.

Edward M. Wurzel, M.D., Executive Director, American Association of Medical Clinics, Alexandria, Virginia.

Prior to each conference, the participants were mailed a series of study questions and data sources compiled by the study staff. A second draft of the questions and a series of probable findings were distributed at the conference and served as a discussion guide.

The program included a brief outline of the origin, history and purposes of the Commission and two panel presentations. Consumer representatives comprised the first panel which concentrated on health care needs of the country. The second panel consisted of a nurse, a physician, and an administrator commenting on health care delivery. It was hoped that these presentations, based on the panelists' personal experience and knowledge, combined with the opportunity for pre-conference review of the study questions, would focus the participants' thoughts and comments for the smaller discussion groups to follow.

The participants were divided into three groups. Within the limits imposed by the composition of the total conference group, each discussion section included representatives from each of the occupational areas and interest groups. Invited participants generally served as the discussion leaders with the staff personnel functioning as observers and occasional resource persons.

Each group was asked to spend the first afternoon and evening discussing, in detail, the questions and findings in one of the three study areas — nursing roles, nursing education or nursing careers. Provision was made for each group to discuss the remaining two areas, in somewhat less depth, on the second day's schedule. To insure that comment and discussion would be as candid and open as possible and would not be confined to the questions and findings compiled by the staff, the outside discussion leaders had free rein to utilize their time as they and the group saw fit.

Typically, the leaders served as facilitators — introducing the questions, moderating discussion and monitoring time to insure that each group's primary study area was covered completely. No constraints were placed on the leader's own participation in group discussion, and efforts were made to ensure that all individuals contributed to the discussion. The proceedings were tape-recorded to facilitate later review by all staff members.

The conference participants were requested to complete a Likert-type scale reaction to each of the preliminary findings in all three study areas. The same material was also sent to the 77 invitees who were unable to attend the conferences. The responses of the total group are included in the analysis in Appendix B.

These reactions, opinions, and comments made a vital contribution to the progress of the study and are reflected not only in subsequent drafts of findings, but in the character and design of the final recommendations and report of this Commission.

APPENDIX F

SUMMARY OF RECOMMENDATIONS FROM
PREVIOUS STATE, REGIONAL AND NATIONAL
STUDIES OF NURSING AND SELECTED STUDIES OF
OTHER HEALTH PROFESSIONS

The study staff became quickly aware that a large number of studies of nursing and nursing education had previously been conducted. It was felt that by reviewing these studies, extracting and categorizing their recommendations, and developing a thesaurus we could determine recognizable trends and earlier proposed solutions for American nursing. No attempt was made to include every single recommendation from each study, but rather a selective screening based on our preliminary questions was employed in order that the most significant and relevant recommendations might be identified and studied. One result of this activity was the accompanying compilation of recommendations from studies of nursing and other health professions.

In undertaking this compilation, each of the fifty state nurse associations was contacted to obtain copies of the most recent studies conducted within their respective states or regions. We generally limited our examination to those studies conducted during and after 1966 but occasionally we received and reviewed a study from the early 1960's. A total of 40 studies from 29 states was received. Additionally, 8 states reported they had no recent studies while 13 states did not reply to our request. The studies reviewed and their dates of publication are:

STATE NURSING STUDIES REVIEWED

ALABAMA   *Assessment of Nursing Education in Alabama.* 1968.

ARIZONA   *Statewide Survey of Clinical Facilities for Nursing Education in Arizona.* 1968.

CALIFORNIA   *Progress Report on Nursing Education in California.* 1968.

COLORADO   *Report — Committee on Planning for Nursing in Colorado.* 1968.

CONNECTICUT   *Nursing Needs and Resources in Connecticut.* 1966.

GEORGIA   *Nursing and Paramedical Personnel in Georgia. A Survey of Supply and Demand.* 1962.
                Georgia's 1966 High School Graduates. 1968.

HAWAII   *Nursing and Nursing Education in Hawaii.* 1962.
                Nursing in Hawaii. 1968.

IDAHO   *A Study of the Nursing Profession in Idaho Medical Facilities.* 1967.
                Nursing in Idaho: A Study of Nursing Needs and Resources. 1969.

ILLINOIS   *Nursing in Illinois — An Assessment and a Plan.* 1968.

INDIANA   *Nurses for Indiana — Present and Future.* 1967.

KANSAS   *Recommendations for Development of Nursing Education in Kansas.* 1968.

MAINE   *Future Development of Nursing Education in Maine.* 1966.

MARYLAND   *Survey of Nursing Needs and Resources in Maryland.* 1966.
                1980 Projection of Health Manpower in Maryland. 1968.

MASSACHUSETTS   *Study of Nursing Education in the Commonwealth of Massachusetts.* 1968.

MICHIGAN   *Nursing Needs and Resources in Michigan.* 1966.
                Plan for Future of Nursing Education in Michigan. 1966.
                Nursing Education Needs in Michigan. 1969.

MONTANA   *Plan to Assist in the Return of Inactive Health Professionals to Active Employment.* 1968.

NEBRASKA   *Nebraska's Nurse Supply, Needs, and Resources.* 1966.

NEVADA   *Nursing in Nevada.* 1964.
                Nevada Health Manpower Program — A Report on Resources and Needs. 1968.

NEW JERSEY   *Nursing Education in Transition: A Plan for Action in New Jersey.* 1968.

NEW MEXICO   *New Mexico's Nursing Needs and Resources.* 1964.
                Reactivation of Health Professionals Project Report. 1968.

NEW YORK   *Study of Nurse Education Needs in the Southern New York Region.* 1967.

NORTH CAROLINA *Nursing Education in North Carolina — Today and Tomorrow.* 1967.

NORTH DAKOTA   *A Study of Inactive Health Personnel in North Dakota.* 1968.
                North Dakota Joint Committee on Nursing Needs and Resources. 1969.

OHIO   *Projected Needs for Nursing Education in Ohio.* 1964.

OKLAHOMA   *Planning for Nursing Education — A Study of Current Resources and Future Needs.* 1965.

SOUTH CAROLINA *Nurses for South Carolina — A Study of Nursing Needs and Resources.* 1967.

TEXAS	*Report on Nursing Resources in Texas.* 1966.
VIRGINIA	*Nursing and Health Care in Virginia.* 1968.
	Nursing in Virginia. 1969.
WISCONSIN	*Re-employment Factors of Inactive Nurses in Wisconsin.* 1967.
	Nurses for Wisconsin's Future. 1970.

In conjunction with the literature search, the staff reviewed 24 studies conducted on a national or regional level during the period from 1923 to 1969. These studies were either directly concerned with nursing and nursing education or else had major sections devoted to these topics. A listing of these studies and their publication dates is:

NATIONAL AND REGIONAL STUDIES OF NURSING AND HEALTH CARE REVIEWED

The Goldmark Report: Josephine Goldmark. 1923.
Nurses, Patients, and Pocketbooks: May Ayres Burgess. 1928.
The Education of Nurses: Isabelle Stewart. 1943.
Nursing for the Future: Esther Lucile Brown. 1948.
A Program for the Nursing Profession: Eli Ginzberg, Ed. 1948.
Nursing Schools at the Mid-Century: West and Hawkins. 1950.
The Education of Nursing Technicians: Mildred L. Montag. 1951.
Collegiate Education for Nursing: Margaret Bridgman. 1953.
Education for Nursing Leadership: Eleanor C. Lambertsen. 1958.
Community College Education for Nursing: Mildred L. Montag. 1959.
A Look at the Future of Education for Nursing: Helen Nahm. 1959.
Liberal Education and Nursing: Charles H. Russell. 1959.
Educational Revolution in Nursing: Martha E. Rogers. 1961.
Nursing Education and Catholic Institutions: Report of the Council of the Conference of Catholic Schools of Nursing. 1963.
Hospital Effectiveness Study: H.E.W. 1967.
Nurse Training Act 1964, Program Review Report: H.E.W. 1967.
Report of the National Advisory Commission on Health Manpower. 1967.
Statewide Planning for Nursing Education: Southern Regional Education Board. 1967.
Technology and Manpower in the Health Service Industry, 1965-75: Department of Labor. 1967.
Future Patterns of Health Care with Emphasis on Utilization of Nursing Personnel: Williamsburg Conference. 1968.
The Problems of Nursing Home Patients — Implications for Improving Nursing Care: Boston College. 1968.
Sickness and Society: Duff and Hollingshead. 1968.
Nurse Career Pattern Study, Part I — Practical Nursing Programs: NLN. 1968.
Nursing in the Upper Midwest: North Dakota Joint Committee on Nursing Needs and Resources. 1969.

The categorizing of the recommendations followed, in general, the format of our study design. Three major divisions were established: nursing education; nursing practice; and a miscellaneous category. Under these three divisions identifiable subtopics were listed. The format was as follows:

I.   Nursing Education

    A.   Practical Nurse Programs
    B.   Diploma Programs
    C.   Associate Degree Programs
    D.   Baccalaureate Programs
    E.   Graduate Education Programs
    F.   Inservice and Continuing Education
    G.   Nursing Faculty
    H.   Nursing Student Recruitment and Financial Aid
    I.   Nursing Education in General

II.   Nursing Service and Practice

    A.   Role and Utilization
    B.   Personnel Policies
    C.   Licensure in Nursing
    D.   Nurses in Planning
    E.   The Inactive Nurse

III.   Miscellaneous Recommendations for Nursing

To complete this analysis of other investigations the decision was to review a sample of studies of other health professions and compile a list of their recommendations which seemed to have significance or relevance for nursing and nursing education. In this activity we reviewed 10 studies covering a period of time from 1961 to 1969 and including the professions of medicine, dentistry, medical technology, public health, and allied health personnel. This endeavor was a further extension of our basic belief that nursing cannot be studied effectively in isolation from the rest of the health care field, but rather must be viewed as an integral part of that total field. Any judgments made concerning the profession must be made in this context. The studies covered in this sample and their publication dates are:

STUDIES OF HEALTH PROFESSIONS REVIEWED

Medical Education Reconsidered. Report of the Endicott House Summer Study on Medical Education. July, 1965.
The Graduate Education of Physicians. Report of the Citizens Commission on Graduate Medical Education. August, 1966.
Lowell T. Coggeshall, *Planning for Medical Progress through Education.* Association of American Medical Colleges. 1965.

Health is a Community Affair. National Commission on Community Health Services. 1966.

Survey of Dentistry. The final report of the Commission on the Survey of Dentistry in the United States. 1961.

The Education of Public Health Personnel. Joint Committee on the Study of Education for Public Health. 1966.

National Correlations in Medical Technology Education. A Report of a Study of Medical Technologists. 1967.

Manpower for the Medical Laboratory. The National Committee for Career in Medical Technology. 1967.

Allied Health Personnel. Ad Hoc Committee on Allied Health Personnel; Division of Medical Sciences; National Research Council; National Academy of Sciences; National Academy of Engineering. 1969.

Association of American Medical Colleges Annual Meeting. Nov., 1968.

The thesaurus of recommendations from previous studies proved to be a valuable resource to the commission and the staff during the conduct of the study. It has been continually employed as a reference, and as a basis for comparison and contrast. The frequency with which certain recommendations appeared and their continuing appropriateness underscore the residual nature of many nursing problems and the consistency with which solutions have been viewed.

Table F-1 contains a complete listing of the recommendations.

TABLE F-1. SUMMARY OF RECOMMENDATIONS

I. Nursing Education
   A. Practical Nurse Programs
      1. Brown '48

The practical nurse should have one year supervised practice after training.

It hasn't been proved where the practical nurse can best be trained — in vocational high schools, hospitals or private training schools.

No system of training for practical nurses is likely to succeed unless the public that creates broad general policy and provides funds, educators who design and operate instructional programs, hospitals and agencies that provide clinical facilities, and nursing associations and state boards of control that set standards and influence recruiting are prepared to manifest an active interest in practical nursing far beyond any interest yet shown.

      2. Ginzberg '48

We recommend the introduction of practical nursing education into the adult and high school vocational system of the country, while making maximum use of the community's hospitals as clinical affiliates.

TABLE F-1. SUMMARY OF RECOMMENDATIONS

3. Bridgman '53	Practical nurse programs belong in vocational school systems, between high school and college. Practical nurses should be on hospital nursing teams, in non-professional home care and in doctors' offices.
4. *Nursing Education and Catholic Institutions* '63	Existing programs of practical nursing in Catholic institutions should continue self-evaluation and improvement.
	Catholic hospitals interested in establishing a program of practical nursing are urged to investigate the possibilities of participating by furnishing a clinical experience field for students in a program of practical nursing under vocational education, provided the vocational education program is on a post-high school level. Because of the length of the program it is doubtful that control of practical nursing programs offers to the Catholic hospital decisive advantages over cooperation with other agencies.
5. Ohio '64	No new practical nurse programs should be established until the findings can be reported of an autonomous commission appointed jointly by ANA and NLN to study the present system of nursing education in relation to the responsibilities and skill levels required for high-quality patient care.
6. Connecticut '66	Practical nurse programs should be continued and expanded to meet regional needs.
7. Maryland '66	The recommendation is made that: 1) The existing programs for the education of the practical nurse be encouraged to: a) Increase enrollments of qualified students; b) Continue to improve the quality of education; and 2) That licensed practical nurses function as members of nursing teams under registered professional nurses at all times.
8. Michigan '66	The present capacity of practical nursing programs should not be increased. However, distribution of facilities should be investigated in relation to regional needs.
	Plan to phase out in an orderly fashion practical nurse schools that do not foresee any possibility of alignment with institutions of higher education.

TABLE F-1. SUMMARY OF RECOMMENDATIONS

9. Alabama '68

Every effort be made to improve the quality of existing practical nursing programs in the State and that establishment of new ones be discouraged.

Specific attention be given by the existing schools for practical nursing education to the qualifications of applicants, and that applicants who qualify for professional nursing programs be urged to attend such programs.

10. Illinois '68

Programs for the LPN should be continued, and, if possible, expanded to produce a 100 percent increase in graduates by 1980.

11. Kansas '68

Additional programs in practical nursing are not warranted.

12. Maryland '68

No new practical nursing schools should be considered until present schools are better utilized.

13. NLN—*Nurse Career Pattern Study* '68

The community must offer an opportunity for steady employment under conditions that will enable the practical nurse to make a real contribution to her community, that will allow her to continue to fulfill her responsibilities as a homemaker, and that will provide an income that will be a meaningful supplement to that of her husband.

Schools and places for educational clinical experience and later employment will need to be convenient in location to the homes of the students and workers. In areas of concentrated population, transportation must be inexpensive and easily accessible. In areas of lesser population, schools will presumably draw from a very limited population because of lack of easy transportation.

Data of this study point to the fact that the high school practical nursing student presents some unique problems. There is a need for a better understanding of a young girl's motivation and interest in choosing nursing in high school. Data also indicate the necessity for help for the student during high school in maintaining satisfactory academic achievement. High school programs offering practical nursing to teenagers need careful depth study in terms of recruitment into nursing, guidance throughout the program, retention in the program, and formulation of career goals.

TABLE F-1. SUMMARY OF RECOMMENDATIONS

13. NLN—*Nurse Career Pattern Study* '68 (continued)

Recruitment of practical nursing students needs considerable study. The findings indicate a need particularly to investigate the role of the guidance counselor. A study should be made of information available to and used by guidance counselors in relation to practical nursing. Also, a study is needed to determine availability and use of guidance facilities by the out-of-school mature woman.

An educational institution should establish a program and determine policies only after careful study of the local community. Three factors are vital in determining educational policies related to students: potential of the population for recruitment of qualified students; the work opportunities available both in nursing and in competitive occupations; a suitable location for the program in terms of the student potential.

The number of men in this occupational group is so small that it is not feasible to plan educational programs or working situations with the needs of this group in mind. Although the few men appear to make a definite contribution, the sparse number precludes any recommendation pertaining to men. It might be presumed that the limited income possibilities of the practical nurse as well as the female image of the nurse in the American culture combine to limit the attractiveness of this occupation. It may well be that only economically depressed areas can expect to recruit any sizable number of men. A study of the factors which prevent men from choosing practical nursing as an occupation might indicate a way to change this situation.

14. Idaho '69

The Department of Vocational Education should continue education of practical nurses in numbers to meet the demand for new personnel in this category.

15. Virginia '69

That the State Board of Examiners of Nurses, the State Department of Education, the State Department of Community Colleges, and the State Council of Higher Education for Virginia encourage the continuation of educational programs for practical nurses, where adequate educational and clinical facilities and sufficient financial support and student enrollment are available.

TABLE F-1. SUMMARY OF RECOMMENDATIONS
B. Diploma Programs
   1. Goldmark '23

The average hospital training school is not organized on such a basis as to conform to the standards accepted in other educational fields; the instruction in such schools is frequently casual and uncorrelated; the educational needs and the health and strength of students are frequently sacrificed to practical hospital exigencies. Such shortcomings are primarily due to the lack of independent endowments for nursing education. Existing educational facilities are on the whole, in the majority of schools, inadequate for the preparation of the high grade of nurses required for the care of serious illness, and for service in the fields of public health nursing and nursing education. One of the chief reasons for the lack of sufficient recruits, of a high type, to meet such needs lies precisely in the fact that the average hospital training school does not offer a sufficiently attractive avenue of entrance to this field.

—therefore—

The fundamental period of hospital training should be reduced to 28 months and unessential, non-educational routine should be eliminated. The course should be organized along intensive and coordinated lines. A hospital institution with financial support and under a separate board or training school committee, organized for primarily educational purposes should attract students of high quality in increasing numbers.

   2. Brown '48

Recommendations Concerning Weak Hospital Schools:

There should be an official examination of every school. A national list of accredited schools should be published and distributed and it should be stressed that any school not on the list has failed to meet the minimum requisites for accreditation or had refused to permit examination.

A broad nationwide campaign should be conducted to rally broad support for accredited schools and to subject slow-moving state boards and nonaccredited schools to strong social pressure.

There should be a periodic reexamination of all schools and the distribution of revised lists of accredited schools, continually.

The public should assume responsibility for a substantial part of the financial burden.

TABLE F-1. SUMMARY OF RECOMMENDATIONS

2. Brown '48 (continued)

Recommendations Concerning Good Hospital Schools:

Improvements should be made if these schools are to continue to exist.

These schools should experiment to increase their strength and social usefulness. The period of training plus improving the course of study should be experimented with. Scientifically controlled tests of the educational value of nursing practice in selected areas of concentration and in diverse environmental situations should be initiated. Transitional steps such as the creation of central schools of nursing and utilization of the teaching resources of junior colleges could be taken.

Recommendations Concerning Distinguished Hospital Schools:

This type of school can only continue to be successful if it is put within the sphere of the university, for only the university can provide the wealth of resources needed.

The transition should be made at the earliest possible moment but also with the wholehearted assistance by the entire nursing profession, medical and hospital associations concerned with nursing, university and hospital administrators, university faculties, administrators and faculties of schools of medicine and public health, foundations, and those members of the laity influential in effecting policy and influencing public opinion.

Recommendations Concerning Schools of Specialized Hospitals:

Hospitals for the mentally ill should relinquish their schools and make their clinical facilities more widely available for affiliating students. The nursing profession, both autonomously and in conjunction with the medical profession and the public at large, attempt to redress the imbalance resulting from long neglect of mental disease by assisting these and other similar hospitals to introduce substantial teaching programs for affiliation or internship and to utilize in-service training for assistant personnel more extensively and

TABLE F-1. SUMMARY OF RECOMMENDATIONS

2. Brown '48 (continued)

effectively. Ways should be sought to stimulate inter-est among the health professions in wider practice in the field of psychiatry as contrasted with other disease, and in wider research in its prevention and cure.

The clinical facilities of public tuberculosis sana-toriums should also be used exclusively for the training of students from other schools that seek affiliations in tuberculosis nursing.

Pediatric hospitals: Their principal problem is that of providing sufficiently varied clinical experiences for their students. Possibly the pediatric hospital should consider the role of providing affiliation rather than attempting to operate small schools, especially since general hospitals are weak in pediatrics.

3. Ginzberg '48

Nursing schools must be removed from hospital jurisdiction and affiliated with universities or colleges.

4. Bridgman '53

Continued efforts to establish uniformly good stan-dards in hospital schools are needed. Both acceleration and the production of better qualified graduates can be accomplished through concentrated emphasis upon educational purposes, more and better teaching, and less repetitive practice. Such improvements involve financial problems and it is doubtful whether hospitals can or should continue to carry this educational responsibility longer than the transition makes neces-sary.

Hospitals should be freed from the expense of providing the formal, preliminary education of nurses so they could furnish excellent facilities for the supervised practice of students.

The diploma programs exist in hospital schools. The better schools should be continued for the present but may be merged ultimately with terminal junior college and baccalaureate programs as educational institu-tions. These nurses are prepared for registered nurse functions.

5. *Nursing Education and Catholic Institutions* '63

The diploma program should be organized as an educational unit and receive from the board of control understanding, acceptance and support necessary to accomplish the school's primary goal of educating the student at this level. The faculty group has the

TABLE F-1. SUMMARY OF RECOMMENDATIONS

5. *Nursing Education and*   responsibility for the planning and implementing of
   Catholic Institutions '63   the total program and must be given the com-
   (continued)   mensurate authority.

                                  Catholic institutions offering effective diploma pro-
                                  grams should continue these programs, striving to
                                  develop them to a high level of excellence as diploma
                                  programs preparing for beginning staff nursing in
                                  hospitals and similar institutions.

                                  Modifications in the curriculum (shorter, etc.) should
                                  be introduced only where thorough study and careful
                                  planning have shown that the change will enhance the
                                  quality of the diploma program.

6. Ohio '64   Nationally accredited diploma programs be continued
                                  for some time. Those which are not nationally
                                  accredited be discontinued. Accredited diploma pro-
                                  grams should phase out in an orderly fashion as basic
                                  baccalaureate programs and AD programs become
                                  established.

7. Connecticut '66   Until such time as adequate numbers are graduated
                                  from AD programs, the strong hospital schools should
                                  be continued and strengthened to accomplish an
                                  orderly and safe transition of the educational shift.
                                  During this transition some hospital schools within a
                                  single region might combine thus sharing costs,
                                  faculty, and facilities.

8. Maryland '66   That hospitals which are not planning to have their
                                  clinical facilities utilized by baccalaureate programs or
                                  associate degree programs, continue the hospital
                                  diploma school programs.

9. Michigan '66   Encourage schools of nursing in hospital settings who
                                  are planning to phase out their programs to offer the
                                  use of their clinical facilities to nursing programs in
                                  institutions of higher education.

10. New York '67   The hospitals offering diploma programs in nursing
                                  must re-assess and extend their resources, and at the
                                  same time improve the quality of their educational
                                  programs.

11. Alabama '68   Diploma programs should continue to provide quality
                                  instruction and recruit students and faculty until such
                                  time as there are sufficient numbers of baccalaureate

TABLE F-1. SUMMARY OF RECOMMENDATIONS

11. Alabama '68 (continued)	and associate degree programs providing adequate numbers of practitioners of nursing to meet community needs.
12. Illinois '68	All hospital programs should seek NLN accreditation at the earliest possible date; accredited diploma programs should continue. When other programs can be developed locally that give clear promise of meeting future needs and, hopefully, expanding the output of nurse graduates, the future of hospital schools in that area should be reconsidered.
13. Maryland '68	No new diploma programs should be opened, but steps should be taken to insure maintenance of current enrollment levels.
14. Williamsburg Conference '68	The Governor's Committee on Nursing should look into the cost of operating hospital diploma nursing programs with a view toward determining the desirability of providing both operational and constructional support to hospitals offering these educational programs. It was emphasized that this recommendation refers to assistance to the diploma schools of nursing presently in operation and not to the establishment of new schools.
15. North Dakota '69	As baccalaureate and associate degree nursing programs become established and/or expand, accredited diploma programs should phase out in an orderly manner.
16. Virginia '69	That existing hospital-diploma schools of nursing:

1) Reduce the length of their programs to two calendar years;
2) Consolidate their programs, where several with small enrollments are located near each other; and
3) Continue cooperative arrangements with nearby two-year and four-year colleges, which could assist in providing instruction in general education and other non-clinical subjects of study; and

That the General Assembly provide sufficient funds for state-supported institutions of higher education to offer academic and non-clinical instruction without charge for students of diploma schools of nursing which are fully accredited by the State Board of Examiners of Nurses.

TABLE F-1. SUMMARY OF RECOMMENDATIONS

17. Wisconsin '70

The Commission recognizes that present hospital schools of nursing, which prepare the largest number of RN graduates in the state, are needed and should be continued, though no additional diploma programs should be established.

The Commission urges that diploma schools not only continue their own self-evaluation, but with others in the community, ascertain their future role in the preparation of nurses. Consultative assistance available from the Board of Nursing and the follow-up agency for the Commission should be utilized in shaping the destiny of diploma schools in the light of evolving trends. The Commission offers to hospitals for consideration these alternatives:

1) Expansion of presently viable schools;
2) Cooperative programming or consolidation with other schools where indicated and feasible;
3) Changing the nature of their participation in nursing education by making clinical facilities available to other education programs.

The Commission suggests that diploma schools evaluate their curriculums and consider the modifications of the length of their current program efforts in light of general societal changes, changing concepts of health care, changing roles and responsibilities of the registered nurse and developments in technology and teaching methodology.

C. Associate Degree Programs
   1. Bridgman '53

The Associate Degree program should take place in technical institutes, in junior colleges and colleges and universities. These nurses would prepare for general registered nurse functions.

If junior college curricula were extensively established to replace hospital school programs, the chief emphasis could be shifted from the service to be obtained from students to the educational goals. Both enrichment and condensation of training would probably result.

   2. Montag '59

The extant confusion about the "short" junior college AD programs must be eliminated. The AD programs are shorter because they are based on more efficient teaching than are the diploma programs. They are *not* merely two thirds of a diploma program. Hospitals

TABLE F-1. SUMMARY OF RECOMMENDATIONS

2. Montag '59 (continued)	which try to attract more students by cutting one year out of current programs will harm their students. Only a *completely revised* program, fitting in all essential training, should be undertaken by interested hospitals.

Experience with the junior-community college plan indicates that long-term planning must precede the formulation of nursing education programs. This planning concerns nurses, educators, administrators of schools and hospitals, and the general community, all of them helping to define the objectives and expected outcomes of the programs.

3. *Nursing Education and Catholic Institutions* '63	Since these programs are increasing in number and since there is a need for more nurses, it is desirable that wherever needed and wherever possible Catholic junior colleges be developed which include a nursing program. Because there are very few Catholic junior colleges, it is desirable that certain Catholic senior colleges with appropriate facilities establish associate degree programs in nursing. There seems to be little future for the two-year single purpose institution.
4. Connecticut '66	Several AD programs should be developed primarily in community colleges. These programs should be distributed geographically and should be designed to graduate students in numbers that are specifically related to regional needs. The Commission believes that AD nursing programs will eventually supply the major percentage of bedside staff nurses.
5. Michigan '66	Cautiously explore establishing new AD programs in nursing in those areas which contain desirable clinical facilities, institutions of higher education, availability of students and with particular emphasis on adequately prepared faculty.
6. Arizona '68	As AD programs develop, it seems logical to expect that the community college will assume much of the responsibility for providing continuing education for the technically-oriented nurse.
7. Kansas '68	Carefully planned associate degree programs which utilize the assets of educational, clinical, and community resources can provide nurse technicians for beginning staff nurse positions.
8. Massachusetts '68	All existing programs, especially in community colleges, should have maximum enrollment before consideration is given to any additional programs. A

TABLE F-1. SUMMARY OF RECOMMENDATIONS

8. Massachusetts '68
(continued)

minimum enrollment of 100 in each class will efficiently use the limited nurse faculty and meet the demands within the community for education of future nurses.

9. Maryland '68

Existing AD programs should expand enrollment as rapidly as possible. However, no new schools should be opened unless a real need can be demonstrated and availability of qualified faculty is assured.

10. Wisconsin '70

The Commission looks to the state's vocational-technical institutions, presently being organized along viable district lines, as the prime vehicle for providing the educational experiences relevant to AD education.

The Commission recognized that the development of associate degree programs in nursing education in the emerging vocational-technical system offers a new direction in the preparation of nurses both to the State and to the rapidly forming vocational-technical districts. The Commission, therefore, offers the following guidelines in order to assist in the development of quality programs:

1) Desirability of "recognized candidate for accreditation" status with the North Central Association of Colleges and Secondary schools;
2) Desirability of AD programs in other fields;
3) Preparatory programs in other health occupations;
4) A qualified registered nurse with a minimum of a master's degree has the authority and responsibility for the development and direction of the associate degree program in nursing education only;
5) Adequate clinical facilities are available for student experiences.

D. Baccalaureate Programs
1. Goldmark '23

The development and strengthening of university schools of nursing of a high grade for the training of leaders is of fundamental importance in the furtherance of nursing education.

2. Brown '48

Nursing schools within institutions of higher learning and those to be created should be autonomous and have the same status as do the other professional schools.

TABLE F-1. SUMMARY OF RECOMMENDATIONS

2. Brown '48 (continued)

The university should provide the school of nursing with physical accommodations and equipment comparable to that provided other professional schools requiring lab and practice facilities; and the university should bring the nursing school as completely as possible within its intellectual and cultural orbit. Furthermore, the university should seek the best clinical facilities to insure sound professional education.

3. Ginzberg '48

Education should be professional, offering a body of cultural materials. A baccalaureate degree should be awarded. Curriculum should integrate the theory and practice of nursing.

Avoidance of repetitive ward duty should enable completion of a professional program in four years, without the need for an internship.

4. Bridgman '53

Faculty members of baccalaureate degree university programs should be employed by the institution on an equal basis with those in other units and share equally all responsibilities and benefits of faculty members.

Supplementary baccalaureate curricula can be taken, for graduate nurses (RN's) leading to a BS degree, in colleges and universities. But soon, this curricula should be provided in connection with basic baccalaureate programs, enabling graduates of hospital schools and terminal junior college programs to meet the same standards for the BS degree as students taking complete basic programs in college.

5. *Nursing Education and Catholic Institutions* '63

We recommend that efforts be continued to insure that the major in nursing be a genuine major, with progressive development from general basic notions to more complex and detailed mastery, and that it be defensible and defended as such in conversations with academic officials in the established colleges and universities.

Since the characteristics of the professional nurse demand breadth of total personal development, the full resources, both curricular and extra-curricular, of an institution dedicated to general as well as specialized education are needed to produce the desired result, and students preparing to be professional nurses should be provided the full range of opportunities available to other students.

TABLE F-1. SUMMARY OF RECOMMENDATIONS

5. *Nursing Education and* There is immediate need to engage in long-range
Catholic Institutions '63 planning, particularly with Catholic universities lo-
(continued) cated where there is access to the clinical facilities of a
medical center (Catholic or other) to work toward the
establishment of additional generic baccalaureate degree programs in nursing. This planning might well
involve investigation of the interest and support for
the program on the part of religious operating
hospitals in the locality of the diocese and should
include plans for the development of highly qualified
faculty.

Existing approved baccalaureate programs are encouraged to continue and to strive for excellence.
Religious communities conducting accredited colleges
with baccalaureate nursing programs should give
wholehearted support to these programs.

Colleges and universities have the right and responsibility to set their own criteria when determining
advanced credit for work completed in other educational institutions. It is understood that the university
or college determines what more, in addition to the
education already received, is necessary for a given
student to obtain a degree. The same consideration
and policies should be applied to nurses as to other
applicants for advanced standing.

6. Ohio '64 Six existing baccalaureate programs expand as much,
and as rapidly, as possible. Expansion of current
programs will make best use of available faculty. These
programs have estimated they can increase admissions
by 40 percent by 1970.

Continuation of four existing programs providing
baccalaureate education for graduates of diploma and
associate degree programs. These programs should be
phased out as their need diminishes. It is not recommended that new programs be established.

7. Michigan '66 Basic baccalaureate programs should expand steadily
to provide facilities for 750 sophomore admissions in
academic year 1969-70. This goal represents 44
percent more sophomore students than were enrolled
in the year ending 10/15/65.

8. Kansas '68 Additional baccalaureate programs are needed as a
foundation for advanced study in teaching, administration, expert practice and research.

TABLE F-1. SUMMARY OF RECOMMENDATIONS

9. Maryland '68

Additional collegiate facilities are needed. The Johns Hopkins School of Nursing, the only diploma school in Maryland associated with a university, should be encouraged to convert to a baccalaureate program. No additional collegiate schools should be opened without proof of need and evidence of availability of qualified faculty.

10. Massachusetts '68

Additional baccalaureate nursing programs must be established. Efforts to expand the number and size of graduate programs in nursing will be fruitless unless there is a corresponding increase in the number of nurses prepared to enter such programs. At present there are only three schools in the public system of higher education offering a baccalaureate nursing program.

11. Georgia '69

It is recommended that Georgia have a total of at least six baccalaureate nursing programs within the next five years. (Presently there are just three).

12. Wisconsin '70

The Commission recommends that institutions of higher education explore and initiate innovative approaches that will reduce the traditional roadblocks, such as time, expense and unnecessary credit and residency requirements, to allow graduates from associate degree and diploma programs to secure a baccalaureate degree.

E. Graduate Education Programs

1. Bridgman '53

Assure the effectiveness of supplementary education for graduate nurses in providing foundations equal to those in basic baccalaureate programs.

2. Rogers '61

Professional-school faculty must be prepared. To this end, doctoral programs must be developed that include substantial doctoral-level content in nursing theory. Doctoral candidates must themselves have full professional preparation.

3. *Nursing Education and Catholic Institutions* '63

One of the problems of educating master nurses at the graduate level is the lack of an adequate number of approved graduate programs in Catholic universities. Much could be accomplished if Catholic universities would cooperate in offering diversified graduate programs planned on a regional basis and according to the resources available. There is an immediate need to provide more opportunities for graduate education in

TABLE F-1. SUMMARY OF RECOMMENDATIONS

3. *Nursing Education and
   Catholic Institutions '63
   (Continued)*

nursing in Catholic institutions, by improvement of existing programs, expansion to other appropriate institutions, and the recruitment of religious and lay students.

New programs should be developed only in institutions which have a generic baccalaureate degree program in nursing, are engaged in graduate work in other areas, are able to obtain adequate graduate faculty, and have access to clinical facilities in which a high level of patient care is maintained, an appropriate variety of clinical situations is available, and experimentation is possible.

Course work in the graduate program should differ from undergraduate courses in kind as well as in extent, emphasizing personal initiative, creativity, depth in a specialty, and genuine research.

Graduate programs should move to a point where the work for a master's degree is centered on a clinical specialty in order to provide the content necessary for teaching and for leadership positions in patient care. Functional preparation for teaching or administration should be in a subordinate position at this level.

4. Ohio '64

Expand the three existing graduate education programs. It is not recommended that new graduate programs be established at this time. Most urgent problem is the need for qualified faculty to teach in existing programs. Next is the need for qualified administrators and supervisors to direct the care of patients in hospitals.

5. Connecticut '66

Professional nursing should provide to the graduates of baccalaureate programs examinations in the area of the behavioral, social, physical and biological sciences. Successful passage of these additional examinations will demonstrate the greater competency of the individual practitioner and enable these competencies to be utilized more effectively.

6. Michigan '66

Universities with master's degree programs in nursing should offer scholarships and financial incentives to baccalaureate degree nursing graduates with outstanding potential for the clinical specialities and teaching.

TABLE F-1. SUMMARY OF RECOMMENDATIONS

7. North Carolina '67	Graduate nursing education programs should be expanded. One of the major obstacles to expansion and improvement of basic education is the lack of a sufficient number of qualified faculty. Master's degree programs should be undertaken only in institutions having adequate baccalaureate programs.
8. Southern Regional Education Board '67	Because leaders, particularly teachers, are so strategic to other developments in nursing, planners should give early attention to graduate education and assign high priority to actions in this field.
9. Illinois '68	Clinical specialization in nursing is now a necessity. It needs to be actively promoted with the medical profession, hospitals and other health agencies and with institutions of higher learning. Just as in medicine — clinical specialization in nursing requires more education — a master's degree.
10. Kansas '68	Primary consideration must be given to immediate expansion of graduate nursing education. Kansas, in cooperation with surrounding states, should develop a comprehensive graduate program which will provide an adequate number of master's and doctorate level nurses. The committee recommends that graduate education be expanded as one of the first steps in meeting anticipated nursing needs for nursing faculty, community health personnel, nursing service directors and supervisors and other highly skilled nurses.
11. Massachusetts '68	The state should explore the possibility of entering into contracts with private institutions to insure that advanced education in nursing is available to all interested, qualified Massachusetts residents until the state itself provides such opportunities. Simultaneously, it might be possible for the state to assume more responsibility for nursing preparation at the baccalaureate level, thus permitting the private institutions to direct more of their resources into graduate level preparation.
12. Williamsburg Conference '68	Clinical specialists need to receive educational preparation in a broader scope in order to reduce fragmentation of health care. Consideration should be given to internship and residency training programs followed by some form of certification. Certification should then take into account differences in training programs which range from a month in duration to those offering degrees as a result of a two-year educational program.

TABLE F-1. SUMMARY OF RECOMMENDATIONS

12. Williamsburg Conference
    '68 (continued)

Another step which should be added for the enhancement of mobility is an increase in the number of
educational opportunities, especially at the graduate
level. Included in this step should be a form of
recognition such as certification by a professional
academy, in order to give an incentive for the nurses
to continue their education.

13. Michigan '69

The Federal program of traineeships for advanced
training of professional nurses under the Nurse
Training Act should be broadened and made more
flexible in order to permit candidates for advanced
degrees in nursing to qualify for aid if enrolled in a
program providing for continuity and sequential
course arrangements, but not necessarily in consec-
utive academic terms. Availability of more flexible
graduate stipends would encourage more schools of
nursing conducting graduate training to develop innovative curricula and adapt programs to fit individual
needs of students.

14. Wisconsin '70

The Commission recommends the highest priority for
development of graduate education at the master's
degree level in nursing science and nursing education
to prepare nurses for positions as:

1) Faculty members at schools of nursing;
2) Nurse administrators;
3) Nurse clinicians.

The Commission suggests that pilot programs at the
post-master's "specialist" level be considered by institutions with recognized BS and MS programs.

The Commission recognizes that doctoral programs in
nursing are important in the overall preparation of
qualified nurse personnel for faculty and leadership
positions, but suggests:

1) A continuation of present interdisciplinary
   doctoral efforts as opposed to the fielding of a
   new doctorate in nursing science (unless some
   long-term financing by the Federal Government
   would make possible such an offering); and
2) Exploration with neighboring states about the
   possibility of cooperative regional effort in
   fielding of a doctoral program.

TABLE F-1. SUMMARY OF RECOMMENDATIONS

F. In-service and Continuing
   Education

    1. Goldmark '23   Superintendents, supervisors, instructors and public health nurses should in all cases receive special additional training beyond the basic nursing course.

    2. Bridgman '53   In-service training for auxiliary nursing personnel should take place in hospitals. Simple general functions and assisting regular nurses would be the role.

    3. Montag '59   Continuing education of graduate nurses is necessary, particularly in specialized fields. This implies a thorough basic preparation in the undergraduate years. Continuing education must actually occur, and not be merely a euphemism for a paper plan.

    4. Nahm '59   Nurse practitioners must accept the obligation of pursuing continuing education throughout their professional lives, in the face of the continuous expansion of knowledge.

Nurses must make use of advances in educational research which may aid in making continuing education truly effective in promoting expanded knowledge and competence.

In planning continuing education programs, we must consider practitioners who drop out of service for reasons of marriage and childrearing. These people should be aided in catching up and keeping up so that more of them might return to practice when the children have grown.

Nurse educators should realize that continuing education may cause identity problems for some nurses who are undergoing it, in that much of such education may consist of turning one's back on an old way of doing something in order to learn a new one. For some nurses, this may be tantamount to turning their backs on their conception of their role as nurses. Educators must be understanding with such nurses, in order to help them towards the desired path of self-discovery.

    5. Connecticut '66   No educational program should be a dead end which discourages the nurse from continuing education and broadening skills. Institutions of higher education

TABLE F-1. SUMMARY OF RECOMMENDATIONS

5. Connecticut '66
(continued)

should develop a system to evaluate the practitioner of nursing in a way which would qualify a nurse to move, with credit, to the next higher educational program.

6. *Hospital Effectiveness Study* '67

Training program opportunities should be the vehicle for advancement in career status, lending visibility to career ladders leading from entry jobs to better positions both within and outside the hospital in other community health services. This may be accomplished by establishing a planned career development which involves both education and training and time off if necessary to pursue both. An essential element is the establishment of a mechanism for relating academic training to job experience the product of which is acceptable as credits for admission to institutions of higher learning where advanced learning is available.

7. National Commission on Health Manpower '67

A program of periodic recertification for licensure should be developed in this country and must have at its base an efficient and effective program of continuing education. Universities involved in health manpower education should be charged with the responsibility and provided full support for the development of an organized system of continuing education.

8. North Carolina '67

It is essential that continuing education programs receive state support for upgrading the knowledge and skills of active nurses. In addition, refresher courses must be expanded to attract inactive nurses back into the profession.

9. *Technology and Manpower in Health Service* '67

Career ladder training projects for health workers should be established on a wide scale both within health facilities and in arrangements between these facilities and vocational schools to facilitate upgrading of health workers.

Career ladder training systems will help to expand the supply of the scarcest group of health personnel — those who require the longest training — more quickly than if the existing system of relying solely on training new recruits is continued.

TABLE F-1.   SUMMARY OF RECOMMENDATIONS

11. Southern Regional Education Board '67	Although continuing education occupies an important place in nursing, it is not a substitute for graduate education, nor can graduate courses be offered piece-meal through continuing education programs. It is also no substitute for in-service education, for which nursing employers must continue to be responsible.
12. Boston College Nursing Home Study '68	In-service education programs for nursing personnel should be directed towards the identification and solution of specific nursing problems present in the particular institution.
13. Illinois '68	There is an urgent need to increase the opportunities in Illinois for nurse practitioners to update and expand their knowledge in order to keep their skills and competencies current. It is recommended that: 1) University of Illinois College of Nursing be charged with developing a state-wide plan for continuing and extension education for nurses; 2) Illinois Nurses Association continue to find ways to strengthen its function of providing opportunities for nurses to update their clinical knowledge and skill; 3) Illinois League for Nursing continue to offer educational opportunities for the development or improvement of supervisory, administrative, and teaching skills of nurses.
14. Georgia '69	It is recommended that the Georgia Regional Medical Program have substantial responsibility in providing continuing education for nurses, particularly in the areas of heart, cancer and stroke. It is recommended that the Georgia State Nurses' Association and the Georgia State League for Nursing continue to sponsor continuing education programs. It is recommended that employers of nurses consider structuring salary scales to reward nurses who complete courses in continuing education.
15. Idaho '69	Continuing education for practitioners of nursing should be vigorously promoted and should become available to nurses in all parts of the state. A division of continuing education with a statewide advisory committee should be incorporated into collegiate nursing programs, should utilize previously mentioned

TABLE F-1. SUMMARY OF RECOMMENDATIONS

15. Idaho '69
    (continued)

studies of specific needs for continuing education of nurses, and should provide direction for courses and conferences.

Institutions and agencies should provide opportunities for in-service and continuing education of nursing personnel. Whenever possible, the employing agency should attempt to subsidize deserving employees.

16. Wisconsin '70

The Commission recommends that employers consider in-service education a necessary factor in the maintenance of a modern nursing service, and provide time and expenses for nurse participation in in-service education on a regular basis.

G. Nursing Faculty
  1. Stewart '43

Nurse educators must have a professional nursing background, and an additional year of study in a school of education is highly advisable. Psychological tests might be used to identify nurses with the potential for teaching.

Nurse educators should actively plan curricula, select and guide students, and generally be responsible for the full range of educational functions.

Nursing educators should be able to plan, revise, and appraise professional and subprofessional education, and to initiate changes in both, as needed. Active research into educational needs should be an ongoing concern.

  2. *Nursing Education and
     Catholic Institutions '63*

Personnel policies for faculty members in hospital schools should be comparable to those in approved educational institutions. They must be developed according to the specific demands of the teaching position and the level of educational preparation required. Therefore, they cannot be constructed on the same basis as policies for nursing service or other hospital personnel.

Faculty members of baccalaureate programs should be engaged by the college under the same policies as operate for the general faculty. They should have the same rights and privileges as the general faculty and should actively participate in faculty affairs.

Faculty members in graduate programs should be, or be in a position to become, recognized authorities in a

TABLE F-1. SUMMARY OF RECOMMENDATIONS

2. *Nursing Education and Catholic Institutions '63* (continued)

specialty within nursing, should have advanced degrees themselves, and should have the graduate habit of mind.

There appears to be a particularly acute shortage of Catholic nurses with preparation in a clinical specialty at the Master's degree and doctoral levels. Steps should be taken to increase the number of religious and lay Catholic nurses with this preparation.

Faculty of collegiate programs in nursing are urged to construct evaluation tools that can be used with higher validity than those now available to identify the degree of professional competency of the associate professional nurse in determining advanced standing.

Each school of nursing and the parent institution should realize that personnel policies for faculty, involving both conditions of employment and salary scales, can be a serious deterrent to attracting students to prepare for faculty positions and recruitment of qualified faculty for a specific institution. (If there is in fact a tendency for graduates of master's degree programs qualified for faculty appointment to avoid positions in hospital diploma schools, the condition may result more from the individual's own observations of limitations on faculty in planning and executing an educational program than from any attempt by the college to discourage such employment.)

3. Michigan '66

Facts and figures in this report indicating that the future supply of nurses in all fields of nursing is contingent upon the availability of qualified faculty should be published and widely distributed to the citizens of Michigan, Governor's Committee on Human Resources, public officials, employers of nurses and medical profession.

Employing agencies, schools of nursing, nursing organizations should all make a conscious effort to identify nurses with potential for teaching and counsel them to prepare for faculty positions.

Salaries for nurse faculty should be comparable to salaries for positions with like responsibilities in other fields of education in institutions of higher learning.

TABLE F-1. SUMMARY OF RECOMMENDATIONS

3. Michigan '66 (continued)	Funds should be provided to enable directors of nursing education programs to acquire modern teaching aids and to utilize new educational media, thus making more effective use of their available nurse faculty.
4. North Carolina '67	The educational attainment of faculty members should be at least one level more advanced than the level of nursing which they teach, but not less than a baccalaureate degree.
5. Alabama '68	Each school of nursing establish an organized plan for faculty improvement through provision of opportunities for advanced education.
	Whenever feasible, similar programs in close proximity share faculty members.
	Liberalize personnel policies to employ increased numbers of part-time faculty.
	Increased attention to faculty research and publishing on a national scale, thereby improving image of nursing education in Alabama.
6. Illinois '68	Increase enrollments in established baccalaureate programs to utilize effectively the scarce supply of qualified faculty.
7. Massachusetts '68	Expansion of part-time employment possibilities.
	Professional nursing associations which have heretofore focused most of their programs on the return of nurses to positions in practice settings should now also direct their programs toward the encouragement and preparation of some of these inactive nurses for teaching positions.
	Curriculum patterns and relationships between schools of nursing must be reexamined in search of ways to use the talents of current faculty members more effectively.
	Courses currently being offered in only one or two baccalaureate or master's programs due to limited number of faculty prepared in a special area should be made available to students enrolled in all such nursing programs. Selected courses in the nursing curriculum of every college and university based nursing program should be open to students from other nursing schools and other nursing programs.

TABLE F-1. SUMMARY OF RECOMMENDATIONS

8. Idaho '69

Adequate budget for qualified faculty must be provided for Idaho nursing education programs to facilitate replacement of faculty members with less than the nationally recommended preparation and to keep pace with increased enrollments.

9. Michigan '69

All possible efforts should be directed toward increasing the number of prepared faculty through strengthening and expansion of graduate programs leading to the master's degree in nursing. These efforts will call for innovative approaches to the organization of faculty and the structuring of curricula as well as for the development of new ways of preparing teachers. Because the baccalaureate graduates constitute the potential pool from which master's degree candidates must be recruited, the number of these graduates must be increased by recruitment of qualified graduates of diploma and associate degree programs into the baccalaureate programs, as well as by initial recruitment of more prospective nursing students into the baccalaureate programs.

The utilization in technical nursing programs of faculty prepared at the baccalaureate level should be explored. This will require curriculum innovation within the baccalaureate programs preparing such faculty, modification of State Board and accreditation requirements, and alteration of faculty staffing patterns in the technical nursing programs themselves.

The shortage of qualified faculty for every level of nursing education represents the most immediate and crucial impediment to the expansion of nursing education; immediate steps should be taken to devise short-range and long-range solutions directed toward:

1) Producing more faculty;
2) Innovation in faculty staffing patterns and teaching methods to facilitate more effective utilization of clinical facilities and personnel;
3) Examination of standards for credentials required of faculty at each level of nursing education.

10. North Dakota '69

An increase in state scholarship or loan funds for the preparation of faculty at the master's level should be implemented.

TABLE F-1. SUMMARY OF RECOMMENDATIONS

10. North Dakota '69
    (continued)
There should be more opportunities for continuing education to assist faculty to improve and upgrade their teaching.

Improved methods of educational technology and cooperation between schools should be explored in order to make it possible for better utilization of adequately prepared faculty.

H. Nursing Student Recruitment and Financial Aids
  1. Brown '48
Nurses everywhere should seek to recruit students and personnel without regard to sex, marital status, economic background, or ethnic, racial, and religious origins. Positive steps should be taken by the profession to create an atmosphere conducive to attracting carefully selected representatives of a true cross-section of the population to nursing.

  2. Ginzberg '48
To improve recruitment prospects, we recommend: greater efforts in smaller communities; larger quotas for training Negro and male nurses; more part-time employment of married nurses; more democratic administration in nursing schools and nursing services.

  3. Bridgman '53
Substantial enlargement of the number of and enrollment in, professional schools of nursing in colleges and universities. The achievement of this purpose involves making these schools equal in fact to other divisions of the institutions, and eliminating the present confusion about their relative significance through interpretation of the distinctive advantages and opportunities they offer.

  4. Nahm '59
Student recruits should be of high intellectual ability, with qualities of character and personality that make for effectiveness in many situations, and with motivation for human service.

  5. *Nursing Education and Catholic Institutions '63*
The scope of opportunities for preparation in nursing should permit the recruitment of the maximum number of men and women differing in interests, abilities, objectives and educational preferences and their preparation for a role which will be useful and satisfying.

Admission policies related to age, race, creed, marital status and sex should be evaluated in the light of social change, and doctrines of the Church and the demanding need for increasing the number of well-prepared nurses.

TABLE F-1. SUMMARY OF RECOMMENDATIONS

5. *Nursing Education and Catholic Institutions '63* (continued)

Changed social conditions as well as sound principles of pastoral and educational counseling indicate that policies discouraging students who wish to marry should be re-examined.

The practice of some hospitals who subsidize one or more students annually for a preservice education in nursing in exchange for a stated length of employment in the institution on graduation should be explored.

Continued effort must be made to clearly define the qualifications, characteristics and purposes of the various types of educational programs, to reach acceptance on these points by nurse educators, and to recruit for each program the student whose abilities are best suited to it. For example, superior students should be encouraged to enter baccalaureate degree programs. Until this is achieved, high school counselors and others who counsel young people will not be able with assurance to guide students interested in nursing to programs in which they may achieve success and may choose to steer them to alternate fields.

Community-wide recruitment programs should be encouraged, designed to reach potential students for any of the educational programs in nursing.

Salaries and conditions of employment for nurses may be a deterrent to recruitment, unless they compare favorably with those in other positions open to women. They should be related to the responsibilities assumed by the graduate, and expense in time and effort to prepare for the position.

All institutions and agencies employing nursing personnel should assume a share of the responsibility for recruitment, especially hospitals which do not contribute to nursing education either as a controlling or a cooperating agency.

Graduates of a two-year liberal arts program in a junior or community college may be a potential recruitment source for baccalaureate degree programs which concentrate nursing courses in the upper division.

TABLE F-1. SUMMARY OF RECOMMENDATIONS

6. Connecticut '66   There should be undertaken:

1) An information program about education for nursing and allied health fields established for all student counselors, educators, and parents; and
2) a continuing campaign to support and advertise all scholarships and loan funds available for those interested in a career in nursing and allied health fields.

7. *Hospital Effectiveness*   Incentives must be established which will encourage
   Study '67   young people to pursue a health occupation. This may be accomplished by imporving the image of the health worker. Perhaps the most common bench mark of "public image" is income. Job security, against periods of economic depression, is another. Increasing income among the health occupations would tend to have greater appeal to a sophisticated public which can no longer afford to be attracted to health occupations solely because they feel a compulsion to help people.

Training opportunities should also be provided including associated financial assistance. The training of health personnel should be a community affair.

8. Indiana '67   Accelerate recruitment activities for students and inactive nurses under the direction of the professional nursing organizations, with the assistance of the employer of nurses.

9. North Carolina '67   Attract more and better qualified students through increases in scholarship and loan funds and efficient dissemination of information about nursing careers. Cooperative efforts should be made by the nursing profession, high school guidance counselors, nursing school faculties and public information media.

10. Nursing Training   The student loan program be continued and the
    Act (Review) '67   maximum amount of loans for baccalaureate and graduate degree candidates be increased to $2,500 per academic year; and the amount for diploma and associate degree candidates be increased to $1,500 per academic year.

Funds be made available to assist private nonprofit and public agencies or institutions for recruitment programs for nursing. Recruitment funds be used to

TABLE F-1. SUMMARY OF RECOMMENDATIONS

10. Nursing Training Act (Review) '67 (continued)	identify talent for nursing among minority and disadvantaged groups and to provide for remedial and tutorial services.
11. Southern Regional Education Board '67	Effective publicity is as important a factor in attracting young people to nursing careers as financial aid and financial reward. The full story of the attractions and satisfactions of nursing has never been told.
12. *Technology and Man-power in the Health Service Industry '67*	Scholarship and living allowance incentives should be made available to qualified candidates for training in critically scarce health occupations.
13. Alabama '68	Lack of qualified applicants is the biggest single factor in preventing existing schools of nursing from increasing their enrollments. To increase the supply of qualified applicants it is recommended that:

> 1) Recruitment practices be reemphasized and reevaluated;
> 2) The amount of remedial work for applicants or new students be increased;
> 3) Public school education be strengthened.

14. Illinois '68	All nurse recruitment efforts in Illinois need reappraisal; there is a need for a more intensive effort in recruitment within the profession focused on leadership development and the specialized fields of nursing; there is also a need for more coordination and sophistication in recruitment efforts at the entry point in nursing.
15. Massachusetts '68	Improvement of Recruitment, Application and Admission Procedures by:

> 1) Purpose and curriculum of each type of nursing program and the nature of each school be described in precise terms that are meaningful and useful to applicant and counselor;
> 2) More cooperative relationships between the profession and high school counselors.
> 3) Board of Higher Education, in cooperation with the professional organization and schools of nursing, initiate a computer program which will identify the schools to which an individual has applied, record outcome of application and report this information to schools involved;

TABLE F-1. SUMMARY OF RECOMMENDATIONS

15. Massachusetts '68 (continued)	4) Schools of nursing adopt procedures to use this information to accelerate the decision making process so the true number of individuals expected as enrollees can be determined as early as possible; 5) Systematic study of dropouts to reduce attrition.
16. Williamsburg Conference '68	Recruitment into and graduation from diploma schools of nursing continues to be a necessity in order to meet the current and future demands for nursing personnel. However, many students today are apparently being discouraged by high school counselors and others from entering diploma programs of nursing because of the public's emphasis on a college education. In addition, of the students who apply for admission to diploma programs, a number are not academically qualified. Consequently, much of the financial aid available to students in the diploma programs is not being utilized. The group recommended that hospitals should encourage qualified students to enroll in diploma programs.
17. Nursing Education in Georgia '69	It is recommended that the Health Careers Council of Georgia, Inc., assume major responsibility for general recruitment for nursing, and provide information for counselors, parents and students. It is recommended that some recruitment efforts be directed toward older women in order to attract them to careers in nursing. It is recommended that recruitment efforts be directed toward individuals who are not presently academically qualified for admission to nursing school, and that a program in remedial and tutorial services be developed to assist these individuals in meeting admission standards.
18. Idaho '69	A State Health Careers Council made up of representatives of organized health professionals, high school counselors, and influential members of selected civic groups should be established to recruit candidates for all of the health professions. Their efforts to be directed toward: 1) The development of recruitment materials aimed at improving the portrayal of the role of the modern nurse;

TABLE F-1. SUMMARY OF RECOMMENDATIONS

18. Idaho '69
   (continued)

2) The involvement in nurse recruitment of more individuals and groups such as district medical and nursing associations, women's medical auxiliaries, and representatives of health institutions and agencies;

3) The provision of scholarships and loans for students entering schools of nursing in Idaho by agencies and service organizations such as the Idaho State Nurses' Association, Idaho Medical Association, the state, and voluntary agencies;

4) Instituting on a local basis such activities as high school essay contests related to nursing that would stimulate reading about and making visits to nursing services and programs;

5) Contacting all high school counselors to inform them about nursing education and career opportunities in nursing;

6) Attracting into nursing more male students, such as men with experience as armed-forces medical corpsmen;

7) Encouraging women in the 35-45 year range to enroll in schools of nursing to prepare to enter or reenter the work force;

8) Improving high school and college counseling in order to reduce the attrition rate and to encourage the most capable students to select careers in the health professions.

19. Michigan '69

Greater efforts should be made by nursing organizations, voluntary, and public health agencies, and schools of nursing to publicize to high school students the career opportunities and challenges of professional nursing.

Informational and educational efforts concerning nursing careers directed to student counselors, both at the secondary and post-secondary school levels, should emphasize the importance of helping the prospective nursing student select the type of training most appropriate to abilities and career goals, and of assuring that the latter have been formulated on the basis of adequate knowledge of the alternative career avenues in nursing.

It should be recognized that economically and educationally disadvantaged persons constitute a potentially important source of manpower for nursing as well as for other health and non-health fields. In order to draw on this resource innovative approaches to the

TABLE F-1. SUMMARY OF RECOMMENDATIONS

19. Michigan '69 (continued)	recruitment of persons from this group should be tested and applied.
20. North Dakota '69	In an attempt to broaden the base of recruitment, emphasis should be placed on:

        1) Recruitment of men;

        2) Recruitment of women over thirty who are established residents of the area.

21. Wisconsin '70 — The Commission suggests that all recruitment of students for initial nursing education programs should place emphasis on:

        1) Development of vigorous programs to attract male students, married women and members of minority groups into nursing education programs;

        2) Elimination of age restrictions if applicants meet admission requirements;

        3) The admission of students who demonstrate that they have the equivalent of a high school education.

I. Nursing Education in General

   1. Goldmark '23 — Standards of educational attainment now generally accepted by the professions and embodied in legislation of the more progressive states must be maintained, and any attempt to lower these standards would be a real danger to the public.

   2. Stewart '43 — Two years of general education and two years of professional education are minimal requirements for educating potential leaders.

Intellectual abilities are to be emphasized over technical skills for professionals. ("education" vs. "training")

Nursing must provide more leaders (of the democratic, education-oriented type rather than the authoritarian, order-oriented type). Broad professional preparation is necessary to provide such leaders. Recognized accreditation agencies should set the standards for such preparation.

Nursing schools should have at least one guidance and coordination specialist, who can aid students and help prevent the faculty from becoming too inflexible and technical training oriented.

TABLE F-1. SUMMARY OF RECOMMENDATIONS

3. Brown '48	Careful consideration should be given to the possible advantages of utilizing the pattern of organizational structure laid down by engineering schools and already introduced in nursing education, rather than the pattern that has characterized most of professional education, when new basic curricula are established within institutions of higher learning. Competing diploma courses should be completely eliminated and advanced programs for graduate nurses be continued only if they do not detract from the time, attention and financial resources that should be devoted to building basic curricula.
	Standards like those formulated by the Association of Collegiate Schools of Nursing should govern the appointment, status, qualification, teaching and administrative load of faculty in professional schools of nursing. The present system of advanced preparation should be examined comprehensively and reorganized to attempt to attract more women of ability and provide more substantial preparation for leadership in nursing education and other nursing specialities.
	Individual persons, groups and private corporate bodies (e.g., foundations and institutions of higher learning) should make the most funds available for the creation and strengthening of good college and university schools of nursing. Also, official groups, local, state and federal, should supply whatever additional resources necessary for adequate support of nursing education on the professional and nonprofessional levels. All contributions and grants should be made on the basis of educational standards maintained by individual schools.
	Effort should be directed to building basic schools of nursing in universities and colleges, comparable in number to existing medical schools, that are sound in organizational and financial structure, adequate in facilities and well distributed to serve the needs of the entire country.
4. Ginzberg '48	Student clinical experiences should include only those that their education requires. Hospital needs are to be fulfilled by hired nurses.
5. West and Hawkins '50	Further self-evaluation of basic programs would help nursing schools determine what specific characteristics might be improved within the school organization.

TABLE F-1. SUMMARY OF RECOMMENDATIONS

5. West and Hawkins '50
(continued)

The schools might be helped by evaluation of current practices within each state by state nursing organizations. Since minimum standards vary from state to state, state nursing education groups could cooperate with state boards in studying strengths and weaknesses toward bringing all schools to a nationally accepted standard.

A clear definition of nursing education standards in objective, measurable terms by the nursing profession would assist state groups and schools in developing new standards to meet current needs.

Further cooperation of state and regional educational groups would be invaluable.

Further study is indicated in several fields touched by the school data analysis: determining the availability of students for all types of nursing programs, with emphasis on more effective recruitment directed toward men and minority groups; determining the most economic and efficient use of clinical and educational facilities, from the point of view of the student as well as the school; and exploring the content and length of program in basic nursing education.

6. Bridgman '53

Nursing Education should be publicly supported under a system planned, supported and conducted solely for educational purposes. Faculties should concentrate upon improving methods, content, and organization of curricula and thus increase the competence of graduates for the nursing services — the end result being a greater supply of better qualified nursing personnel. Every consideration seems to point in the direction of a gradual integration of nursing education into the national system which already provides, for every other occupational group requiring it, opportunity for post-high school education in institutions founded and supported for that purpose.

Nursing education at all levels should be available equally to every qualified person — equality of opportunity.

Establishment of curricula in nursing in junior colleges and lower-division units of four-year colleges and universities on an equal basis with terminal-occupational courses in other fields.

TABLE F-1. SUMMARY OF RECOMMENDATIONS

6. Bridgman '53
(continued)

In a university setting, the same policies must be applied to nursing as are consistent with the general standards of colleges and universities. Nursing students must recognize the benefits of a genuine college education and nursing degrees must be truly representative of the completion of an upper-division major in the degree-granting institution.

Nursing education must be supplied on the college level to prepare sufficient potential candidates for specialized functions such as the clinical specialists, public health nurses, supervisors, administrators, teachers, researchers, writers and staff for professional organizations and planning agencies. Thus, the most important and immediate demand for the maintenance and improvement of health services is for larger numbers of better qualified personnel for the highest range of functions (teachers, administrators, etc.).

7. Lambertsen '58

A professional nurse should be a liberally educated person who can share social and professional responsibility with others. To attain this end, a multi-discipline approach to nursing education seems advisable. Nursing educators should work with other educators of professionals to identify more precisely the general competencies which all college educated men and women should possess.

Professional education should prepare the student for continuous learning and growth even as the principles learned are being applied. The product of a professional education program should be a beginning practitioner, not an accomplished one. The emphasis is on the discipline of problem solving rather than on the accumulation of facts and technics.

The professional curriculum should reflect the philosophy and ideals of the profession. It should teach what the profession ideally could do as well as the current state of practice.

8. Montag '59

Objectives of each type of nursing education (AD, diploma, BS, etc.) must be clearly stated; so that the end product of each can be clearly defined as to preparation and functions to be performed:

1) The decision as to whether there is a place for the *professional* practitioner in nursing must be made, and specific programs for educating these professionals must be provided;

TABLE F-1. SUMMARY OF RECOMMENDATIONS

8. Montag '59
(continued)

2) The "ladder" concept of nursing education (i.e., having different stopping points in one overall program for practical nurses, technical nurses, RN's, professional nurses, etc.) is not defensible if clear differentiation of function is made. Different functions imply the need for differences in preparation, rather than a split-up continuum of nursing education.

Student nurses must be viewed as *students*, not as part-time ward workers, if full advantage is to be taken of recent curriculum revisions. These revisions make it possible to include a great deal of teaching material in a comparatively short time. Thus, if students are expected to do work, this part of their "experience" must be separated from their actual nursing "education", which should consist of theoretical work and learning laboratories.

New teaching methods and a refinement of older methods are needed if nursing programs are to train an increasing number of students with a limited number of qualified instructors. Specifically, further studies are needed on the student-teacher ratio.

9. Nahm '59

Nursing education programs should be established for graduates of liberal arts colleges. Such programs, geared to high-ability students who could be prepared for leadership positions in nursing, could be based on these students' liberal background.

All programs of nursing education must undergo constant re-evaluation, in light of seeking to produce the ideal graduate: one who is flexible and capable of constantly enlarging her own body of knowledge and depth of understanding.

Many time-honored methods of education and the assumptions underlying the use of these methods should be critically examined. Analysis should be done of developing new methods which are based on changing concepts of human behavior and of the learning process.

10. Russell '59

One-half of all nursing school coursework should be in liberal arts courses. (i.e., 60 hours of a 120-hour program). The remaining one-half of the program should be devoted to courses designed for practical, direct application to the professional field.

TABLE F-1. SUMMARY OF RECOMMENDATIONS

10. Russell '59
(continued)

Liberal arts and professional courses should be offered *concurrently* as much as possible. (while admitting that scheduling problems often make this a difficult goal to achieve)

11. Rogers '61

Nurses must recognize that the primary purpose of professional education is to provide students with the principles and theories prerequisite to practice. Curricula must be designed to reflect this aim.

Those who plan the professional curricula, identify the theoretical concepts, and teach the teachers must also write the college-level texts and the scholarly references. They must spearhead the development of a body of literature geared to professional nurse readers.

12. *Nursing Education and Catholic Institutions '63*

A Catholic school of nursing should not plan to discontinue its program, develop a new one, or make radical changes in length or design until a thorough study has been made of all aspects of the situation and consultation secured from appropriate sources. As a general principle, an existing program which is good should not be changed unless something which is better can be developed.

Educational costs should be separated from other costs, and tuition charged which is realistically related to the educational costs. Consideration should be given to measures which would reduce educational costs without jeopardizing quality of programs such as:

1) Realistic utilization of faculty; the ratio of faculty to students should be based on demonstrated need in relation to the goals or objectives of the program;
2) Preparation of religious and their retention in faculty positions for which they are qualified;
3) Sharing of faculty and resources;
4) Charging students the tuition and other costs, such as transportation, involved in course affiliations for clinical subjects;
5) Students should pay for incidental education and living expenses, including uniforms, supplies, laundry, maintenance and textbooks.

TABLE F-1. SUMMARY OF RECOMMENDATIONS

12. *Nursing Education and Catholic Institutions '63* (continued)

In order not to exclude able and worthy students because of financial limitations, the following methods of assistance are suggested:

1) Encourage scholarships from all sources;
2) Provide opportunity for self help i.e., part-time work such as college students engage in;
3) Loans where available;
4) The possibility of accelerating the program for students with ability might be explored.

In planning to begin a new school or the expansion or renewal of facilities of an existing school, serious thought should be given to the establishment of a day school. Where residence is provided, a charge should be made to the student which is realistically related to the cost of providing the residence accommodations.

The existence of an educational program in nursing makes a valuable contribution to patient care. When costs of nursing education programs are realistically established and the appropriate portion charged to the student, the cost to the institution will be relatively minor.

The costs of nursing education should be accurately identified. Care must be taken to avoid overemphasis or exaggeration of the cost, which results in deterring continuation, growth or development of nursing education programs. In determining costs of operating a hospital school of nursing, it is suggested that the "avoidable cost" formula be investigated.

In order to maintain our voluntary system of education we should appeal more forcefully to industry, nationally or locally, for educational funds or trusts. Potential donors should be encouraged to contribute to a fund for faculty salaries and school expenses as well as for scholarships. The concept of "living endowment" could be used.

13. National Commission on Health Manpower '67

Formal education of all health professionals, graduate as well as undergraduate, be conducted under the aegis of universities. This is not to say that a college degree should be required of everyone entering the field of nursing, however, it is felt strongly that the university must take the overall responsibility for development and coordination of the various educational programs within the field of nursing.

TABLE F-1. SUMMARY OF RECOMMENDATIONS

14. New York '67

The establishment of educational programs that will assist — within the confines of the law — out-of-country nurses to become licensed as registered professional nurses in New York State, should be encouraged.

It is recommended that institutions conducting National League for Nursing accredited programs (or programs of quality that would warrant NLN accreditation) use the urban centers operated by the community colleges to aid otherwise eligible applicants who are in need of remedial assistance with such basic skills as reading and arithmetic.

It is further recommended that the services of urban universities be expanded to provide specific secondary school courses that will enable otherwise eligible applicants to meet the entrance requirements of nursing programs.

15. North Carolina '67

The finding that the ratio of students' to faculty members is unrelated to educational preparation of the students suggests that the cheapest way in time, money, and effort to increase educational opportunities is through expansion of existing programs having adequate hospital resources and faculty. Programs with inadequate resources should not be expanded. Since a high percentage of students from these programs do not pass the State Board Examination, the expansion of these programs would not aid significantly to the existing supply of nurses.

Enrollment in a nursing program should insure a ratio of at least five patients to each student receiving clinical experience in a given area or department of the training hospital at a given time.

16. Nurse Training
    Act (Review) '67

Construction of educational facilities for diploma, associate degree, baccalaureate, and graduate degree nursing programs should be continued under a single authorization with increased funds to provide for new construction and renovation of facilities and to substantially increase first-year places in schools of nursing.

TABLE F-1. SUMMARY OF RECOMMENDATIONS

16. Nurse Training
Act (Review) '67
(continued)

Basic support grants be given to all types of accredited nursing programs and these grants include:

1) A fixed sum for each type of program;
2) Additional funds based on full-time enrollment according to type of educational program and its costs to the institution;
3) Assurance that the present level of support allocated to the nursing program by the institution not be reduced.

Special grants be given to colleges and universities with no medical centers to assist them in starting new programs in nursing education.

Grants for improvement of nursing education be continued and expanded to cover total costs of projects to public and private nonprofit hospitals, institutions, and agencies, as well as to nursing education programs in universities and senior colleges, junior and community colleges, and hospital schools for the improvement, expansion and extension of their educational programs and services.

Grants be made to accredited nursing programs for studies to determine the long-range role and goals with regard to nursing education; and to facilitate cooperative agreements among agencies and institutions for orderly transition from one type of nursing education program to another.

Grants be given to nursing programs to assist them to reach high quality standards (i.e., accreditation).

Grants to public and private nonprofit institutions and agencies be made to assist in the planning, development, and establishment of new or modified programs for nursing education. This would include such projects as:

1) Acceleration of establishment of sound programs to prepare certain categories of professional nurses that are in short supply;
2) Establishment of centers where RN's could obtain baccalaureate education necessary to professional practice and graduate study;

TABLE F-1. SUMMARY OF RECOMMENDATIONS

16. Nurse Training
Act (Review) '67
(continued)

   3) Development of programs by which disadvantaged minority groups of students with
potential could realize a career in nursing;

   4) Development of programs to update the skills
of inactive nurses who wish to return to the
field but who feel inadequate because of the
changes in nursing practice.

Grants be made to those universities with medical and
health science centers that have programs in health
professions to study the feasibility of establishing a
nursing program; if such a study reveals the university's ability to finance the program, to recruit
qualified faculty and students, and to provide adequate resources and administrative support, then funds
will be extended over a five-year period for the
establishment of a nursing program.

Professional Nurse Traineeship Program be expanded
and modified to:

   1) Provide traineeship for advanced training of
professional nurses in administration,
supervision, teaching, and clinical nursing practice;

   2) Provide traineeship for diploma and associate
degree graduates to obtain the baccalaureate
preparation prerequisite to advanced training.

Funds and support be made available to private
nonprofit or public agencies for statewide or regional
planning for nursing.

17. Southern Regional
Education Board '67

The qualitative and quantitative gaps in nursing
services will become more threatening to the well-
being of people, and will continue to cause economic
loss unless planned action is taken at once. The first
point of attack must be nursing education: quality, its
capacity, and the balance among the components of
the nursing education system.

Planning for improved, expanded nursing education
must be done on a statewide basis.

An official state body must be responsible for planning and action to improve and expand nursing
education.

TABLE F-1. SUMMARY OF RECOMMENDATIONS

17. Southern Regional Education Board '67 (continued)	A clear understanding of the requirements and potentialities of each type of program (diploma, AD, baccalaureate) is needed in order to understand trends in nursing education, and to make decisions about which trends should be reinforced to produce the number and kinds of nurses needed in each state. Decisions about creating new programs, and modifying or closing others, also rest on a clear understanding of each type of education and institution.

Statewide planning must deal comprehensively with all types of nursing education, and must aim at the preparation of the various kinds and levels of personnel needed, each in proper balance with the others. Balance among the kinds of nursing personnel available has a great influence on the quality of nursing care. When the number of aides and practical nurses is out of proportion to the number of RN's, the quality of care is diluted and supervision is skimpy. In addition, when the number of RN's and nurses with advanced training is proportionately few, there is a shortage of leadership for improvement.

Planning for nursing education should be flexible enough to allow experimentation and justified changes, yet stable enough to resist capricious action to meet very temporary or local needs.

In general, the nursing programs should be distributed throughout the state in a manner which parallels the distribution of the population, keeping in mind that one large program is likely to produce better results than two small ones in the same general locale.

In spite of the high costs involved, planning bodies should see to it that facilities for nurses are large enough to accommodate growing enrollments in nursing, and that limited facilities do not become obstacles to the growth of programs. Per capita costs are higher when enrollments are small. |
| 18. Alabama '68 | The State Board of Nursing approach the State Board of Education relative to the employment of a state consultant for paramedical programs in junior colleges. Such a consultant could assist new programs in their establishment and implementation. |

TABLE F-1. SUMMARY OF RECOMMENDATIONS

19. California '68	Nursing programs should be large enough to accommodate growing enrollments in nursing. Limited facilities should not become obstacles to the growth of programs. Per capita costs are higher when enrollments are small.

Disparity of curriculum within and between programs indicates need for an in-depth curriculum study.

20. Illinois '68	Organized nursing in Illinois promote the principle of general subsidization of operating costs of the total educational enterprise recognizing the lack of such assistance as a great deterrent to the expansion and development of baccalaureate and higher degree programs in nursing in private universities.

The two year curriculum for the AD program will establish the mode for all other programs preparing technical nurses. Hospital schools already are shortening their curricula: this process will continue. One by-product of this change will be an increasing number of nurse graduates. Another by-product will be increased responsibility for employers to provide adequate clinical orientation and in-service education for the nurse graduates they employ.

21. Massachusetts '68	A temporary delay in the establishment of new nursing programs at less than the baccalaureate level. To bring into better balance the number of nurses with baccalaureate and master's preparation to supply faculty for all types of programs and to provide the leadership in nursing service. Until this balance is achieved none of the personnel or financial resources needed to accomplish this objective should be drained off into new programs at the AD, Diploma, or LPN level.

All schools of nursing in an area designate a certain portion of the clinical curriculum in which students from different types of programs will be assigned to the same patients and/or families and discussions regarding the care of these patients will be carried out with students and faculty from these different programs.

It is recommended that nursing programs in community and state colleges establish a transfer policy for students after one year of preparation. To implement this policy, procedures must be set up to:

TABLE F-1. SUMMARY OF RECOMMENDATIONS

21. Massachusetts '68
    (continued)

1) Identify students with the potential and desire for baccalaureate preparation;
2) Counsel them to this effect; and
3) Assist them in making this transfer.

22. Williamsburg Conference '68

In order that the schools will be more attuned to community needs, there should be more liaison between schools of nursing and those services in which nurses are employed, especially in hospitals which do maintain schools of nursing.

For all health education programs, there should be a core curriculum which is patient-oriented.

The present standards for entrance into the various nursing programs should not be lowered.

Education cannot be isolated from the utilization and development of the health services. Responsibility for clinical and educational aspects of nursing education should be centrally coordinated.

There is need to educate the public about health care education in an attempt to eliminate the mass confusion that presently exists.

There must be more comprehensive research in the area of health care needs.

Steps to encourage and facilitate advancement should be instituted in all health professions. This is particularly true in nursing. It was felt that one step would be flexibility in the academic requirements in nursing schools in order to ease the problems involved in upward transition of various levels. Such flexibility would also encourage the entry of military trained medical specialists, or corpsmen, into the civilian health care field upon release from active military service.

23. Georgia '69

It is recommended that the official state educational agencies, the State Department of Education and the Board of Regents, have primary responsibility for providing the nursing education programs necessary for the state.

TABLE F-1. SUMMARY OF RECOMMENDATIONS

23. Georgia '69
    (continued)

It is recommended that the appropriate unit of the University System of Georgia take leadership in exploring the concept of sharing faculty members among the Georgia schools of nursing, and that sufficient budget be provided to develop and implement the plan.

It is recommended that consideration be given to the inclusion of nursing education courses in the vocational education curriculum or that collegiate study in nursing be recognized as the equivalent of vocational education for certification purposes.

It is recommended that expanded planning and consultative services be provided for schools of nursing through the two State Examining Boards, and that sufficient budget be allocated to the Boards to provide for these consultative services.

24. Michigan '69

In light of existing federal grant programs for schools of nursing, the first priority of budgetary support at the state level should be to provide for the greatest possible expansion of enrollments in *existing* nursing programs leading to the associate degree in nursing, the baccalaureate, and higher degrees, as the first phase of state planning to expand nursing education in Michigan.

Community college districts should be encouraged and assisted to develop reciprocity agreements which would facilitate regional recruitment of nursing students and the development of regional and statewide planning for nursing education.

Institutions of higher learning with potential resources for the development of associate and baccalaureate degree programs should be encouraged through consultative services and financial assistance to develop these programs.

The State Board of Education, under its constitutional mandate, should assume primary responsibility for the implementation of the State Plan for Nursing Education. The State Board of Education should work closely with the State Board of Nursing in discharging this responsibility.

TABLE F-1. SUMMARY OF RECOMMENDATIONS

24. Michigan '69
    (continued)

Effective implementation of state planning will require that private educational institutions and professional associations be consulted in the planning for health services, health manpower, and health facilities. They should be involved from the beginning in the development of the State Plan for Nursing Education. The professional associations, in particular, should undertake a leadership role in gaining acceptance and implementation of recommendations relating to such aspects of the state plan as utilization of nurses in various health settings, in-service training recruitment, and reactivation of nurses.

The State Board of Education will need to make decisions as to the relative merit of expanding existing programs of nursing education versus establishment of new programs. Because of the immediate critical shortage of nursing faculty, the proliferation of programs should be avoided. The Advisory Committee therefore recommends first priority be placed on expanding existing programs where appropriate.

A systematic approach needs to be devised for facilitating transfer or progression from one educational level of nursing to another, for example, RN to BSN or aide to LPN. This will require experimentation by educational institutions in designing curriculum, the support and encouragement of the State Boards of Nursing and of Education in fostering such experimentation, and appropriate evaluation procedures. The experience gained by nursing educators in the planning, development and evaluation of ADN programs might provide guidelines.

For the immediate future, primary emphasis must be given to expansion of existing schools of nursing. Those schools which, by virtue of geographic location, potential for student recruitment, and quality of program, have the potential for expansion should be encouraged to utilize every possible means of increasing enrollments. This requires development of innovative methods of teaching, utilization of multimedia, and the economical and effective use of clinical facilities.

25. North Dakota '69

We support the trend of placing responsibility for nursing education programs in institutions of higher education with cooperating responsibility in health care institutions providing adequate clinical facilities.

TABLE F-1. SUMMARY OF RECOMMENDATIONS

25. North Dakota '69
(continued)

Since two levels of nursing practice and preparation are the goals for nursing, we recommend that the North Dakota Board of Higher Education assume responsibility for placing nursing education into the general system of higher education. Nursing education should be included in the master plan for higher education in North Dakota.

We recommend that programs unable to meet the national accreditation standards due to lack of prepared faculty, inadequate clinical facilities, inadequate student enrollment, and inadequate financing be discontinued.

26. Virginia '69

That, in developing plans for adequate and coordinated educational programs for nurses in Virginia, the Committee on Education for the Health Professions and Occupations of the State Council of Higher Education:

Give immediate attention to the formulation of a policy whereby challenge or equivalency examinations will be used in the various nursing education programs throughout the Commonwealth of Virginia as a means for nursing students to receive credit for specific courses in which they may prove competent without the necessity of their actually being enrolled in each course in the curriculum.

That all schools of nursing in the Commonwealth of Virginia grant credit toward completion of requirements for graduation of their students for previously acquired competency and knowledge on the basis of equivalency examinations.

That the state-supported institutions of higher education provide, without charge, academic and nonclinical instruction to students of diploma schools of nursing fully accredited by the State Board of Examiners of Nurses and that there be appropriated for the state institutions of higher education a sum sufficient to defray the cost thereof.

27. Wisconsin '70

The Commission recommends that the Board of Nursing encourage hospitals and other health care institutions and community action agencies that have adequate clinical facilities and that are located in proximity to educational agencies offering nursing education programs, to evaluate their educational role

TABLE F-1. SUMMARY OF RECOMMENDATIONS

27. Wisconsin '70
    (continued)

and interest, meet requirements for becoming an extended unit and offer facilities for use in the preparation of nurses — if not now affiliated or participating.

II. Nursing Service and Practice
A. Role and Utilization
    1. Goldmark '23

The role of the nurse in public health is one of health work and health teaching in families; thus, public health people should be capable of giving general health instruction, as distinguished from instruction in any one specialty; furthermore, these persons should be capable of rendering bedside care at need and should, therefore, complete basic nurses' training. All employers of public health nurses should require basic hospital training followed by a postgraduate course including both class work and field work in public health nursing.

The development of nursing service adequate for the care of the sick and for the conduct of the modern public health campaign demands as an absolute prerequisite the securing of funds for the endowment of nursing education of all types. It is of primary importance, in this connection, to provide reasonably generous endowment for university schools of nursing.

    2. Stewart '43

Nurses should concentrate on essential nursing functions, leaving other (housekeeping, accounting, etc.) functions to other groups.

    3. Ginzberg '48

Practical nurses should be formally trained and licensed, and used only under professional nurse supervision.

The tasks which appropriately fall within the sphere of nursing care and nursing administration are being performed increasingly with the assistance of practical nurses. By shifting some portion of the performance of nursing care to practical nurses, it is possible to reduce requirements for professional nurses. This step is desirable not only as an emergency measure to ease the shortage, but also as a contribution to improving the basic structure responsible for providing nursing services.

TABLE F-1. SUMMARY OF RECOMMENDATIONS

4. Montag '51

Recommendations Concerning the Technical Functions of Nursing

Because no specific provision is made for the large middle group of nursing functions (on either side of the middle are simple and complex functions), a *new* worker in nursing is being proposed: a Nursing Technician who should have semi-professional or technical functions.

The Nurse Technician should be called upon to use skill and some judgment but should not be expected to function at the complex end of the function spectrum.

Recommendations Concerning Programs for Nursing Technicians

Preparation of nursing technicians should be carried on in any post-high school level institution such as junior colleges, technical institutes and the most ideal setting being the community college. But programs can be offered by both public and private institutions.

Federal, state and local funds should be provided for these nursing programs.

The curriculum should be experimented with and if possible, ultimately shortened from 3 to 2 years.

The curriculum should be integrated throughout with both general and technical subjects.

The development of technical skills should be emphasized and the educational experience should be practical and applied. The program should lead to the AD degree and to licensure (there should be *one* licensure for nurses — one which sets the minimum requirements for the safety of the public).

The programs must become integral parts of higher educational institutions so the programs will be financially secure enough to permit experimentation so that the most effective organization can be determined.

More emphasis should be placed upon the educational experiences which the clinical services offer, rather than on service needs; thus, clinical experiences should

TABLE F-1. SUMMARY OF RECOMMENDATIONS

4. Montag '51
(continued)

be regulated by the educational institution so that nurses won't be exploited by hospitals — so that they can be students rather than workers.

Recommendations Concerning Professional Personnel

Programs should be established in graduate institutions (eg: Columbia Teacher's College), on or beyond the masters level, to prepare professional nurses to administer and teach the nursing technician programs.

The programs should be experimented with first, before they are implemented.

5. Bridgman '53

Nursing's single purpose is all-inclusive care for patients; however, functions must be distributed among several contributors instead of being concentrated in one person.

Improve nursing service by expansion of in-service training.

6. Lambertsen '58

Research into the determination of the roles of the professional nurse and all nursing team members is needed. These roles should be separately identifiable.

Only professional nurses should be responsible for the performance of the nursing team, and only professional nurses may delegate nursing or quasi-nursing functions to other team members.

7. Montag '59

RN's should do actual bedside nursing, not merely supervision of nurses' aides and students who are doing the actual nursing. Nursing services must see that the RN's actually nurse, partly to serve as role models for students.

Graduate nurses must be oriented to the setting in which they will work, including exposure to the physical plant and their expected duties. The nursing shortage makes inevitable the fact that new graduates will have to assume responsibilities for which they are ill prepared, but the graduates in such situations cannot be censured for failure.

The profession is responsible for defining the role functions of the various "nurse" practitioners, and for defining the preparation expected of each level. Additionally, the profession should be concerned over

TABLE F-1. SUMMARY OF RECOMMENDATIONS

7. Montag '59 (continued)	the preference of so many RN's to do supervisory and managerial work in preference to bedside nursing.
	Statements of functions, such as those prepared by several sections of the ANA should be taken seriously. The profession should educate practitioners and students as to the content of such statements. The statements should become curricular guides for nursing schools.
8. Nahm '59	Continued research is needed in defining the role of the nurse; for determining where nursing ends and medicine and social work begin.
9. Rogers '61	Nursing must be composed of professional, technological, and vocational workers, with each of these levels clearly focused on different roles.
	Only professional nurses should direct, supervise, and make decisions concerning nursing practice.
10. Connecticut '66	Concerted effort should be made by all institutions and agencies throughout the state to prepare persons to do the many non-nursing tasks which are now performed by nurses but could be done as well or better by individuals with other special skills.
	There should be a significant increase in communications and joint planning between the educators in nursing, on the one hand, and the administrative and supervisory nurses who are responsible for patient care, on the other.
11. National Commission on Health Manpower '67	Specially organized ambulatory care centers be established especially in geographic areas of need (slums, rural areas, etc.). Twenty-four hour services including the disciplines of public health nursing and social work would be provided.
	The establishment and rapid and widespread application of automated diagnostic and laboratory services for mass medical screening of large populations and for diagnostic workups for non-emergency hospital admissions. These services would employ highly trained technicians and nurses but few physicians.

TABLE F-1. SUMMARY OF RECOMMENDATIONS

12. Southern Regional Educational Board '67	Goal setting should not be hampered by fears that goals cannot be reached. A planning body must know how many nurses are needed in order to achieve the full benefits of nursing services for the people of the state. Goals must reflect this actual need, and should not take into account a state's ability to produce the nurses needed. Compromises with reality should be made in the second stage of planning when action to meet stated goals is designed. Planners will have to distinguish between demands for nursing personnel and real needs.
13. Arizona '68	There is need for more standardization of nomenclature in reference to nursing personnel in order to improve communications among hospital workers. Nurse consultants able to spend time helping nurses identify nursing problems and seach for solutions are greatly needed. Nursing consultation requires graduate preparation and a practical understanding of the work setting. It seems desirable that this consultant service should be separated from any type of licensing procedure. Whether consultant nurses should be based in the State Department of Health, the SNA, or one of the universities is a matter that might require some study.
14. Boston College Nursing Home Study '68	RN's currently employed in nursing homes should be prepared to assess patients, and to develop goal-directed nursing care plans. The current system of delivering nursing services in nursing homes should be modified in light of the unique needs of this patient population. Decisions about nursing service should be based on accurate data germane to nursing rather than on other variables which cannot determine the kind and amount of nursing required. The scope and limitation of the nursing service available in a nursing home should be a key factor in deciding on the admission of patients. The number and kinds of nursing service personnel employed be determined by the needs of the patients.

TABLE F-1. SUMMARY OF RECOMMENDATIONS

14. Boston College Nursing Home Study '68 (continued)	The findings of this study be used to develop guidelines for determining the costs of nursing services in nursing homes.
15. Illinois '68	Continuous effort is needed to improve the career incentives and economic appeals of nursing and to open lines of communication between nursing and management in these subjects. Because of acute problems of recruitment and retention in mental health nursing, a special study be undertaken to identify what economic and other career incentives are needed to relieve this situation. The appropriate role of the RN is not well defined in most employment situations and existing definitions are not well accepted. Delineation of the role provides the tools for measuring what effective utilization is. But it is the consensus of the Commission that efforts to improve nurse utilization cannot await the "last word" on roles and functions. Enough is known now about what is good and what is not good nurse utilization to permit immediate efforts toward improvement.
16. Maryland '68	Experiments with new work patterns for more effective utilization of nurse personnel should be made. These new work patterns should be part of prospective studies of patient care to determine the type of personnel best fitted for specific responsibilities.
17. *Sickness and Society* '68	Continuing senior medical leadership focus on the care of patients in each patient-care division: It is possible that a senior medical director of each division could pull together fragments of medical, personal, and social data from patients, family members, practitioners, nurses, and house staff to provide more adequate care of patients. We believe such an innovation offers promise of improved patient care and increased satisfaction for nurses who then might have sufficient medical leadership and protection to assume more responsibility for both the technical and personal care of patients. (In so doing, she also might find herself elevated to a new, stable position as a medical auxiliary with built-in career opportunities. This would contrast sharply with her current blocked mobility).

TABLE F-1. SUMMARY OF RECOMMENDATIONS

17. *Sickness and Society* '68
    (continued)

Nurses be responsible largely to this medical leader-ship:Originally we thought the "problems of nursing" were those of low morale and personnel shortages. Data demonstrate that these problems did exist; they were serious and chronic. However, we no longer think these and other issues that involve nurses can be solved within the profession of nursing. The RN's and ancillary staff were under the partial control of physicians. Their roles were defined as administrative, technical, or routine. They could not concentrate upon individual patients for lack of time; they were not encouraged by physicians to do so and at times were not even permitted to do so. The patients identified with physicians and often repelled the efforts of nurses to help them. Recognizing the importance of the nurse in the routine running of the hospital, in providing for sick persons, and in satis-fying patients and physicians in their current patterns of defining and dealing with patients, we have no specific recommendations regarding the reorientation of hospital-paid nurses unless medical leadership changes as mentioned above. However, with such changes medical and administrative authorities should allow and require nurses to assume roles of close relationship with patients and offer them, along with physicians, suitable career opportunities in that role.

We believe the private-duty nurse should be incorpo-rated fully into the hospital's nursing services; her direction, supervision, and continuing development as a nurse should be formally controlled by the hospital. The performance of the private duty nurses was costly, wasteful and problematic. Their tendency toward obsolescence was marked. Their efforts were not concentrated where the greatest need existed. Private duty nurses denied, discounted, or ignored these problems. Their aim was to maintain themselves as private entrepreneurs.

18. Williamsburg
    Conference '68

Any conclusions concerning nursing in the future must include more specialized care. There will be more emphasis for the need of the nurse-clinician or clinical nurse specialist with a master's degree. Despite other resulting difficulties nursing must be organized to remove non-patient care duties from nursing by developing such systems as the unit manager system and by freeing the nurse's time from clerical and administrative tasks.

TABLE F-1. SUMMARY OF RECOMMENDATIONS

18. Williamsburg Conference '68 (continued)	The kinds of patients treated in the various hospitals will determine the type of personnel needed. Nursing personnel will need to be flexible and adaptable. This fact reinforces the necessity of offering good educational backgrounds to nurses. More extended care facilities staffed principally by auxiliary nursing personnel will be used in the future. Hospital beds will correspondingly be released and patient costs will be reduced. Other developments will be the use of self-care facilities for ambulatory patients within the general hospital complex, minimal care units staffed with clerks and no nurses, as well as motel type facilities for convalescent care and diagnostic studies.
19. Idaho '69	In view of the vital role performed by members of the nursing profession, vigorous efforts should be made to portray accurately the role of the modern nurse in today's society. Utilization studies of all categories of nursing service personnel should be undertaken by the Idaho State Nurses' Association in conjunction with representatives of allied interests. These studies should be based on an identification of tasks best performed by each level of nursing personnel. The Statewide Coordinating Committee on Nursing Education should serve as the mechanism through which faculty of baccalaureate, associate degree, practical-nurse, and continuing education programs can work with administrators of institutions and nursing-service directors in the joint promotion of effective utilization of nursing-service personnel.
20. Michigan '69	Quantification of projected nurse manpower needs should be derived from analysis of the data collected on supply, current utilization and emerging patterns of development and utilization of nurses, rather than by the application of arbitrary standards such as practitioner-population ratios. Comprehensive and current data should be collected on the supply and distribution of Michigan's nurse supply and utilization patterns of various levels of nurse manpower in major fields of employment.

TABLE F-1. SUMMARY OF RECOMMENDATIONS

20. Michigan '69
    (continued)

Existing research and studies on new and innovative patterns of nurse utilization, on changing concepts of nursing practice and on emerging fields of nursing employment should be analyzed and evaluated as a basis for predicting future demand for nurse manpower.

The organization and administration of health and hospital services should be studied and modified in order to provide for more effective utilization of all personnel, with specific attention given to relieving nurses from tasks not directly related to nursing care.

The results of pilot and demonstration programs in the organization of patient care need to be more widely disseminated. Additional testing and demonstration of innovative approaches to the rational organization of patient care services are also needed.

Qualified nurses should participate actively in planning and implementing direct patient care. In addition, qualified nurses must take responsibility, in cooperation with hospital administration, in developing patterns for providing nursing services to large groups of patients.

21. North Dakota '69

Employers (including the physician-employer) and nurses should continue to study and implement ways to relieve the nurse of duties that can be delegated to less prepared and/or non-nursing personnel in order to allow more time for activities related to direct patient care.

Directors of nursing services should have preparation beyond basic nursing and adequate experience in order that newer concepts and ideas regarding nursing care and utilization of personnel be implemented.

22. Virginia '69

The Virginia Nurses Association, the Virginia League for Nursing, the Virginia Hospital Association, the Virginia Nursing Home Association, the Medical Society of Virginia, and the Old Dominion Medical Society, jointly stimulate interest among their members in the implementation of well-planned and coordinated programs of investigation to determine the proper functions of nursing and nursing responsibilities in the various settings of nursing service.

TABLE F-1. SUMMARY OF RECOMMENDATIONS

22. Virginia '69
    (continued)

Such programs of investigation be conducted in collaboration with other health professions, organizations, institutions, and agencies to attain required cooperation and interest and to avoid duplication or unnecessary overlapping of research efforts.

Commonwealth of Virginia should encourage development of research in nursing practice and the effective utilization of nursing personnel through direct subsidization of programs which are appropriately planned, staffed, and directed.

Organizational mechanisms be established through which nursing may maintain active, appropriate, and effective communication with institutional managements, as well as with the medical and other allied health professions with respect to matters which may affect the practice of nursing.

Health care organizations institute systems of patient care and service which will facilitate efficient and effective utilization of nursing personnel and resources.

Health care structures and equipment be designed to facilitate effective and efficient practice of nursing and proper utilization of health care personnel.

Health care organizations make budgetary provisions for the types and appropriate numbers of support workers required to achieve optimal utilization of nursing personnel.

Health care organizations institute systems of health care and service which recognize the proper role of each professional and non-professional worker, and properly assign functions and responsibilities on the basis of education, training, licensure, and other qualifications.

B. Personnel Policies
   1. Michigan '66

Employers should devise various means to encourage part-time nurses to work more days per week.

Significant pay differential for nurses working less desirable hours and weekends and holidays.

Employers should continue to study and implement ways to relieve nurses of duties that can be delegated to others.

TABLE F-1. SUMMARY OF RECOMMENDATIONS

1. Michigan '66
   (continued)

   Employers should use every possible means to strengthen their in-service education programs for nurses-use of nursing faculty 12 months, cooperation between nursing service and nursing education administrators to develop ways to make use of new educational media such as television and to share educational programs for their nursing service or instructional staffs.

   Employers should provide financial resources so that directors of nursing services and nursing education programs may secure the services of qualified nurse consultants to assist with analysis of problems and with plans for improvements or change.

2. *Hospital Effectiveness Study '67*

   It is recommended that hospitals be encouraged to provide care centers for young children to accommodate staff nurses on all shifts. The result would be an increase in the active nurse population of all communities.

   It is recommended that hospitals provide nurses on the evening and night shifts with an escort or shuttle services to and from the parking lot. If transportation schedules do not satisfy hospital employee needs, the hospital should consider providing its own service.

3. Indiana '67

   Employers should recognize past experience and demonstrated excellence of performance and develop salary schedules which reflect this.

   Employers should offer significant pay differentials for less desirable hours, weekends, and holidays.

4. Illinois '68

   Employers give sufficient economic and professional recognition to nurses with higher levels of preparation and responsibility, career incentives essential to promote their permanent attachment to the profession and their commitment to continuing professional growth and improved practice.

   In Illinois, in the future, nursing salaries and benefits maintain a level that will allow for effective competition with the growing number of other career opportunities for women; that they relate to the nurses educational attainment, and that they adequately recognize years of service and experience.

TABLE F-1. SUMMARY OF RECOMMENDATIONS

5. Idaho '69

A graded salary scale reflecting levels of education, years of experience and participation in continuing education should be developed by the Idaho State Nurses' Association.

Because the services of working mothers with professional or technical education are needed by the community, adequate programs of care for the children of working mothers should be accepted as a community responsibility and should be developed wherever sufficient need exists.

6. Michigan '69

Attention should be given to ways of incorporating job satisfaction into all levels of nursing practice. Opportunities for career progression in areas of nursing other than administration should be opened up. Recognition of increasing competence in direct patient care should be given in terms of increased status and salary.

7. North Dakota '69

Every effort should be made to improve the economics, working policies and job satisfaction for nurses in North Dakota in an attempt to reduce the out-migration of nurses, to interest men, and to attract inactive nurses back into practice.

8. Virginia '69

Each health care facility in the Commonwealth of Virginia, which has not otherwise made such provision, develop a written statement of personnel policies, practices, and procedures for its nursing staff and other employees.

Each statement of personnel policies, practices, and procedures be reviewed periodically, and in the process of review nurses of that health care facility, including general duty nurses, and representatives of other health professions and services of that health care facility be involved.

Periodically, at least once a year, each health care facility in the Commonwealth of Virginia review its salary administrative program for its staff of nurses.

Such review be conducted in consultation with representatives of the nursing staff of the health care facility.

TABLE F-1. SUMMARY OF RECOMMENDATIONS

8. Virginia '69
   (continued)

In the development of compensation policies for nurses, recognition be given to differentials in pay for:

1) Degree of individual responsibility;
2) Length of service;
3) Proficiency; and
4) Length of tours of duty, as well as night, weekend and holiday duty.

Each health care facility in the Commonwealth of Virginia periodically review the working conditions for nurses, appropriate to the individual facility, including such factors as:

1) Assignment of responsibilities consistent with the education, experience, and ability of the individual nurse;
2) Financial compensation which is adequate in relation to the education, experience, responsibilities, and performance of the individual nurse;
3) Insofar as they are consonant with personnel policies, flexible working hours for nurses who are available to work part-time;
4) Regular provisions for continuing education and refresher courses for both practicing and inactive nurses;
5) Provisions for leave of absence with remuneration for practicing nurses to enroll in regular and formal study;
6) Retirement and other benefits, comparable with other employment opportunities; and
7) Other factors, such as nurseries and kindergartens for children of nurses, adequate lounge and dressing room space for members of the professional staffs, and availability of protected car parking space and transportation, especially during evening and night hours.

C. Licensure in Nursing
   1. Goldmark '23

Steps should be taken through state legislation for the definition and licensure of a subsidiary grade of nursing service. The subsidiary type of worker should serve under practicing physicians in the care of mild and chronic illness, in convalescence and possibly, assisting under the direction of the trained nurse in certain phases of hospital and visiting nursing.

TABLE F-1. SUMMARY OF RECOMMENDATIONS

1. Goldmark '23 (continued)	When the licensure of a subsidiary grade of nursing service is provided for, the establishment of training courses in preparation for such service is highly desirable. Such courses should be conducted in special hospitals, in small unaffiliated general hospitals, or in separate sections of hospitals where nurses are also trained. The course should be of 8 or 9 months duration, provided the standards of such schools be approved by the same educational board which governs nursing training schools.
2. *Hospital Effectiveness Study* '67	Licensure requirements frequently differ from state to state which tends to impede mobility of some health specialists. Such requirements should be examined to set uniformly high standards that preserve quality of service but also permits a more free movement among states with great need. Licensure requirements relating to the career ladders concept must be changed to provide work equivalency credits which could be used in promoting personnel from one level of licensed responsibility to a higher one.
3. National Commission on Health Manpower '67	A national uniform licensing code should be developed for each category of health manpower requiring licensure to practice: In several states there is now no mandatory regulation of the practice of nursing; citizens in those states are not protected against the practice of "nurses" who fail the licensing examination, who have never been educated or whose nursing education has been terminated prior to its completion. The permissive laws in those states restrict the use of the term RN, not the practice. A national uniform licensing code would allow for the greater mobility and freedom of choice necessary if health workers are to respond to positive inducements for correction of geographical maldistribution. Entrance to the uniform licensing examination should be granted upon certification by the applicant's school that he or she is adequately qualified for examination rather than a strict definition of minimum education and experience requirements: Nursing has had some success in altering licensing procedures in an effort to increase the mobility of its practitioners. Although each state jurisdiction retains the right to designate hours of study and specific required coursework, in

TABLE F-1. SUMMARY OF RECOMMENDATIONS

3. National Commission on Health Manpower '67 (continued)

actual practice most states accept certification by the schools that their graduates are ready for examination. A uniform exam is used nationally, however, each state board sets the score below which candidates for certification fail the examination.

4. Virginia '69

That the General Assembly adopt a mandatory licensure law for both professional nursing and practical nursing for the purpose of promoting the safety and welfare of those requiring nursing care and assisting in the desirable regulation of those who hold themselves out to the public as having special education, training, or skill in nursing care.

That, in order to make clear its intent, the licensure law be drafted so as expressly to provide that it does not in any way prohibit or limit the performance by any person of acts in the physical care of a patient when such acts do not require the knowledge and skill required of a professional under order or direction of a licensed physician, licensed dentist, or professional nurse.

That the law be drafted so as also to provide that persons performing such acts should not be allowed to designate themselves or be designated by the word "nurse," but may use the term "nursing" in connection with a word to distinguish their occupation, including but not limited to "nursing attendant," "nursing assistant," or "nursing aide".

That the law provide that nursing students in accredited education programs may be employed for compensation in off-duty time in a "nursing assistant" capacity.

That during its 1970 legislative session, the General Assembly enact a new nurse practice act, which, among other provisions, changes the name of the State Board of Examiners of Nurses to the Virginia State Board of Nursing and delineates its role as the official licensure board for those seeking to perform nursing duties and as the state accrediting body for all types of nursing education programs leading to licensure.

5. Georgia '69

It is recommended that when an acceptable proposal is presented, mandatory nurse practice legislation should be supported.

TABLE F-1. SUMMARY OF RECOMMENDATIONS

6. Wisconsin '70

The Commission recognized it is desirable for the Wisconsin Board of Nursing to seek modifications in the licensing laws to reflect the type of practice the nurse is prepared to perform.

The Commission recommends that the Board of Nursing establish a policy requiring refresher courses or some type of evaluation procedure for nurses returning to active practice after a given period of inactivity before the license is renewed.

D. Nurses in Planning
1. Brown '48

Appropriate nursing bodies should initiate planning on a statewide basis for the distribution of the kinds of schools that are designed to meet state needs. Planning should be undertaken on a regional and nationwide basis for those higher forms of nursing education that require fewer units but consequently greater selectivity of resources and location. Representatives of education and the health services, whether official or unofficial, representatives of channels of communication and others in position to influence public opinion should give generous assistance to professional nursing associations in this socially important undertaking.

2. Michigan '66

There should be community and regional planning for orderly expansion and sound development of nursing education facilities. This planning should be initiated by nurses, and all interests in the community should be brought together to participate in this planning. Such a group should include representatives of the consumer public, employers of nurses, schools of nursing, and nursing organization bodies.

3. Indiana '67

A state level nursing education planning body be established to be composed of the administrators of nursing schools and appropriate nursing service representation. Planning would be toward: expanded enrollments and educational facilities for nursing; the number and kind of needed educational programs in nursing; the availability of the quantity and quality of needed clinical facilities, including the wise and cooperative use of such facilities.

Nursing organizations in the state should seek ways to involve nurses in leadership positions and other inter-

TABLE F-1.   SUMMARY OF RECOMMENDATIONS

3. Indiana '67
(continued)

ested nurses in planning for community health through appointment to local and state agencies and state planning groups.

4. Southern Regional
Education Board '67

Participation in statewide planning should include leaders from public and private institutions; leaders in each kind of nursing education and service; leaders of related health professions and in various other fields of health work; leaders in technical, vocational, and higher education; leaders in secondary education; and leaders among students of nursing.

Effective planning will always be a judicious combination of long-term and short-term study and action. While planners must study the nursing situation in their state, as well as related trends, they must also be able to pinpoint the most strategic problems immediately and go to work on these at once.

Some problems will require short-term action while long-term solutions are being set in motion. While long-term action to acquire more nurses with advanced training is being planned, for example, planners can launch continuing education programs to upgrade teachers, or start short programs to prepare needed specialists.

Planning must be founded on a clear understanding of existing conditions and future trends in:

1) Nursing;
2) Higher education; and
3) Other health services and professions.

5. Illinois '68

There is too little involvement of nursing in health planning, both locally and at the state level; such involvement is much needed and will benefit the planning process. Active involvement of nursing leadership in comprehensive health planning is needed and nurses should be appointed to Illinois Hospital Licensing Board as well as to other health service licensing boards.

Relationships between nurses and physicians in the patient care setting are frequently strained and a cause for both job dissatisfaction and concern among nurses. Therefore, medical staffs of hospitals should be urged to formally include hospital nurses in all of their staff committee activities that involve nursing in any way.

TABLE F-1. SUMMARY OF RECOMMENDATIONS

6. Michigan '69

The orderly development of nursing education programs to meet Michigan's needs for nurse manpower in the years ahead requires the construction of a state plan for nursing education in Michigan. The planning process should be instituted without delay.

The State Board of Education, as part of its duty to plan for and encourage the orderly development of a comprehensive state system of post-secondary education, should assume primary responsibility for developing a state plan for nursing education.

The nursing profession should participate in the planning process from its initiation.

The cooperation and participation of the Comprehensive State Health Planning Commission and the State Board of Nursing should be obtained from the start of the planning process.

7. Virginia '69

Health care organizations involve nursing representation in the planning of facilities, selection of equipment and supplies, development of organizational structure, establishment of training programs, staffing patterns and in all other matters which may have direct or indirect influence on the practice of nursing.

That increased attention be given to the assignment and referral of patients to appropriate facilities; that one method in the pursuance of this objective be greater use of utilization committees and that provision be made for more adequate information on referral of patients, in order to provide proper continuity of care in various types of health care facilities.

E. The Inactive Nurse
1. Alabama '68

All possible means be explored and every effort made to facilitate the return of inactive RN's to active status. That the State Nurse Association, the State League of Nursing and the State Board of Nursing give assistance and consultation to any group in helping them to resolve any unique problems which are deterrents to the return of inactive RN's in a particular community.

TABLE F-1. SUMMARY OF RECOMMENDATIONS

1. Alabama '68
(continued)

Current refresher programs for inactive nurses be evaluated by the State Nurse Association to determine points of strength and ways to make these programs available to more nurses.

2. Montana '68

Inadequate administration, total and nursing service, of health care facilities, was a reason given by inactive nurses for not returning to employment. Examples given were: the lack of written personnel policies; inadequate salaries; lack of orientation and in-service programs; insufficient number of adequately trained nursing personnel. The Montana Nurses' Association and Montana Hospital Association are jointly sponsoring a workshop for Directors of Nursing Service to assist them in developing administrative skills which will assist the participants in meeting accepted standards for nursing service departments.

3. Nevada '68

Although there is a reservoir of inactive and interested personnel in most areas, many of the rural communities cannot support organized refresher classes even for RN's. The number of candidates is so small that standard procedures are economically infeasible. They do not have qualified instructors available or adequate resource materials and teaching equipment.

4. North Dakota '68

In order to create interest for the nurse to return to the labor market, refresher courses must be made available to her in order to help her overcome the barriers of returning to nursing.

Working conditions must fit into the pattern of the home so that the mother can secure a job, if only on a part-time basis.

Some salaries must be increased in order to make it worthwhile for the inactive nurse to work.

On-going in-service education programs must continue to assist the reactivated nurse.

Continued studies on the health occupation's needs and resources should be made in order to determine health manpower shortage.

TABLE F-1. SUMMARY OF RECOMMENDATIONS

III. Miscellaneous Recommendations for Nursing

A. Burgess '28

If nursing is to retain its high idealism it must make sure that its members are free from undue economic pressure. Therefore, nursing should try to insure that the number of graduate nurses admitted to the profession bears a close relationship to the amount of adequately paid work available to them.

While many positions remain unfilled, there is currently (1928) no lack of applicants, but these applicants are often of insufficient quality. The "shortage" is quality, not quantity.

So, there is (in 1928) an "overproduction" of nurse graduates, and not enough adequately paying positions for them to fill.

B. Nahm '59

Individual differences make it difficult to judge in advance who will make the better nurse and who will not, especially where qualities of leadership are concerned. Perhaps a study of the career patterns of nurses who today are making major contributions to the profession would uncover information to be used in selecting and educating students for the future.

Better communication and understanding among patients, students, and nursing groups is the first essential component needed if changes in nursing and nursing education are to be effected.

C. National Commission on Health Manpower '67

A federally administered program be developed which would allow health manpower students to distribute the costs of their education over the period of their income-producing life. The proposed program would be the converse of the Social Security System: payment would be made initially by the government and repayment by the individual would be spread over the period of his financial productivity.

More grants to health manpower schools for teaching and service to balance against research.

D. New York '67

Career incentives should be provided. It is recommended that each hospital in the Southern New York region identify registered nurses with potential for supervision, administration, teaching, and research and assist them in obtaining preparation in graduate programs by educational leaves, fellowships, and

TABLE F-1. SUMMARY OF RECOMMENDATIONS

D. New York '67
   (continued)

monetary incentives that will encourage them to complete the program and return to the institution following completion.

E. Nurse Training Act
   (Review) '67

Federal funds be substantially increased for all mechanisms of support to accelerate and advance:

1) Research into all aspects of nursing practice, the organization and delivery of nursing services to the patient, nursing as an occupation, and ways of communicating research findings;
2) Research training as a necessary adjunct to prepare nurses to do independent research, to collaborate in interdisciplinary research, and to stimulate and guide research important to nursing.

The unit which now provides a federal focal point for nursing, the Division of Nursing, be strengthened, supported, and that it be given the visibility and organizational placement necessary to develop it into a truly national center for nursing where the essential elements of education, service, research and practice will be kept together, where total national needs will be reviewed and assessed, and where adequate resources will be available for allocation to assure balanced program to meet these needs.

F. Southern Regional
   Education Board '67

Educational programs for all the fields of health work have much in common including courses in the health sciences, expensive laboratories, and the need for clinical practice. Coordinated planning may result in proposals for sharing scarce teaching personnel, equipment, or clinical facilities.

G. *Technology and Manpower*
   in the Health Service
   Industry '67

Research programs are needed to fill gaps in statistics on the number of persons actually employed and the number of job vacancies in individual health occupations among various types of health establishments; or the number and kinds of employees required in relation to existing and new methods and standards of health care and in relation to differences in technological and other characteristics of health facilities; on characteristics of inactive former health workers. Data now available on some of these subjects is very incomplete or lacks the up-to-dateness or frequency of recurrent collection needed for guidance in planning health manpower programs.

TABLE F-1. SUMMARY OF RECOMMENDATIONS

H. California '68

Needs for nursing personnel should be determined regionally and related to statewide developments in health and education and in terms of expected population and economic growth of the state.

I. *Sickness and Society* '68

Medical auxiliaries to eventually replace nurses and be given more responsibility and career opportunities in patient care. Although the nursing profession has recognized the need for men in the field, recruitment has been minimal. We suggest a new career in the health field — the medical auxiliary. Should not suitable schools be opened to prepare men and women for careers in the health field which involve direct care of patients? Should such schools replace nursing schools? We think that either nurses or others should develop a career under a title which will attract both men and women. A title so uniquely feminine as nurse will not suffice as an appeal for men to enter a field so vital to health care.

Since it is necessary that men meet societal expectations of family support, suitable career and economic advances must be offered to ensure success of recruitment and stability within the role. In our view, such a new role could be satisfying to men and women, but to be sufficiently popular to attract many, and thus possibly reduce the manpower crisis in the health field, attractive career opportunities are essential. Such a condition, in our view, is more likely to exist if the suggested auxiliaries are strongly linked to patients and physicians and avoid roles which should be taken only by administrators and their assistants.

J. Williamsburg Conference '68

In the future, planning emphasis should be placed on phasing out most of the small hospitals with bed capacity under 100 since larger hospitals are more economical. More attention should be given to outpatient care. There should also be more attention to new construction and less to renovation and remodelling.

Expensive facilities should be limited to those patients actually requiring intensive care. Less costly facilities and equipment are adequate for long-term extended care and intermediate care patients. Furthermore, motel type facilities are proving satisfactory for ambulatory patients who, for example, need brief but repeated medical treatments.

TABLE F-1. SUMMARY OF RECOMMENDATIONS

K. Georgia '69

It is recommended that no additional undergraduate nurses (individuals who have attended nursing school for 12 months or more but who have not completed a course of study in nursing) be licensed in Georgia. In proposing discontinuance of this licensure category, it is recommended that all persons licensed as undergraduate nurses retain their status as long as they maintain current licenses.

IV. Recommendations from Studies of other Health Professions

(Selected Recommendations from studies of other health professions which might have relevance, or serve as a model, for our recommendations in nursing and nursing education.)

A. *Medical Education Reconsidered.*

Report of the Endicott House Summer Study on Medical Education. July, 1965.

There was a general belief that the medical schools must engage in redefinition of their roles. To a large extent, the schools now offer an all-purpose medical education apparently predicated on the assumption that all its graduates will be all-purpose physicians. In fact, their graduates will proceed to careers that will differ substantially among themselves. A small and decreasing proportion will be general practitioners and will remain general practitioners throughout their careers. Others will specialize almost immediately, some in the various medical or surgical specialties, some in medical research, some in the management of medical affairs. To each of those groups the medical school must be prepared to offer a coherent course of study that recognizes from the outset the diversity of goals.

Among the suggestions that were made was one that proposed that the training of medical research scientists be shared between the medical school and the graduate school of science. A student contemplating a career in medical research might begin with a year at medical school and proceed to the graduate school of science to complete his training. Upon graduation, he might receive both a Ph.D. and a M.D. degree.

There appeared to be something of a consensus that much of the education now offered — and required — in medical school should be moved back into the undergraduate years. In particular, there has been recently a movement toward far more sophisticated secondary-school education in the natural sciences and mathematics; this has led to a general improvement of undergraduate courses. In many universities and in the better colleges, an undergraduate now encounters the

TABLE F-1. SUMMARY OF RECOMMENDATIONS

A. *Medical Education Reconsidered.*
(continued)

natural sciences and mathematics in a form far more sophisticated than that of parallel courses offered in medical schools. Two conclusions might be drawn from this: first, the colleges can be relied on eventually for much of the education that is now presumed to take place in medical school: second, those aspects of science education that must inevitably remain for medical schools must be prepared and presented in a form far more mature and pertinent than that which now prevails.

There was consensus that the compression of education now taking place in secondary schools and colleges now makes it possible to consider three years of undergraduate education, properly spent, adequate preparation for medicine. To effect this, it was considered necessary that steps be taken to assure that the third years of undergraduate education be oriented toward the needs of the medical school. In many colleges and universities, courses of extremely high quality in the natural sciences, the behavioral sciences, and mathematics are now offered to undergraduates; such courses, as they stand, provide far better preparation for medical studies than most of those now offered in medical schools. In other undergraduate institutions, there is a reserve of excellent teachers but appropriate premedical courses are not now offered; it is certainly possible for faculty in medical schools, working in conjunction with university faculty, to prepare the appropriate courses.

Consideration was given to the feasibility of adopting procedures that would enable medical schools to accept students at the close of their second year in college, deferring their actual entry into medical school until they had completed a third year of college and making that entry contingent upon their selection of undergraduate courses during the interim year. Students applying from undergraduate institutions that could not provide the requisite third-year courses might be asked to transfer, for that year, to an institution that could do so.

Most of the participants clearly believed that the medical student should be introduced as quickly as possible to the facts and the atmosphere of disease. Such a procedure has important implications for the

TABLE F-1. SUMMARY OF RECOMMENDATIONS

A. *Medical Education Reconsidered.* medical school curriculum. It implies that the initial
(continued) course in anatomy, for example, should be designed to
deal at once with the abnormal as well as the normal,
and to have at its starting point the position of the
doctor confronting a patient rather than of the
student confronting a model.

It was suggested also, as an extension of the need for a
more immediate association of the student with the
real nature of medicine, that even during the third
year of undergraduate instruction the clinical faculties
of the schools of medicine associate themselves with
the preparation and presentation of materials for
courses in science and mathematics. Again, the most
effective utilization of the years prior to entry into
medical school was being sought.

There was almost unanimous agreement that means
must be found of bringing internships and residencies
under direct control of schools of medicine. A similar
emphasis is to be found in the Coggeshall Report to
the American Association of Medical Colleges, and
steps in that direction would certainly be firmly
supported by that organization. In general, it is
proposed that by agreement with hospitals, the
medical school be able to stipulate the range of
activities in which the graduate is to engage during his
internship and residency and empowered to monitor
his progress. Where the range of activities in a given
hospital is considered by the medical school to be
inadequate, arrangements might be made through
which the graduate could assume limited duties for
limited periods of time in hospitals directly associated
with the university.

The need for curriculum reform in the behavioral
sciences was particularly stressed, it was stated that
this was perhaps the greatest deficiency in the education both of premedical and medical students. Many
felt that a multi- disciplinary study should be devoted
to this subject alone.

Where the matters under consideration lend themselves to direct experimentation, such a procedure
should be adopted as expeditiously as possible. The
process of curriculum reform, for example, can be
undertaken and pressed on a piecemeal basis. Experimental courses can be introduced where there is a

TABLE F-1. SUMMARY OF RECOMMENDATIONS

A. *Medical Education Reconsidered.* (continued)

temper to test them, and can be refined progressively until they meet with general acceptance. It was certainly the consensus of the meeting that such activity in the behavioral sciences is an urgent need.

As change becomes more pervasive, however, it necessarily must involve the reshaping of institutions on a broad scale, of a sort that cannot well be provided by a single institution or even by a small group of institutions. Thus, an alteration in the mode of accepting medical students imposes obligations on the colleges and unversities from which those students are drawn. Alterations in the relationship between the university and the practitioner require the approval of the medical profession as a whole. Actions that might be taken in the education of specialists call for the cooperation of the specialist societies and certifying boards.

B. *The Graduate Education of Physicians.* Report of the Citizens Commission on Graduate Medical Education. August, 1966.

Because educational programs properly differ from one institution to another, we recommend that each medical school faculty and each teaching hospital staff, acting as a corporate body, explicitly formulate, and periodically revise, their own educational goals and curricula. To do so would be a healthy exercise for medical educators and a fundamental step toward the solution of many of their educational problems.

Simple rotation among several services, in the manner of the classical rotating internship — even though extending over a longer period of time — will not be sufficient. Knowledge and skill in the several areas are essential, but the teaching should stress continuing and comprehensive patient responsibility rather than the episodic handling of acute conditions in the several areas. Some experience in the handling of emergency cases and knowledge of the specialized care required before and following surgery should be included. There should be taught a new body of knowledge in addition to the medical specialities that constitute the bulk of the program. There should be opportunities for individual variations in the graduate program. The level of training should be on a par with that of other specialties. A two-year graduate program is insufficient.

We recommend that each teaching hospital organize its staff, through an educational council, a committee on

TABLE F-1. SUMMARY OF RECOMMENDATIONS

B. *The Graduate Education of Physicians.* (continued)

graduate education, or some similar means, so as to make its programs of graduate medical education a corporate responsibility rather than the individual responsibilities of particular medical or surgical services or heads of services.

We recommend that the internship, as a separate and distinct portion of medical education, be abandoned, and that the internship and residency years be combined into a single period of graduate medical education called a residency and planned as a unified whole.

We recommend that state licensure acts and statements of certification requirements be amended to eliminate the requirement of a separate internship and to substitute therefore an appropriately described period of graduate medical education.

We therefore recommend that graduation from medical school be recognized as the end of general medical education, and that specialized training begin with the start of graduate medical education.

We recommend that hospitals experiment with several forms of basic residency training, and that the specialty boards and residency review committees encourage experimentation by interpreting liberally those statements in the residency requirements that now inhibit this form of educational organization.

We recommend that the specialty boards, in amending their regulations concerning eligibility for examination for certification, not increase the required length of residency training to compensate for dropping the requirement of a separate internship. This can be done by retaining present wording concerning length of residency training and deleting statements concerning internship training.

We recommend that programs of graduate medical education be approved by the residency review committees only if they cover the entire span from the first year of graduate medical education through completion of the residency.

We recommend that programs of graduate medical education not be approved unless the teaching staff, the related services and the other facilities are judged

TABLE F-1. SUMMARY OF RECOMMENDATIONS

B. *The Graduate Education of Physicians.* (continued)

adequate in size and quality, and that, if these tests are met, approval be formally given to the institution rather than to the particular medical or surgical service most directly involved.

We recommend that staff members of university medical centers and other teaching hospitals explore the possibility of organizing an intensive effort to study the problems of graduate medical education and, where such development appears feasible, they seek to arrange for the development of improved materials and techniques that can be widely used in graduate medical education.

We therefore recommend that a newly created Commission on Graduate Medical Education be established specifically for the purpose of planning, coordination, and periodically reviewing standards for graduate medical education and procedures for reviewing and approving the institutions in which that education is offered.

C. Lowell T. Coggeshall, *Planning for Medical Progress Through Education.* Association of American Medical Colleges. 1965.

Need to devote increasing attention to the requirements of the nation.
The need of the future will be for the field of medical education to assume responsibility for meeting the quantitative as well as the qualitative needs of the nation. Those responsible for medical education will, in decades ahead, need to devote careful attention to appraising the needs of society for health care and health personnel and to developing and implementing plans to meet those needs. If those responsible for medical education fail to assume and act on a responsibility that is now clearly theirs, it will be assumed by others. The reemergence of medical schools of marginal quality outside the jurisdiction of the university is a clear likelihood. The intervention of government to see that emerging needs are met and to provide the means of meeting them is an even greater likelihood.

Need for more and better prepared physicians.
The number of physicians that will need to be produced in the years ahead cannot be projected with precision. There is yet no adequate measure of "need" for health care. Nevertheless, it seems likely that the nation will be able to use the services of all the physicians that existing, expanded, and planned medical schools will be able to educate in the foreseeable future.

TABLE F-1. SUMMARY OF RECOMMENDATIONS

C. *Planning for Medical Progress Through Education.* (continued)

New schools will be needed. The new schools should be established as integral parts of mature universities with well established graduate programs. They should not be established as appendages to institutions of higher learning that are at a distance from them, are prepared to take but limited responsibility for setting or overseeing their standards of scholarship, or are themselves just developing programs in the sciences at the graduate level.

Whenever possible, new schools should be planned and developed as four-year schools. Lack of continuity, environmental changes, and the lesser ability to establish good and continuing student-faculty rapport are all among the factors that make two-year schools less desirable than four-year schools.

Need for more persons for related health professions and occupations.
Well-trained persons have long been used under the physicians leadership to provide needed care and augment the physician's skills, time, and capabilities. It seems certain that more persons with specialized skills will need to be trained to buttress the physician-led team and compensate for the fact that fewer physicians will be available than might be desirable.

More trained persons will be needed to take full advantage of scientific advances. The team approach to health care cannot be perfected unless there is a balanced team available to the physician and he clearly takes responsibility for its leadership.

The role of the medical school in the years ahead should be that of seeing that persons needed for related health professions and occupations are trained, that their training is appropriate, and that they are trained to participate effectively in the physician led health care team. The medical school should not, of course, have to assume direct responsibility for their education.

A major advantage of meeting health needs of the nation by preparing more persons for related health professions and occupations is that an increasing percentage of the educational need can be met by institutions other than medical schools. Universities, colleges, junior colleges, and other institutions can be expanded more easily and less expensively than schools of medicine.

TABLE F-1. SUMMARY OF RECOMMENDATIONS

C. *Planning for Medical Progress Through Education.* (continued)

Need to improve delivery of health services.

The trend toward greater specialization, greater reliance on a team approach to health care, and growing institutionalization of health care have all arisen quite spontaneously and their development has been largely without planning or structure. A great need of the future is for the rational development of improved organization and methods for health and the delivery of health care.

Schools of medicine should be taking the lead in studying the ways medical care is delivered to patients. Their concern should be with comprehensive family care as well as with specialty care. The university-sponsored medical school is in an unequalled position to draw upon the resources of many disciplines to study the way in which comprehensive health care is provided. The need is for careful study of how health care can best be made available — including how medicine can best be practiced — and for the development of more effective plans of organization and delivery of health care.

Need to view medical education as a continuum.
The sharp separation between pre-professional and professional education should be minimized by including appropriate "professional" subject matter in the pre-professional curriculum and continuing liberal education into the professional years.

It should be recognized that the physician can no longer master all areas of the basic biomedical sciences — he cannot even be acquainted with all of them. Nor can he be competent in all technologies associated with his own speciality. He must be increasingly dependent upon personnel trained in related fields.

The physician must now assume the role of team leader having the broad familiarity and competence to marshal the appropriate expertise and resources beyond his individual skill. This ability to use technical assistance and to work cooperatively in a team should be the essence of professionalism. Basic principles required for intelligent decision making should compose the curriculum, with emphasis placed on problem-solving and the use of human technological resources.

TABLE F-1. SUMMARY OF RECOMMENDATIONS

C. *Planning for Medical Progress Through Education.* (continued)

At present the M.D. degree is earned at about the mid-point of the formal education of the physician. It is recognized that the doctor is not fully qualified to practice at this point, but it is here that the traditional medical school abandons him and relinquishes responsibility. In the future, professional physician education should continue in a coordinated sequence, under the sponsorship and guidance of university medical schools, through internship and residency programs.

It is increasingly clear that the need of the future is for the university to assume comprehensive responsibility for medical education. While universities cannot, in the forseeable future be expected to exercise control over all intern and resident training programs, the greatest possible effort should be made to move in this direction.

Only the university can integrate instruction and research. The university alone comprises all the fields of knowledge and disciplines related to health. However, the universities cannot extend their facilities to produce all the large numbers of health service personnel required by society. The universities should educate the teachers, research workers, and administrators for the allied health professions and occupations, and should develop and accredit educational programs in these disciplines for colleges and junior colleges to train the majority of practitioners. The recent expansion of junior college nursing schools has demonstrated the excellent potential of these institutions for training certain types of health personnel. Community hospitals in affiliation with medical schools should also be regarded as part of the training base for the practicing allied health personnel.

D. *Health is a Community Affair.* National Commission on Community Health Services. 1966.

All arrangements for organization or delivery of comprehensive personal health services should be based on a firm and continuing relationship between the individual patient and a personal physician. This personal physician is responsible for bringing the individual into the integrated program of comprehensive personal health services, and for providing or securing needed health care. In order to make the most efficient use of limited physician manpower, health care functions not requiring medical training should be delegated by the physician to other members of the health care team to the maximum extent that is practical.

TABLE F-1. SUMMARY OF RECOMMENDATIONS

D. *Health is a Community Affair.* (continued)

The community should provide and the personal physician should utilize a full range of community health services, within and outside the hospital. Every hospital should have a service for personal physicians, and conversely, every qualified personal physician should have a staff appointment in one or more accredited hospitals with privileges in accordance with his capabilities, and each personal physician should have access to a program of continuing medical education. The personal physician should work as part of a team in which the special abilities of the different members are integrated for a common purpose — the health and well-being of the patient.

Emphasis should be given to the stimulation of those forms of association among physicians which would facilitate overcoming undesirable fragmentation of health services, maintenance of high standards of quality of care, and payment mechanisms that reduce economic barriers to preventive services and to prompt diagnostic and therapeutic services. The group practice of medicine, as a specific way of integrating the service of physicians, has demonstrated that it can provide an effective and efficient method of furnishing comprehensive medical care of good quality. Such organization of services should be stimulated and encouraged as one of the best routes toward comprehensive personal health services.

E. *Survey of Dentistry.* The final report of the Commission on the Survey of Dentistry in the United States. 1961.

The dental schools give students more experience in working with auxiliary personnel, especially with dental assistants. Students should understand completely the importance that effective utilization of such personnel plays in the practice of dentistry.

Dental schools have active hospital affiliations, and dental students receive instruction and experience in hospital procedures.

Universities assume more responsibility for the development of close relations among their dental schools, other health science schools, and graduate departments in order to promote exchanges of knowledge and ideas.

It would appear that the dental hygienist is overtrained for the limited function she is allowed to perform. It appears inconsistent to require two years

TABLE F-1. SUMMARY OF RECOMMENDATIONS

E. *Survey of Dentistry.*
(continued)

to train a dental hygienist primarily to perform oral prophylaxis and conduct health education, while an RN, performing a very wide range of responsible clinical duties, can also be trained in as little as two years.

Every possible approach — expanding dental schools, increasing training facilities for dental hygienists and assistants, development of new methods of using auxiliary personnel, and the widespread application of preventive procedures must be pursued with vigor if adequate dental service is to be available to the American public in 1975.

The profession give greater recognition to the importance of developing administrative skills; encourage formal training for those who may become engaged in administrative dentistry; and encourage outstanding dental students and dentists to enter the field.

A large number of carefully supervised dental internships be developed in hospitals and clinics and dental students be encouraged to enter internships following their graduations.

In the interest of total health care of patients, both hospitals and dental societies should work for the establishment of more hospital dental departments, and encourage dentists to participate in hospital service.

An effective relationship between state licensing boards and the Council of the National Board of Dental Examiners be developed, and all states accept the results of the National Board examinations.

Reasons given by dental hygienists for not favoring educating males for practice:

1) Women are better adapted to dental hygiene work than men;
2) Hygienists would not want male competition;
3) Men might be mistaken for dentists or might practice dentistry illegally;
4) Income is too small to support a man;
5) Men should become dentists;
6) Men lack patience and gentleness;
7) Male ego is too great and the profession would not appeal to them;

TABLE F-1. SUMMARY OF RECOMMENDATIONS

E. *Survey of Dentistry.*
(continued)

8) Patients prefer woman assistants;
9) Most dentists prefer woman assistants.

All state boards of dentistry accept the results of the National Board Dental Examinations in lieu of their own written examinations, thereby restricting their evaluation to technical and clinical procedures.

Dental schools should place much greater emphasis upon educational research. Such research should include experimentation with the organization of the dental curriculum and with methods of training auxiliary personnel and of teaching dental students and auxiliary personnel how to function as a team.

Another improvement that should be made in each school is the establishment of an honors program for the better students. Each school, therefore, should develop a method by which better students can pursue in depth areas of special interest to them. Some might wish to obtain research experience, some, greater clinical experience..in advanced methods of treatment, and some greater knowledge in a basic science. In this way, many of the better students might receive the impetus to become teachers and researchers.

Repeatedly, dentistry through three previous major surveys of dental education, has been urged to give increased emphasis upon the biological sciences and their correlation with clinical practice. This has not occurred seemingly because there is the implication that by such action, the technical skills of the dentist would be reduced to some unknown extent.

Although many dentists are willing to accept the statement that dentistry is the equivalent of a recognized specialty of medicine, they know also that dentistry is a profession in itself. In either case they see the possibility that the recommendations for more emphasis on the basic sciences would result in making the dentist more like the physician — something that they do not believe necessary. They have not been shown clearly enough how dental practice would improve by an increased emphasis on basic science or how the American public might be expected to benefit from such changes.

TABLE F-1.   SUMMARY OF RECOMMENDATIONS

E. *Survey of Dentistry.*
(continued)

If the dental schools were to make a significant change in the manner in which their graduates will practice, the public would have to be advised of the new image of the dentist. This would require a program of public education, and it would have to be planned carefully so as to help the younger dentists without hurting the older ones.

What American dentists and dental schools appear to need is a philosophy that would permit the basic sciences to be integrated more clearly into the pattern of dental practice and dental education.

As one contemplates the future practice of dentistry and the direction in which dental education should move in the years ahead, it seems most appropriate that the dental schools should seek to develop curricula, by 1970 at least, which will educate dentists who are much more periodontically and biologically oriented than today's graduates.

If dental schools were to begin teaching under a new philosophy, the present clinical teachers would have to be retrained by in-service programs, and graduate and post-graduate programs would have to be created to prepare new teachers capable of teaching from the suggested viewpoint. Since clinical teachers are drawn from the ranks of the profession, they tend to teach their students in the same tradition and philosophy as they were taught. To accomplish a significant change in dental teaching; therefore, dental education must break this circle, and it can only do so by changing the concepts of its teachers at some point in its future.

For a long time, the dental schools have been faced with challenge to correlate the basic sciences and clinical dentistry — it is now time for them to act. Dental education should be made more truly a university discipline and the public should be given the advantages of more complete dental services.

Dental schools should seek to have their own teachers do more and more of the teaching in refresher courses. Although initial impetus may be given to the continuation program by securing outstanding practitioners or teachers from other schools, a sound educational program can be developed best by placing the responsibility for teaching upon the regular faculty. Teachers improve significantly through the

TABLE F-1. SUMMARY OF RECOMMENDATIONS

E. *Survey of Dentistry.*
(continued)

experience they gain in giving lectures and demonstrations to practicing dentists and through exchange of ideas with them.

F. *The Education of Public Health Personnel.* Joint Committee on the Study of Education for Public Health. 1966.

It is recommended that the schools of public health greatly strengthen their teaching and research programs in public health practice, giving full consideration to current problems in the field and the anticipation of future needs.

It is recommended that the schools of public health provide both the broad professional preparation needed by community health leadership personnel and specialists in the various academic fields related to public health and that a clear distinction be made in the curricula designed to prepare the two types of personnel.

It is recommended that the standard of admission to a one-year MPH or DPH program of study be the possession of a master's or first professional degree in a field relevant to public health.

It is recommended that the schools of public health actively recruit high quality students immediately after they gain the bachelor's degree for graduate work in special academic fields in the school of public health.

It is recommended that in the interest of allowing for more than one year of graduate preparation of the student who leaves a job in the field to attend a school of public health on a training grant, some combination of the following suggestions be investigated:

1) The granting agencies extend their training grants to cover longer periods of time for students in the schools instituting two-year MPH programs;
2) The schools of public health work out a schedule for the student's program of study which would permit him to return periodically to his job so as to minimize the dislocation his absence might produce in the employing agency;
3) The public health agency allow more than one year's leave for such a student, working in concert with the school of public health as suggested in 2) above.

TABLE F-1. SUMMARY OF RECOMMENDATIONS

F. *The Education of Public Health Personnel.* (continued)

It is recommended that the school of public health take the initiative, working with other groups of health professionals as necessary, in maintaining an active recruitment program for students in the health professions.

It is recommended that the schools of public health strive, in their faculty staffing patterns, for a better balance between the two prototypes of faculty members: the academician prepared in depth in a constituent discipline of public health, and the experienced practitioner thoroughly familiar with the problems of the field and the means for applying current knowledge and skills to the solution of community health problems.

It is recommended that the schools of public health devote immediate and concentrated attention to developing, at both the master's and post-master's levels, programs of study designed to prepare qualified persons to assume leadership roles in community health, concerned with all types of services - public and private, preventive and curative. It is further recommended that the U.S. Public Health Service give serious consideration to providing grants to schools of public health for the specific purpose of helping them strengthen their departments of public health practice.

It is recommended that research funding agencies and especially the U.S Public Health Service give greater encouragement and financial support to the schools of public health to establish research ties with the field of program operations in public health and that in particular they consider more active support of administrative research and evaluation.

It is recommended that the schools of public health review their curricula with a view of building them on some unifying concept which will give them consistency and coherence. The following are offered as suggestions of a way this might be done. In this instance the curriculum would be built on the basis of several specific determinations of the faculty:

1) The societal needs which the field of public health should fulfill in the foreseeable future;
2) The different competencies or specializations which will be required by the field to fulfill these needs;

TABLE F-1. SUMMARY OF RECOMMENDATIONS

F. *The Education of Public Health Personnel.* (continued)

3) The role of the school in helping the field fulfill these needs, including the kinds of research and teaching competencies which will be necessary in the school;

4) The specific ways in which each major instructional unit in the school (e.g. Environmental Health, MCH, etc.) contributes to the realization of 3) above (these will then become the specific, clearly enunciated goals of the individual instructional unit);

5) The specific goals of each course, and how they contribute to the realization of the goals of the instructional unit of which it is a part, as in 4) above.

It is further recommended that the instructional program — i.e., the materials selected for study in seminars, lectures, laboratory, field trips and other learning experiences — be geared to the realization of the stated goals of the course, and that the evaluation (or testing) of the students be aimed specifically at determining how well the student has mastered these goals.

It is further recommended that, as a part of these considerations, the concept of a "core" of instruction for all students in a given program (e.g. the MPH) be reexamined and, if found necessary, the specific course content which should go into it be spelled out.

It is recommended that state and sizable local departments of public health investigate the possibility of setting up special training programs to prepare personnel for those positions in departments of public health which do not require university instruction. It is further recommended that where advisable a school of public health help with the training program and that the U.S. Public Health Service consider giving financial assistance to the enterprise.

It is recommended that in the interest of achieving closer coordination between the instruction in public health subjects in schools of public health and other schools, either or both of the following be considered:

1) The Association of Schools of Public Health, or another appropriate group, obtain funds for a project to experiment with ways in which better coordination could be brought

TABLE F-1. SUMMARY OF RECOMMENDATIONS

F. *The Education of Public Health Personnel.* (continued)

about. This would include identification of areas where such coordination would be desirable, the mechanics for working it out, and the actual development of coordinated programs, with joint curricula developed by both institutions;

2) Grants be sought from the U. S. Public Health Service sufficient to pay the salary and expenses of a person who would be attached to the school of public health and would work for such coordination between the school and appropriate institutions in the area.

It is further recommended that the Committee on Professional Education of the APHA consider the accreditation of such programs, thus lending the prestige of its approval to these endeavors.

It is recommended that the Association of Schools of Public Health assume an active and strong leadership role in determining the direction of public health in the United States and Canada, and in the preparation of the necessary leadership personnel for the future. To this end it is further recommended that the Association seek financial assistance to obtain sufficient staff to carry out such a program.

G. *National Correlations in Medical Technology Education.* A report of a Study of Medical Technologists. 1967.

AMA accreditation standards for schools of medical technology be amended to require:

1) College or university affiliation;
2) A minimum staffing requirement of 10 medical technologists possessing bachelor's degrees; and
3) A minimum capacity of eight students.

Pre-clinical education programs for students of medical technology be strengthened through increased emphasis on bacteriology, biochemistry, physics, and mathematics.

Clinical education programs in schools of medical technology be strengthened through additional instruction in all aspects of quality control, instrumentation, practical application of laboratory test results.

TABLE F-1. SUMMARY OF RECOMMENDATIONS

G. *National Correlations in Medical Technology Education.* (continued)

The certification examination administered through the Board of Registry of Medical Technologists (ASCP) be reviewed to include additional evaluation of knowledge, judgment and proficiency in instrumentation, technical problem solving, quality control and mathematics.

Further studies, incorporating site visits and interviews, be undertaken to determine:

1) If the curricula and content of pre-clinical education programs leading to the degree of BS in Medical Technology vary significantly from other pre-clinical programs;

2) If the curricula and content of clinical education programs embody factors contributing to the success of medical technology students and their proficiency in subsequent laboratory practice;

3) The utilization of quality control practices in medical laboratories, the extent to which medical technologists are prepared to exercise judgment, and the contribution of both to the performance of laboratory work;

4) The degree of latitude employed by laboratory supervisors in judging performance of technologists relating to both technical and nontechnical aspects of laboratory work, and if technologists generally fail to perform within the expectations and demands of their supervisors.

H. *Manpower for the Medical Laboratory.* The National Committee for Careers in Medical Technology. 1967.

There is urgent need for a study to determine and define skills and manpower requirements for present and future medical laboratory practice, with consideration of anticipated changes in laboratory methodology, demands for laboratory services, and organization, administration, and delivery of laboratory services.

Findings of the study of necessary skills should be employed to reassess and realign laboratory career categories and the educational and technical levels required for the categories.

To measure and project manpower needs accurately, a uniform laboratory workload reporting system should be formulated and adopted nationwide.

TABLE F-1. SUMMARY OF RECOMMENDATIONS

H. *Manpower for the Medical Laboratory.* (continued)

An analysis should be made of the need for new specialties and disciplines in the clinical laboratory, and of the curriculums and training to be developed to prepare personnel for the new roles.

Allied health careers should be promoted by directing information on laboratory as well as other health careers to science teachers, guidance counselors, librarians, parents, and students starting as early as upper elementary grades.

Recruitment efforts should be directed to new sources of manpower.

Laboratory professionals should cooperate with educators and science education groups to help upgrade the quality of science education in elementary and high schools.

Assistance and guidance should be provided junior colleges and vocational schools in developing educational programs leading to medical laboratory careers.

Colleges and universities should be encouraged to strengthen baccalaureate curriculums for medical technology education, and the current 3-year college plus 1-year clinical training system should be reviewed.

Graduate education for medical laboratory personnel should be strengthened and expanded.

Continuing education programs for medical laboratory personnel should be expanded and strengthened, and better methods for coordinating and evaluating them developed.

New curriculums and teaching methods should be explored, with experimentation encouraged, and self-instruction in laboratory education should be utilized more effectively.

Career opportunities in medical laboratories should be improved and financial rewards provided at the top that will attract and retain more professional administrators and other specialists.

TABLE F-1. SUMMARY OF RECOMMENDATIONS

H. *Manpower for the Medical Laboratory.* (continued)

Representatives of medical laboratory disciplines should initiate efforts with educational testing specialists to develop equivalency tests to provide increased mobility between levels and categories of laboratory careers.

The agency administering a licensing program for clinical laboratory personnel should have an advisory board of representatives of the scientific disciplines involved as well as knowledgeable representatives of the public.

Accrediting and certifying agencies should explore possibilities and ways of offering their services to all schools requesting evaluation, and to graduates of non-accredited programs applying for certification.

I. *Allied Health Personnel.* Ad Hoc Committee on Allied Health Personnel; Division of Medical Science; National Research Council; Nation Academy of Sciences; National Academy of Engineering. 1967.

Those in positions of leadership in civilian medicine re-examine the ranges of services rendered by the many categories of health-care personnel, and re-structure these services in ways that increase the effectiveness of the delivery of health care by both professional and supporting personnel.

Leaders in civilian medicine counsel with leaders in military medicine to learn from the military experience better ways of training and using supporting personnel in civilian health care systems, hospitals, clinics and private practice.

Experiments be conducted in the training of new categories of supporting health personnel and their integration into health-care teams, and in desirable changes in the skills of presently recognized personnel categories to meet changing requirements. The VA is suggested as a logical system in which such experiments might be tried.

Career patterns for supporting health-care personnel be so structured that a person can rise from one classification to another in his present specialty or enter a related field while receiving adequate credit for prior training, experience, and education.

Adequate attention be given to methods of recruiting and retaining ex-corpsmen in the civilian health care system; to pilot programs for developing adequate methods of evaluating the ex-corpsmen's existing

TABLE F-1. SUMMARY OF RECOMMENDATIONS

I. *Allied Health Personnel*
(continued)

skills, and programs for increasing those skills to meet specific technical and other job requirements, and to seeking the necessary changes in accreditation and licensing regulations and laws that at present often prevent the technically qualified person from meeting employment requirements.

J. *Association of American Medical Colleges Annual Meeting.* Nov., 1968.

Create a much larger number of comprehensive, hospital-based health care centers, ensuring that the consumer of health care along with physicians and businessmen of the community are involved in the design of the health care facility and in planning pertinent aspects of the program.

Greater flexibility in the admission policies of existing four-year medical schools. More students might be taken at the end of two or three years of college if there is evidence of maturity and commitment. The medical school experience should also be adjusted to the needs of the student and might vary in length from three to six years.

Medical schools should individualize the education of the physician to fit the student's varying rates of achievement, educational background, and career goals. The individualization should include the length of time utilized to satisfy the requirements for the M.D. degree as well as content of curriculum. Alteration of content must not be accomplished by compressing existing content, in existing sequences into smaller numbers of instructional hours.

It was recognized that emergency room visits have been increasing over the past two decades and that there should be provision for more adequate, and probably specialized services. A specific recommendation was made that specialized training for emergency room and ambulatory services be developed.

It was recommended that more attention be given to the training of specialists in the supervision of members of the health team in order to stretch the services of the professional staff without any reduction in the quality of services.

There must be continued participation of students and faculty in joint committees to evaluate the learning experience of the students. This learning experience is

TABLE F-1. SUMMARY OF RECOMMENDATIONS

J. *Association of American Medical Colleges Annual Meeting.* (continued).

the prime measure of the validity of curriculum reform.

There must be increased financial support for and recognition of teaching. This will permit rearrangement of faculty time to meet the demands of increased flexibility and individualization in the new curriculum. The Dean's office must also be strengthened in the areas of student advisement and curriculum supervision.

There must be increased efforts by clinical teachers to meet the charges leveled for years of lack of humaneness in their teaching. The teaching of the scientific aspects of medicine must be maintained; but it must no longer be, and never should have been, at the expense of the demonstration of real concern with the personal and social problems of patients.

APPENDIX G

AN ANNOTATED BIBLIOGRAPHY OF RECENT PUBLICATIONS IN NURSING AND RELATED HEALTH FIELDS

The annotated bibliography that follows is the result of a literature search which includes items from a sample of 20 national and international publications, issue by issue, for the years 1967, 1968, and 1969.*

By examining the different magazines concerned with the health care field (nursing in particular; the health related fields in general), the staff hoped to become familiar with the ideas, developments and issues in nursing and nursing education over the very recent past. This extensive search of the literature was only one of several methods used by the staff to uncover information about nursing practice, (roles and functions), nursing education, and nursing careers — the three major divisions used in defining the limits of the study.

Not only did the literature contribute to baseline data for the report, but the articles scrutinized also yielded references that were used to procure large quantities of unpublished reports. In addition, this general search of the literature served a valuable purpose in providing the staff a foundation and orientation toward both nursing and the entire health care field.

---

*The journals and publications used for each area appear in a list at the end of this introduction.

211

As a first step, a data retrieval system was organized for sources relating to nursing practice. Some 900 bibliographic citations that seemed to bear at least indirectly on our objectives were extracted. This number was then subjected to further critical review and when duplication and quality standards were invoked, the staff annotated and organized the remaining 160 references. We then repeated this process with the areas of nursing education and careers, with the final product being an annotated bibliography of approximately 540 items.

Our initial inquiry into nursing practice, when searching published material, was guided by certain questions to which we hoped to find some answers and even more, some consensus of opinion. In general, these questions concerning nursing practice in relation to the health scene were: what are the major trends in the patterns of patient care which will significantly affect future roles of nursing personnel; what changed or new responsibilities and functions will these future patterns require nursing personnel to undertake and perform; what changes in nursing performance and behavior will be needed to carry out future responsibilities and functions successfully; what skills and capabilities should nurses either possess or share with other health care personnel; what differences exist between innovative practices, current practices, and current institutional expectations of nurses and how can these differences be resolved to adequately and economically meet future patient care needs; does delineation of nursing into technical and professional roles improve patient care; and finally, are there factors affecting the application of innovations which make some more likely to gain acceptance than others, and how will such factors affect nursing personnel?

The final bibliography concerned with nursing practice included approximately 165 references gathered from 13 journals — references that were then organized into specific areas: trends and changing patterns in health care settings; capabilities, attitudes and skills needed of nursing personnel; health care needs which could require nursing attention and effort; and the development, introduction and evaluation of innovations in health care affecting nursing.

This same procedure for extracting material regarding practice was used in the areas of nursing education and careers. After defining needs for nursing practice, we then were in a position to look at education for that practice; consequently, published material was sought which dealt with the issues of nursing education. Four major areas were soon defined and references categorized under the following headings: the discernible trends in the institutional patterns for the preparation of nurses and the short and long-term answers to the most pressing problems of nursing preparatory institutions; the strengths, weaknesses and trends among nurse faculty and students and the effects of these on future institutions educating nurses; changes in other health schools that will affect the future of nursing education; and the trends, changes and needs in the basic nursing curriculum, advanced (graduate or specialized) curriculum, and continuing and in-service education for nurses.

Initially, some 212 items bearing heavily on these concerns were collected from 15 journals and were later organized and combined with the list from the other two areas.

To complete our search of material, it was then necessary to look specifically at nursing in relation to manpower requirements in the health scene and to the economics of those requirements and their effects on nurses and the consumers of nursing and health care. We reviewed the literature with the following topics in mind: manpower requirements in the health care field and their relationship to nursing education and functions; the economic factors influencing present and future nursing functions and resultant manpower planning; the "shortage" of nurses and the possible answers to that problem; licensure and accreditation as affected by federal and other legislation and manpower needs for nursing.

After reviewing 13 journals for a three-year period, we refined and organized our references for nursing careers into the following areas: significance of economic factors for nurse manpower planning; factors affecting the supply of nurses such as career mobility, educational mobility, men in nursing, etc; manpower and the institutions responsible for the education of nurses; laws, licensure and accreditation; issues and relations between medicine, health administration, the consumer-public and nursing; the planning of health services and the role of the nurse; and nursing and cost control. The final number of references was 172.

All in all, 20 different journals were scanned, resulting in an annotated list of references of 540 items relevant to the ideas and developments of nursing and nursing education over the past three years. The staff, of necessity, had to be selective and, consequently, extrapolated those articles that seemed to relate to our initial probable findings. We then eliminated duplications among the three areas. This, incidentally, was quite extensive since it was difficult to look at any single area without considering the other two. The interrelations among nursing practice, education and careers are so complete that almost any given article yielded information concerning all three areas.

At each stage of development, the separate bibliographies were given to the members of the Commission and our two advisory panels for their review and consideration. In the final analysis, this extensive review of the literature was invaluable as one source of information that influenced the final recommendations of the Commission.

Journals reviewed for information in all three areas:

American Journal of Nursing
Nursing Outlook
Nursing Research
Canadian Nurse
Modern Hospital
Hospital Progress
Hospitals

American Journal of Public Health
Journal of the American Medical Association

Additional journals reviewed for Nursing Practice:

Geriatrics
Journal of Practical Nursing
International Nursing Review
Nursing Clinics of North America

Additional journals reviewed for Nursing Education:

Journal of Medical Education
Journal of Nursing Education
Nursing Forum
Canadian Hospital
International Nursing Review
National League for Nursing Publications

Additional journals reviewed for Nursing Careers:

Journal of Nursing Education
Medical Economics
New England Journal of Medicine
Journal of Medical Education

ANNOTATED BIBLIOGRAPHY

Abdellah, Faye G. "The Nature of Nursing Science," *Nursing Research*, 18 (September-October 1969), 390-393.
    The progress the profession makes in developing a scientific base for nursing depends largely on the research that provides facts from which generalizations and laws can be applied to the solution of nursing problems.
Abraham, Gertrude E. "Promoting Nursing Research in an Organized Nursing Service," *American Journal of Nursing*, 68 (April, 1968), 818-821.
    The V. A.'s effort to increase participation in nursing research makes identification of nursing problems the role of the clinical practitioners, while selection and design of studies is done by nurses with research training. Four Regional Research Support Centers are available to assist in implementing research ideas and to supply services such as statistical analysis.
Adams, Robert E. "Hospital's Learning Center Uses Multimedia Approach," *Hospitals*, 43 (March 16, 1969), 52-56.
    A well-designed educational facility boosts morale and provides meaningful and efficient training for hospital personnel.
"Administrators Speak Out on the Role and Future of Hospital Schools of Nursing," *Modern Hospital*, 109 (August, 1967), 95-96, 103-105.
    A policy change is needed now if we are to avert a disastrous shortage of nurses in the years ahead. Some of the administrators are Robert E. Adams, Richard Highsmith, etc.

Aichlmayr, Rita Hoeschen. "Cultural Understanding: A Key to Acceptance," *Nursing Outlook*, 17 (July, 1969), 20-23.

   The nurse must not only recognize and understand cultural values different from her own, but must gear her work activities with other ethnic groups in a way that will foster their trust and acceptance. Students and an instructor reach the "unreachable" Indians by reinforcing Indian cultural values in their nursing actions.

Aldag, Jean and Cherryl Christensen. "Personality Correlates of Male Nurses," *Nursing Research*, 16 (Fall, 1967), 375-376.

   The study was designed to investigate more thoroughly the personality characteristics of male students of nursing.

Alfano, Genrose J. "The Loeb Center for Nursing and Rehabilitation: A Professional Approach to Nursing Practice," *Nursing Clinics of North America*, 4 (September, 1969), 487-493.

   A unique staffing pattern and organizational structure is based on the belief that nursing is a therapeutic force in recovery and rehabilitation. All direct patient care is the responsibility of the professional nurse.

Allyn, Nathaniel C. "College Credit by Examination," *Nursing Outlook*, 17 (April, 1969), 44-46.

   A college-level examination program can save time and money, and save the student the boredom of pursuing courses of study that he has already mastered. The program should be one of both general and specific subject examinations, permitting measurement of knowledge acquired in other than the conventional ways.

American Journal of Nursing. "Do Beginning Jobs for Beginning Graduates Differ?" *American Journal of Nursing*, 69 (May, 1969), 1009-1011.

   An informal *Journal* survey reports what distinction directors of nursing in hospitals make in orientation supervision and nursing assignments for newly graduated nurses from diploma, AD and BS programs.

American Medical Association Committee on Nursing. "285,000 Inactive Registered Nurses Could Turn the Tide," *Journal of American Medical Association*, 200 (May 29, 1967), 779-780.

   Inactive RN's should be encouraged to return to practice by a community-wide educationally sound, cooperatively supported and sponsored refresher course program (6 weeks), planned on a continuing basis, in order to alleviate the nurse shortage.

American Nurses' Association. "Statement Regarding Nurses in Regional Medical Programs," *Nursing Outlook*, 17 (February, 1969), 23.

   The ANA supports the development of RMP's and it urges state and district nurses associations to strive for official representation in these programs.

Amicarella, Henry. "The Rewards of Sustained Recruitment Effort," *Hospitals*, 41 (June 1, 1967), 91-94.

   The author suggests more effective recruitment programs, and cooperative activities with local schools and other health organizations.

Ammer, Dean S. "Hospital-Oriented Nursing School No Guarantee of Full Staff, Study Shows," *Hospitals*, 42 (May 1, 1968), 55-57, 110.

   Hospitals that operate schools of nursing suffer nursing personnel shortages as severe as hospitals that don't operate such schools, according to a recent study of hospitals in the greater Boston area. The author reports on the findings of that study and relates the statistics on shortage rates to such factors as geographic location, incidence of nursing schools, wage incentives, and hospital size.

"Among Other Things, Prescribing Nursing Care," *Nursing Outlook*, 15 (February, 1967), 64-65.

In a Vermont mental hospital, registered nurses work only with patients. All administrative and managerial tasks are done by LPN's. Each nurse has a specific caseload and works closely with one physician as a team.

Andreali, Kathleen G. and Eugene A. Stead, Jr. "Training Physician's Assistants at Duke," *American Journal of Nursing*, 67 (July, 1967), 1442-1443.

Authors discuss the role of the "Physician Assistant."

Anello, Michael. "Responsibility for Change and Innovation in Professional Nursing," *International Nursing Review*, V. 16, No. 3 (1969), 208-219.

The author stresses the need for a core curriculum in professional nursing.

Archer, Sarah E. and Marilyn A. Jarvis-Eckert. "Health Classes on Wheels," *Nursing Outlook*, 16 (April, 1968), 52-54.

Students from nursing, medicine, dentistry and pharmacy at West Virginia University Medical Center shared a new kind of experience in community health studies by participating on a team that assessed the health needs of three Appalachian communities.

"Are Men Nurses Really Accepted?" *Nursing Outlook*, 15 (May, 1967), 27.

This editorial states that we need men in nursing and a great deal more effort should be expended on the recruitment of men nurses.

Ayers, Rachael, Rowena Bishop and Fay Mass. "An Experiment in Nursing Service Reorganization," *American Journal of Nursing*, 69 (April, 1969), 783-786.

Report of experiment in California in which recognition of clinical competence is equal to that of administrative competence. Care has improved, nurse job satisfaction is higher and nursing service costs are down.

"B. C. Nursing Schools Adopt 2-Year Plan," *Canadian Hospital*, 44 (May, 1967), 68.

The six hospital schools of nursing in British Columbia have unanimously agreed that their three-year training programs should be reduced to two years.

Barritt, Evelyn and J. F. Ohliger. "Continuing Education," *American Journal of Nursing*, 69 (October, 1969), 2170-2171.

College programs in nursing have a responsibility to provide continuing education programs for nurses. The authors report findings of a questionnaire asking such schools how many and what types of courses are offered.

Barry, Mildred C. and Cecil G. Sheps. "A New Model for Community Health Planning," *American Journal of Public Health*, 59 (February, 1969), 226-231.

A description of the process by which the Cleveland Metropolitan community developed a health goals plan is presented. The three basic elements that made up the framework of this project were a concept of health, involvement, and utilization of knowledge. Included in planning or counseling were health professionals and consumers.

Bates, Barbara. "The Better the Doctor Does His Job, The Better the Nurse Can Do Hers," *Modern Hospital*, 108 (January, 1967), 72-75.

The nurse becomes the victim when physicians fail to communicate, and both patient care and staffing problems can be improved by doctors.

―――― and M. Sue Kern. "Doctor-Nurse Teamwork: What Helps? What Hinders?" *American Journal of Nursing*, 67 (October, 1967), 2066-2071.

The authors conclude that freer communication between the medical and nursing professions is the first step toward the collaborative practice which should benefit patients.

Batman, Robert H. and Veronica A. Binzley. "Group Meetings With Charge Aides," *Nursing Outlook*, 16 (June, 1968), 38-40.

An inservice program which had partially failed in the beginning provided the impetus for a new approach that may have contributed significantly to changes in ward programs and nursing practice at Cleveland State Hospital.

Baumgart, Alice J. "Preparation for Health Team Practice," *The Canadian Nurse*, 64 (September, 1968), 42-43.

The developing Health Services Centre at the University of British Columbia has been conceived with the goal of providing common educational experiences by integrating health science disciplines. The university has created an interprofessional curriculum committee.

Baumgartner, Leona. "How Will We Get Well and Keep Healthy?" *Nursing Outlook*, 16 (March, 1968), 40-42.

The author suggests that by the beginning of the Twenty-First Century, dazzling social and scientific changes will necessitate a more formal, better organized system of delivery of health care services than we have today.

Bayer, Alan E. "Nurse Supply: It's Better Than We Thought," *Modern Hospital*, 109 (July, 1967), 75-79.

More nurses than were previously expected may be available in the years to come, but there will still be a shortage for which planning must begin now.

——— and Lyle F. Schoenfeldt. "Student Inter-changeability in Three-Year and Four-Year Nursing Programs," *The Journal of Human Resources*, V:71-88, 1969.

This paper reports analyses of measures of interests and personality, scores on aptitude and achievement tests, and data on personal and background variables from a national longitudinal survey. Result: implications for diploma programs and the future number of young people entering the nursing field.

Baziak, Anna T. "Nurses Told to Select Priorities," *Hospital Progress*, (August, 1969), 66.

The author feels that nurses are too task-oriented and their job of "nurturance" has fallen by the wayside. Nurses should nurse the ill!

Beebe, Joyce E., Elaine M. Pendleton and Elizabeth Kenz. "Bench Conferences in a Large Obstetric Clinic," *American Journal of Nursing*, 68 (January, 1968), 85-87.

Clinic waiting time is utilized by nurse-wifery students for informal prenatal teaching when women would not attend formal classes held elsewhere in the clinic building.

Beloff, Jerome S., Parnie S. Snoke and Richard E. Weinerman. "Yale Studies in Family Health Care," *Journal of the American Medical Association*, 204 (April 29, 1968), 63-68.

Detailed report of organization and administration of family health care delivery system includes general outline of role of public health nurse.

——— and Marion Willet. "Yale Studies in Family Health Care," *Journal of the American Medical Association*, 205 (September 2, 1968), 663-69.

Review of two and one-half years of study with emphasis on make-up of health team and utilization of consultants. (Most used were MSW, psychiatrist and nutritionist). A new experiment will assign new families to the public health nurse functioning as prime assessor of health.

——— and Richard E. Weinerman. "Yale Studies in Family Health Care," *Journal of the American Medical Association*, 199 (February 6, 1967), 383-389.

Objectives of, and planning and project design for, a health care delivery system which will be utilized by medical education for student experience in community health. Health team concept is stressed.

Benz, Edward G. "Nursing Service," *Hospitals*, 43 (April, 1969), 157-162.
    Review of 1968 literature indicates automation is accelerating, more administration by non-nurses, improved patient care by study of nursing functions, and research on new patient care roles, including clinical specialization. Good basic reference list.
Bergman, Alice C. "A Do-It-Yourself Refresher Program," *American Journal of Nursing*, 69 (April, 1969), 792-795.
    By marshalling her own talents, taking advantage of professional consultation and resources and utilizing available published guides and texts, the author emerged from a self-directed refresher course as an able and confident practitioner.
Bergman, Rebecca. "Education of Paramedical Personnel," *International Nursing Review*, 16 (April, 1969), 161-165.
    Paramedical workers must sometimes assume leadership roles with auxiliaries of their own discipline. Details six essential components of the educational programs.
Berkowitz, Norman H. and Mary F. Malone. "Intra-Professional Conflict," *Nursing Forum*, VII: No. 1 (1968), 50-71.
    Task of this generation is to bring nursing service and nursing education back together again. Article discusses where graduates of what nursing institutions go for jobs, etc. The author delineates the differences that arise as nursing moves away from its former relationships and attempts to establish itself as a profession.
Biggart, John H. "The Challenge of Nurse Education," *International Nursing Review*, 15, No. 4 (October, 1968), 292-304.
    The author, an MD faculty member from Belfast, proposes such things as: joint appointments in schools of nursing *and* an initial training or educational program for *all* nursing students.
Bitzer, Maryann and Martha C. Boudreaux. "Using A Computer to Teach Nursing," *Nursing Forum*, VIII:3:234-254, 1969.
    The authors write of the contributions to nursing education of computer-based education, particularly used at Mercy Hospital School of Nursing in Urbana, Illinois.
Boorer, David J. "Men Nurses in Britain," *Nursing Outlook*, 16 (November, 1968), *24-26.*
    Although the status of men nurses in Britain has improved considerably, it is unlikely that any great numbers of men will enter the profession for some time to come.
Bowden, Edgar A. "Nurses' Attitudes Toward Hospital Nursing Services," *Nursing Research*, 16 (Summer, 1967), 246-251.
    The article discusses implications for job satisfaction and transfers between services. There should be a specific conscious recognition and acceptance of differentiated roles.
Bowles, Jr., Grover C. "Continuing Education May be Required for Pharmacist License," *Modern Hospital*, 113 (October, 1969), 130.
    Some states consider inservice education so important that they require it for license renewal: Florida and Kansas.
——: "Extending Pharmacists' Duties Helps Alleviate Nurse Shortage," *Modern Hospital*, 108 (January, 1967), 106.
    The pharmacist's potential outside the confines of pharmacy must be recognized to relieve nurses of pharmacy chores.
Breslow, Lester. "Political Jurisdictions, Voluntarism, and Health Planning," *American Journal of Public Health*, 58 (July, 1968), 1147-1153.
    This article addresses itself to questions such as, what roles shall governmental and voluntary agencies take in health planning, etc.

Brockmeier, Marlene J. "Nursing in The Community Health Settings," *Nursing Outlook*, 16 (April, 1968), 54-58.

How the role of the nurse differs from that of other health care workers is often more difficult to delineate in the mental health field than in others. Author offers five elements which make that role a unique one.

Brodie, Donald C. "Trends in Pharmaceutical Education," *American Journal of Nursing*, 68 (September, 1968), 1948-1951.

Discussion of the problems and practices in pharmacy provides a basis for greater nurse-pharmacist understanding. Professional isolation is incongruous with the health care concept. Present education fails to prepare the pharmacist for his emerging clinical role.

Brooks, Sr. William Mary. "A Pattern for Unit Management," *Hospital Progress*, 48 (May, 1967), 124-128.

Good review of the progress of unit manager program in nine hospitals, including individual adaptations and responsibilities in each organization.

Brophy, Margaret and Evelyn Leech. "Nurse Refresher Program Offers Immediate Staff Positions," *Hospitals*, 42 (September 16, 1968), 73-74, 78.

Rather than taking a course, inactive nurses enrolling in this program become salaried members of nursing teams.

Brown, Howard J. "Changes in the Delivery of Health Care," *American Journal of Nursing*, 68 (November, 1968), 2362-2364.

Adding more money or personnel will not end the chaos in our health care system. Drastic changes must come — and will come. The author tells what to expect and suggests how nursing can prepare for the changes.

Brunet, Jacques. "Laval University Accepts a Challenge," *The Canadian Nurse*, 65 (August, 1969), 44-45.

In 1968, a new program was initiated — a baccalaureate program in health sciences.

Bryan, Doris S. and Thelma S. Cook. "Redirection of School Nursing Services in Culturally Deprived Neighborhoods," *American Journal of Public Health*, 57 (July, 1967), 1164-1170.

At the end of one year of study there is evidence that (1) a planned program of personal contact between school nurse and parents will increase parental actions to maintain and promote health, (2) non-nurse assistants can take over routine managerial functions, and (3) time released will be used by nurses for the exercise of specialized nursing knowledge and skills.

Buckles, Joan V., Leah G. Cashar and Linda N. Olson. "Learning Purposeful Nursing Intervention," *American Journal of Nursing*, 68 (December, 1968), 2578-2580.

Each patient contact becomes a learning experience for students using the 'Guides for Nursing Intervention' developed by three psychiatric nursing instructors at the University of Washington in Seattle.

Bulbulyan, Ann, Rose Marie Davidetes and Florence Williams. "Nurses in a Community Mental Health Center," *American Journal of Nursing*, 69 (February, 1969), 328-331.

Nurses join the three traditional disciplines of medicine, psychology and social work and are now serving as therapists for patients and consultants for other health professionals.

Burgess, Michael M. and Margery Duffey. "The Prediction of Success in a Collegiate Program of Nursing," *Nursing Research*, 18 (January-February, 1969), 68-72.

A total of 58 intellective, interest, personality, and educational variables were examined as potential predictors of GPA on two independent student samples in a collegiate program of nursing. Results: it is possible to significantly predict collegiate nursing GPA using 20 or even five predictors.

Burnside, Helen. "Practical Nurses Become Associate Degree Graduates," *Nursing Outlook*, 17 (April, 1969), 47-48.

At Cuyahoga Community College in Cleveland, the career mobility of practical nurses is enhanced by a policy that allows them to apply for "credit by examination" in subject areas they have already covered.

Burtz, Gudrun S. "A Fifth Year for School Nurse Preparation," *Nursing Outlook*, 17 (October, 1969), 38-40.

Baccalaureate graduates are offered a 30-credit program to better prepare them for school nursing in California at San Francisco State College.

Callahan, Barbara. "Regional Medical Programs Taking Giant Steps," *Hospital Progress*, (March, 1967), 78-83, 108.

Includes a chart showing planning grants for the RMP's approved and funded as of December 31, 1966.

Campbell, Emily B. "Not Education, Not Service, But Nursing," *American Journal of Nursing*, 67 (April, 1967), 990-994.

A venture into joint appointment as assistant professor and supervisor of medical-surgical nursing meant an extended orientation period and eventually a role model for both students and staff who could both "teach and do."

"Can We Afford Small Schools?" *The Canadian Nurse*, 63 (December, 1967), 48.

The author quotes an NLN cost study (1964) and relates it to Canada, raising the question of cost of small diploma programs.

"Canada Urged to Experiment With Nursing Patterns," *Canadian Hospital*, 46 (June, 1969), 51.

Dean Dorothy Smith of the University of Florida, in a recent speech, stated that "faculty nurses should stop teaching disease and practice nursing." Students should observe the instructor as a role model instead of the instructor watching the student.

Carb, Genevieve R. "Tutoring Project is Gateway to Nursing Careers for Underprivileged Girls," *Hospitals*, 41 (September 1, 1967), 59-61, 154.

Author describes a tutorial project offering remedial education to high school students who are underachievers but who have expressed interest in professional nursing careers. She discusses the recruiting and screening procedures and the outcome of this intensive 8-week summer session that required residential living: Chicago.

Carlson, Sylvia, Rona Kaufman and Madeline Schwaid. "An Experiment in Self-Determined Patient Care," *Nursing Clinics of North America*, 4 (September, 1969), 495-506.

Report of a New York hospital's attempt to bridge the gap between theory and practice by creation of a climate in which the nurse assists the patient to mobilize his own coping mechanisms. Methods of implementation include new visiting policies, reorientation of charting procedures, and reorganization of personnel utilization.

Case, Robert W. et al. "Automated Narcotic Control System Saves Time for Pharmacy and Nursing," *Hospitals*, 41 (May 16, 1967), 97-98.

Time consuming routine of "counting narcotics" can be virtually eliminated from nurses' duties.

Casella, Carmine. "Need Hierarchies Among Nursing and Non-Nursing College Students," *Nursing Research*, 17 (May-June, 1968), 273-275.

Study tested view that psychological needs are operative in vocational and professional choices. Results were more a measure of homogeneity between the two groups than otherwise.

Castle, C. Hilmon. "Intermountain Program Focuses on Community Hospitals," *Hospitals*, 42 (July 1, 1968), 49-51.
> A case study of the Intermountain Regional Medical Program.

Cathcart, H. Robert. "Nursing Education: An Appraisal and a Forecast," *Hospitals*, 42 (August 16, 1968), 108-116.
> The author suggests that the community hospitals are charged with the responsibility for raising standards and acquiring support for nursing education in hospital schools.

Chambliss, Virginia L. "Steps to Learning," *Nursing Outlook*, 17 (May, 1969), 46-47.
> Deaconess Hospital School of Nursing in Evansville, Indiana, received a Public Health Service grant (two-year) to develop a project titled, "Nurse-Teacher Development and Use of Selected Audio-Visuals for Teaching Clinical Nursing." The objectives are to develop and improve the faculty's knowledge and skills by involving them in the preparation of audio-visual teaching tools.

"Characteristics of Baccalaureate and Graduate Education in Nursing," *Nursing Outlook*, 16 (July, 1968), 36-37.
> These characteristics were accepted by the Council of Baccalaureate and Higher degree programs. The article lists some general assumptions regarding baccalaureate education in nursing.

Chow, Rita. "Postoperative Cardiac Nursing Research: A Method for Identifying and Categorizing Nursing Action," *Nursing Research*, 18 (January-February, 1969), 4-13.
> Video-tape monitoring of first four hours of post-operative care in cardiac surgical intensive care unit was used to gather data on behaviors. A conceptual model for classifying behaviors is utilized.

Christie, Jean E. "Central Service: A Key to Nurse Efficiency," *Modern Hospital*, 108 (January, 1967), 100.
> Central Service can help meet the nursing shortage by encompassing all of the factors related to provision and control of supplies and equipment.

Christman, Luther. "The Nurse Clinical Specialist," *Hospital Progress*, 49 (August, 1968), 14-16, 24-28.
> Author defines specialization as the deliberate and thoughtful application of science to the care of patients within the confines of the specialty area in an attempt to expand the dimensions of expert nursing practice. Factors which encourage and those that inhibit nurse specialization are discussed.

———: "Specialism and Generalism in Clinical Nursing," *Hospitals*, 41 (January 1, 1967), 83-86.
> Review of historical basis for present nursing structure. A proposal to delegate non-nursing functions to unit managers allowing better utilization of nurses is advanced.

———: "The Role of Nursing in Organizational Effectiveness," *International Nursing Review*, 16 (June, 1969), 248-257.
> Nursing time is diluted by being physician's assistant, administrative assistant and by use of managerial nursing care. Reorganization with nurses doing nursing is essential. New roles (specialist) will disturb the status quo. How soon we achieve progress depends on whether nurses and administration choose comfortable status quo or uncomfortable change.

——— and Richard C. Jelinek. "Old Patterns Waste Half the Nursing Hours," *Modern Hospital*, 108 (January, 1967), 78-81.
> The authors propose a fresh look at nursing service and suggest a model to double nursing utilization, including the use of more clinical specialists.

Clare, Sister M. Virginia. "Toward a More Effective Program of Operating Room Administration," *Nursing Clinics of North America*, 3 (December, 1968), 575-589.
    Responsibility for surgical suite rests jointly on nurse clinical specialist, the unit manager and medical chief. Author foresees fewer, but better prepared, professional nurses and more technicians in O. R. areas.
Cleland, Virginia S. "Effects of Stress on Thinking," *American Journal of Nursing*, 67 (January, 1967), 108-111.
    A discussion of some implications for nursing practice which emerge from a study of RN's performance under four conditions of environmental stress. Nursing's problem is that no nurse can give comprehensive nursing care in the ordinary busy medical-surgical unit under present staffing patterns.
Clover, B. H. "A New Nurse Therapist," *American Journal of Nursing*, 67 (May, 1967), 1003-1005.
    Three-stage experiment conducted at University of Wisconsin to train nurses to be independent psycho-therapists; supervised, but not directed by psychiatrists. This role is similar to that of the psychologist and the social worker who function as therapists.
Coates, Mary E. "Imaginative Development Programs Make the Most of Personnel Resources," *Hospitals*, 43 (June 1, 1969), 67-72.
    The administrator of a small Detroit hospital explains management techniques that inspire improved performance, including paying LPN's to get their RN's.
Committee on Nursing Service, Canadian Nurses' Association. "Recommendations from the Committee on Nursing Service," *The Canadian Nurse*, 64 (May, 1968), 39-40.
    The committee recommends that nursing needs can best be met by RN's; clinical specialists should be used; nursing service should participate in the formulation of the objectives of the health service agency; the administration, supervision and carrying out of non-nursing activities should be done by other departments, etc.
Conant, Lucy H. "Closing the Practice-Theory Gap," *Nursing Outlook*, 15 (November, 1967), 37-39.
    Nursing, because it is a practice discipline, will retain the need for intuitive activity which may precede knowledge. The practitioner has a vital role in pinpointing areas of research and corroborating findings.
Conley, L. Ann. "Editorial: For the People or With the People?" *Nursing Outlook*, 17 (April, 1969), 27.
    The author wants more of the public represented on the NLN Council on Community Planning for Nursing — citizen participation.
Conley, Veronica L. and Stanley W. Olson. "Regional Medical Programs," *American Journal of Nursing*, 68 (September, 1968), 1916-1926.
    Cooperation from all health resources, a focus on specific needs in an area, and putting knowledge from research into practice — these are the keys to the approach now underway in improving health care under Regional Medical Programs. Author cites various programs.
Cooper, Signe S. "Activating the Inactive Nurse: A Historical Review," *Nursing Outlook*, 15 (October, 1967), 62-65.
    Inactive nurses are a hidden resource that we cannot afford to ignore. A review of the history of reactivating nurses reveals the lack of a systematic, coordinated plan to prepare them for reentry into the profession.

———: "Continuing Education: An Imperative for Nurses," *Nursing Forum*, Vol: No. 3 (1968), 289-297.

Author urges all institutions to offer inservice and continuing education courses for nurses.

Costello, C. G. and Sister T. Castonguay. "Two-Year Versus Three-Year Programs," *The Canadian Nurse*, 65 (February, 1969), 62-64.

A Canadian study showed that students in a three-year diploma program performed better generally than those in a two-year program. However, with some modification of the two-year program, the difference in favor of a three-year program may disappear and the study findings reversed. Conclusion: make a good two-year program.

Coye, Dorothy H. "Programmed Instruction for Staff Education," *American Journal of Nursing*, 69 (February, 1969), 325-327.

Experiment proved two things: programmed instruction increased the probability that personnel will learn what is being taught and that the time and cost of preparation is such that the method may have to be used selectively for content that is crucial to patient care and necessary for all staff members to know.

Coye, Robert D. and Marc F. Hansen. "The 'Doctor's Assistant'," *Journal of American Medical Association* 209 (July 28, 1969), 529-533.

Report of a survey of expectations of Wisconsin physicians regarding physician's assistants. If adequate nurses were available as "helpers" physicians would see no need of this new category of worker. Authors question whether the nurse should not be the physician's professional associate rather than his assistant.

Crocker, Goldie. "Nursing in a Sociological Perspective," *Nursing Outlook*, 16 (April, 1968), 65-67.

As she begins to assume her responsibility in society, the baccalaureate nursing student, participating in the special course (acquaintance with social systems and with their influences on the patient and on themselves as individuals and nursing students), considers human relationships and social environment in an ever-changing society (Northeastern University in Boston).

Cummins, A. B. "Doctors Need Nurses to Manage the Care," *Modern Hospital*, 108 (February, 1967), 107-108.

New understanding of nurse's role is needed to make best use of medicine. Nurses are in the best position to operate medical care systems, but they need doctors' understanding to make such a system work.

Currey, Jean W., John D. Swisher and Lorane C. Kruse. "Improving Human Relations Skills Through Programmed Instruction," *Nursing Research*, 17 (September-October, 1968), 455-459.

Study tested the effectiveness of a programmed instructional sequence, 'The Management Improvement Program' in increasing the human relations skills of nurses (Ohio State University). Results: the program had significant impact on these skills of nurses.

Dahlstedt, Joan M. "Rearrangement to Enrich Bedside Nursing," *American Journal of Nursing*, 69 (June, 1969), 1254-1257.

On 28 bed study unit in Phoenix, RN's are utilizing nursing history, care plan and orders; are being relieved of tasks, such as passing medications, in an effort to upgrade patient care and increase nurse satisfaction.

Danzig, Ronald and H. J. C. Swan. "Practical Experience in a Coronary Care Unit," *Geriatrics*, 24 (June, 1969), 95-101.

Both intensive care and observation units are used in care of myocardial infarction patients in a community hospital. The nurses role has been expanded into treatment realm with definite evidence of lessening patient mortality.

Darley, Ward and Anne R. Somers. "Medicine, Money and Manpower — The Challenge of Professional Education," *The New England Journal of Medicine*, 276 (June 1, 1967), 1234-1238.

Outmoded licensing laws and professional mores prevent RN's, LPN's, etc. from the upgrading of jobs and skills that would benefit patients and employees. Physicians continue to perform many tasks that could be done as well or better by other personnel. There is little career mobility between even closely related groups.

———: "Medicine, Money and Manpower — The Challenge to Professional Education; Increasing Personnel," *The New England Journal of Medicine*, 276 (June 22, 1967), 1414-1423.

The authors stress the need for the ranges of the RN's responsibility to be increased in size and complexity; recruitment of inactive nurses and the upgrading of RN's skills.

———: "Medicine, Money and Manpower — The Challenge to Professional Education; New Training for New Needs," *The New England Journal of Medicine*, 276 (June 29, 1967), 1471-1478.

The professional nurse should be upgraded for greater responsibility and core curricula should be introduced.

David, Janis H. "Liaison Nurse," *American Journal of Nursing*, 69 (October, 1969), 2142.

Description of a new nursing role being developed at a Southern California rehabilitation center.

Davidson, Richard J. "Education and Hospitals," *Hospitals, 43 (April 1, 1969), 79-82.*

Author discusses: a new philosophy on training and development of personnel; internships, seminars, work-study programs to lure young recruits and minority groups; new job categories such as "physician's assistant" as a hope for the future and the growing importance of multi-media tools.

Davis, Anne J. "Self-Concept, Occupational Role Expectations, and Occupational Choice in Nursing and Social Work," *Nursing Research*, 18 (January-February, 1969), 55-59.

Most nursing students make the decision to become a nurse in high school — thus, implications for recruitment.

Davis, Katherine G. "Give Nurses the Chance to Explore These Routes to Better Care," *Modern Hospital*, 111 (October, 1968), 82-85.

Twelve areas in which nurse-initiated research could produce more efficient methods of patient care include computerization, family intensive care, nursing audits, discharge routines, etc.

DeChow, Georgeen H., Vivian Malmstrom and Ruth P. Ogden. "Education For Registered Nurses," *Journal of the American Medical Association*, 203 (March 18, 1968), 1051-1053.

Authors compare and contrast the three types of nursing programs and stress the idea that the employer of nurses must have and gear an orientation program to that specific type of nurse.

Deegan, Mary, Clarence D. Dieter and Catherine Voelker. "An Audio-Tutorial Approach to Learning," *Nursing Outlook*, 16 (March, 1968), 46-48.

The use of the audiotutorial lab for the teaching of an integrated science course enables students to learn at their own rate of speed. This school in Pennsylvania (Washington Hospital School of Nursing) found not only that more students could be educated, but they could accelerate the program from three to two years.

DeLora, Jack R. and Dorothy V. Moses. "Specialty Preferences and Characteristics of Nursing Students in Baccalaureate Programs," *Nursing Research*, 18 (March-April, 1969), 137-144.

Purpose of the study is to ascertain the specialty preferences and to develop criteria predictive of such choices. The results are very interesting: many implications for nursing education including improving the image of geriatric care, etc.

DePaul, Alice V. "The Nurse as a Central Figure in a Mental Health Center," *Perspectives in Psychiatric Care*, VI (February, 1968), 17-24.

Community after-care clinic at Worcester State Hospital, Massachusetts, utilizes four nurses, a psychiatrist and clinical psychologist for long term supportive therapy. Primary care contact is nurse who is involved in medication review and change, consultant role in hospital and community.

Derian, Paul S. "The Creation of the Medical Therapist," *Journal of the American Medical Association*, 206 (December 9, 1968), 2524-2525.

In a letter to the editor, the author suggests the creation of this new health worker, sandwiched in between the doctor and the nurse, with a salary ranging from $12,000 to $20,000, after a five to six year educational base.

DeSanders, Nancy. "Computer's Basic Plans Help Doctors Initiate Rehabilitation Regimen," *Modern Hospital*, 113 (November, 1969), 97.

A Texas rehabilitation unit schedules treatment services to patients instead of patients to services. The physician's individualization of the admission basic care plan permits treatment to begin in 10 minutes rather than the one hour it formerly required.

DeStefano, Mrs. Grace M. "Management Program Increases Nursing Service Effectiveness," *Hospital Progress*, (December, 1968), 54-60.

A three-year study of nursing service brings about better utilization of personnel and participative management.

deTornyay, Rheba and Mary W. Searight. "Micro-Teaching in Preparing Faculty," *Nursing Outlook*, 16 (March, 1968), 34-35.

Micro-teaching labs provide an excellent setting for practice teachers to teach, reteach and be critiqued by student subjects and other student teachers —·a different use of TV; the 5-minute teaching lab presentation used at the University of California school of nursing, San Francisco Medical Center.

Diedrick, Geraldine R. "Nursing in a Bureau of Social Work," *Nursing Outlook*, 17 (March, 1969), 50-51.

Unique role of public health nurse in Bureau of Social Work in California which supervises community placement of mentally handicapped. Public health nurse assists the community facility in providing optimal care by planning and evaluating care program and instructs in specific techniques of care. Also serves as consultant to the bureau's social workers in nursing problems arising in other community placement agencies such as family care program. Public health nurse is involved in student education — both nursing and social work.

Dineen, Mary A. "Current Trends in Collegiate Nursing Education," *Nursing Outlook*, 17 (August, 1969), 22-26.

The author warns against a rapid increase in the number of new programs — there is not necessarily a correlation between quantity and quality — indeed, quantity may dilute quality.

DiPietro, May Holmes. "An Undergraduate Course in Nursing Research," *Nursing Outlook*, 15 (May, 1967), 52-53.

At the Boston University school of nursing, a two semester-hour course, taught as a seminar, attempts to help the student acquire knowledge of developments and trends in professional nursing as demonstrated through the use of research studies in nursing.

Doderer, Minette. "Health Services at All Levels of Government; Desirable Structure and Relationship — On the State Level," *American Journal of Public Health*, 58 (December, 1968), 2202-2206.

The author stresses cooperative governmental health planning with full and active lines of communication. The lines of communication should include specialists drawn from all levels in an advisory capacity, and for counseling purposes from federal to state to local level, and in some cases in the reverse order.

Dolora, Sister M. "A Team Leader Development Program," *Hospital Progress*, 48 (October, 1967), 104, 108.

Description of a seven-week leader development course at St. Mary's Hospital, Grand Junction, Colorado.

Doyle, Margaret. "An Environment for the Clinical Practice of Nursing," *Nursing Clinics of North America*, 4 (September, 1969), 521-525.

Report of Vanderbilt study, utilizing changed organizational patterns to create an atmosphere in which individualized care is possible.

Drummond, Rev. E. J. "The Hospital School — As School," *Hospital Progress*, (February, 1969), 45-48, 64.

The author contends that the hospital school must determine more sharply what kind of school it is to be. He discusses the fact that the regional accrediting associations do *not* accredit single purpose institutions.

Dudas, Susan. "The RN in the Baccalaureate Program," *Nursing Outlook*, 16 (July, 1968), 51-53.

The author believes that nursing educators should assist RN students in collegiate programs by counseling and by giving them the opportunity to challenge some courses.

Dunn, Helen. "Facing Realities in Nursing Administration Today," *American Journal of Nursing*, 68 (May, 1968), 1013-1018.

A director of nursing tells how she deals with three problems — one being controlling the absorption of medical techniques into nursing practice.

Dunne, John B. "Where the Action Is — RMP," *Nursing Outlook*, 17 (February, 1969), 31-32.

Author urges nurses to be on the committees for regional planning — to pull her weight! RMP needs nurses and nurses need RMP.

du Plessis, D. J. "Challenge to the Nursing Profession," *International Nursing Review*, 14 (January-February, 1967), 41-48.

The question of academic vs. technical education for nurses and that of generalist vs. specialist in nursing as seen from the viewpoint of a South African Professor of Surgery.

Dustan, Laura C. and Thomas Hale. "The Iowa Debate: Education For Nursing: Apprenticeship or Academic? Wanted: Nurses to Nurse Patients," *Nursing Outlook*, 15 (September, 1967), 26-32.

The report of a debate, in Marshalltown, Iowa, on educational preparation for nursing, as seen through the eyes of a nurse educator and a physician — hospital administrator.

Dutrisac, Claire. "Mind Your Own Business," *The Canadian Nurse*, 65 (August, 1969), 46-48.

The author feels that nurses should be represented on committees and boards which make decisions affecting them. This article reviews new additions to the Quebec Hospitals Act with respect to nursing.

Edwards, Carl N. and Gretta Gribble. "Nursing as a Career: How Students Perceive It," *American Journal of Nursing*, 69 (June, 1969), 1223-1225.

A survey of senior students in twenty schools of nursing indicates that a majority of students in all types of programs desire a life style which combines marriage with work after their children are older. This and other perceptions of the future may vary, however, depending upon the type of program attended and the extent to which the program facilitates the student's own particular objectives.

Egolf, Marion C. "Unit Management Program Provides More Effective Use of Personnel," *Hospitals*, 43 (July 16, 1967), 77-81.

Details a wide spectrum of non-nursing functions assumed by a very highly skilled and trained ward manager. Includes necessary qualifications and possible sources of supply of ward managers. (Persons retired from upper enlisted ranks of armed services' medical departments.)

Ellis, Rosemary. "The Practitioner as Theorist," *American Journal of Nursing*, 69 (July, 1969), 1434-1438.

Defines theory as a conceptual structure built for a purpose. In nursing, unlike other sciences, that purpose is practice. Practitioners must develop and test theories for nursing as they practice.

"Establishing Standards for Nursing Practice," *American Journal of Nursing*, 69 (July, 1969), 1458-1463.

A *Journal* interview with nurses working on the Committees on Standards of the five ANA Divisions on Nursing Practice. They discuss the work now under way to develop standards for practice in geriatric, medical-surgical, psychiatric-mental health, maternal-child health and community nursing practice.

Evans, Robert L. "Hospitals and Regional Medical Programs: A Plea for Coordinated Action," *Hospitals*, 41 (December 16, 1967), 52-58, 114.

Establishing a foundation of continuing education is the first step toward closing the gap between medical research and care — continuing education for physicians and other health personnel.

Fagin, Carl. "Pharmacists' Role Expands in the Neighborhood Health Center," *Hospitals*, 42 (December 16, 1968), 70-72.

Office of Economic Opportunity medical care demonstration unit in the South Bronx exemplifies the best in health team practice. Pharmacist is cast in the role of educator of both professionals and patients in the field of medications, a function all too often relegated to nurse, ill-prepared for such a role.

Fagin, Clair. "The Clinical Specialist as Supervisor," *Nursing Outlook*, 15 (January, 1967), 34-36.

The clinical specialist in her role as practitioner, teacher, investigator, and role model has great potential for influencing the quality of patient care through staff development.

Farago, Peter J., Elizabeth W. Seigel and John E. Robinson. "Hospital-College Program Taps New Manpower Source," *Hospitals*, 43 (September 1, 1969), 73-76.

   A Chicago hospital joins forces with a junior college to train for occupations in allied health fields. Career ladders and greater job mobility are inherent in the program. An AA degree (two years) can be gained in nursing.

Farrisey, Ruth M. "Clinic Nursing in Transition," *American Journal of Nursing*, 67 (February, 1967), 305-309.

   Comprehensive review article on the development of expanded role for OPC nurse. This 1967 article still sees many managerial tasks (maintaining medical supplies) the realm of the nurse but the *process* of change seems useful and is outlined well.

Farthing, Frances. "Associate and Baccalaureate Degree Faculty in the South," *Nursing Outlook*, 17 (November, 1969), 56-58.

   A survey reveals that promising students and young graduates need encouragement to enter teaching positions.

Fein, Rashi. "The Doctor Shortage: An Economic Dx," *Medical Economics*, (September 4, 1967), 270-279.

   This economist suggests that the doctor shortage be regarded as a shortage of doctors' services and therefore, physicians' productivity should be increased. One possible method is to use ancillary paramedical personnel.

Feldman, Eugene and Norman C. Hirsch. "Night Administration Must Meet Daytime Standards," *Modern Hospital*, 110 (January, 1968), 80-83.

   Whatever the staffing system, the responsible person at night should be a regular participant in hospital policy making. The author stresses the various techniques of providing night administration — leaving the nurse free for bedside care.

Feldman, Herman. "Learning Transfer From Programmed Instruction to Clinical Performance," *Nursing Research*, 17 (January-February, 1968), 51-54.

   Study reports the construction and use of a criterion performance test to measure the transfer of practice to knowledge gained through the use of a programmed text in medical asepsis. Subject: AD students and a group of non-nursing college students. On two out of six procedures, there was a significant difference on post-test scores for the experimental group.

Fenninger, Leonard D. "Education in the Health Professions," *Nursing Outlook*, 16 (April, 1968), 30-34.

   A discussion of the serious gap in the health occupations' available resources and the way in which they are organized and used, and the expectations — in fact, demands — of those who use them.

Feuer, Helen Denny. "Operation Salvage," *Nursing Outlook*, 15 (November, 1967), 54.

   At the N. Y. Hospital for Joint Diseases and Medical Center, a 15-month course of study was formulated and implemented to enable practical nurses to become RN's.

Fielding, Vera V. "New Team Plan Frees Nurses to Nurse," *Modern Hospital*, 108 (May, 1967), 122-124.

   Pittsfield General Hospital has gotten nurses out of clerical work and back to the bedside while reducing the required nursing staff by about one-fourth.

Filosa, Lawrence. "New Information System Uses Less Staff, Provides More Data, More Dollars," *Modern Hospital*, 112 (June, 1969), 87-89.

   By this system, nurses have been released from clerical work and it is now up to hospital administration to make sure the time saved is spent on patient care.

Ford, Loretta C. and Henry K. Silver. "The Expanded Role of the Nurse in Child Care," *Nursing Outlook*, 15 (September, 1967), 43-45.

At the University of Colorado School of Nursing, a post-baccalaureate demonstration program prepares nurses to make independent nursing judgments in giving comprehensive care to children.

Fosberg, Gordon C. "Teaching Management Skills in a Team Nursing Setting," *Nursing Outlook*, 15 (April, 1967), 67-68.

Management is a part of nursing and worthy of being included in the basic curriculum. Nursing service should not be expected to train the new graduate for this role.

Foster, John T. "Nurses' Strike: Many Faces, Many Voices," *Modern Hospital*, 108 (April, 1967), 103-106, 194, 196.

A wide range of issues and viewpoints appeared when nurses at this Illinois hospital took their fight for recognition to the picket line.

French, Jean G. "A Delicate Balance," *Nursing Outlook*, 16 (August, 1968), 52-53.

A small study points out that nursing educators must recognize the importance of maintaining a balance between the behavioral and the physical-biological sciences in the curriculums of basic collegiate programs.

Funkenstein, Daniel H. "Implications of the Rapid Social Changes in Universities and Medical Schools for the Education of Future Physicians," *The Journal of Medical Education*, 43 (April, 1968), 433-454.

The author proposes that paramedical personnel take on some family physician roles — personnel such as specially trained nurses like the pediatric nurse practitioner.

Gammon, Ola M. "The Texas Plan," *Nursing Outlook*, 15 (May, 1967), 58-59.

From a statewide curriculum project conducted by the state board of nurse examiners evolved a master plan for all diploma programs in nursing — the new curriculum is designed for 126 weeks instead of 156 weeks.

Gascoyne, Rosemarie A. "Supervisors of Nursing are Superfluous," *The Canadian Nurse*, 64 (January, 1968), 25.

Nursing is the only profession that employs persons specifically to supervise the work of its members.

Gee, Molly S. "Sharing Experiences," *American Journal of Nursing*, 69 (May, 1969), 1038-1040.

Report of a community health project in Michigan where the multi-disciplinary team included two nursing students, two medical students and one health education student.

Geitgey, Doris A. "A Study of Some Effects of Sensitivity Training on the Performance of Students in AD Programs of Nursing Education," *National League for Nursing Publications Catalog*, 23-1344 (1968).

Results of a project involving 103 students in three California junior colleges.

———: "Some Thoughts on Team Teaching in Nursing Education," *Nursing Outlook*, 15 (October, 1967), 66-68.

The shortage of qualified faculty and urgency of high caliber educational opportunities for students are among the elements that should make nurse faculty take a thoughtful look at the potentials of team teaching as an effective method.

———: "The Teacher in Associate Degree Nursing Programs," *Nursing Outlook*, 15 (February, 1967), 30-32.

Philosophy of the college, purpose of the program, heterogeneity of students, curriculum design, teaching load — all make the teaching in AD programs different from that in other kinds of nursing programs.

Gerard, Sr. Mary. "Recognizing the Nursing Service Director as An Administration Team Member," *Hospital Progress*, (March, 1969), 100-110.

The author summarizes the results of a study in which administrators, indicated to what degree nursing service directors act as administrative assistants. The author feels that a nursing service director should be recognized as a valuable component of the administrative team.

Gerber, Alex. "The Medical Manpower Shortage," *Journal of Medical Education*, 42 (April, 1967), 306-319.

Author states that the nursing pool is *not* a potent source of personnel to alleviate the doctor shortage — because of nurse shortages. Also, nursing has relied on a program of augmented use of paranursing personnel, etc. to the virtual exclusion of an increased output of graduates — so still a shortage.

Germain, Carol P. Hanley. "Nursing Role Variations in Coronary Care," *Hospitals*, 43 (September 1, 1969), 147-151.

With the advent of specialized patient care units (such as intensive coronary care) the nurses role is both altered (in her professional relationship with physicians, for instance) and expanded (in being a co-author of advance planning for, and ongoing policies of care), within such a facility.

Gerrish, Madalene J. "The Family Therapist Is a Nurse," *American Journal of Nursing*, 68 (February, 1968), 320-323.

Case study involving RN as family therapist in a Boston hospital. Some of the advantages of the nurse over the physician in this role are outlined.

Gillam, Robert. "The Use of Computers in Nursing," *International Nursing Review*, 15 (October, 1968), 308-313.

Includes what a computer does, how it works and ways in which it can be utilized to assist the nurse. The question of how to insure that freed nursing time is actually utilized for patient care is raised.

Gillan, Dale E. "Improved Methods Program Brings Savings in Money, Manpower," *Hospitals*, 43 (August 16, 1969), 77-81.

Use of consultants and implementation of an improved methods program have created significant savings for a Kansas hospital, especially in nursing service. The author is convinced of the advisability of hiring outside consultants for such a project.

Ginsberg, Frances. "Like it or Not, Surgical Technicians are Here to Stay," *Modern Hospital*, 112 (April, 1969), 114.

The attrition of professional nurses from the operating room and the dim prospects for attracting new nurses have forced the introduction of this category of worker.

———: "The Attitude of Nursing Educators Contributes to Operating Room Nurse Shortage," *Modern Hospital*, 108 (January, 1967), 102, 104.

The author argues for post graduate courses in O. R. nursing — or at least introducing the course in the basic curriculum, because of the shortage.

———: "The Case for Operating Room Technicians," *Nursing Clinics of North America*, 3 (December, 1968), 613-619.

Surgical technicians are here to stay. To safeguard the consumer, a national certification plan is advocated. This requires standardization of course content, faculty qualifications and applicant prerequisites.

Ginzberg, Eli. "A Manpower Strategy for Public Health," *American Journal of Public Health*, 57 (April, 1967), 588-592.

The author states that the physician isn't necessarily the natural leader of the health team; in some areas, others are likely to be more competent.

————: "Nursing and Manpower Realities," *Nursing Outlook*, 15 (November, 1967), 26-29.

Ginzberg feels the nursing profession should work on methods of certification for their specialists.

Glover, B. H. "A Psychiatrist Calls for a New Nurse Therapist," *American Journal of Nursing*, 67 (May, 1967), 1003-1005.

This author believes that nurses can become psychotherapists and outlines a program to prepare them for this role, at the University Hospitals, Madison, Wisconsin. He feels the competencies of the psychiatric nurse without an academic degree must be tapped. This program is an inservice one.

Good, Shirley R. "Considerations for Nurse Recruitment," *The Canadian Nurse*, 63 (December, 1967), 31-32.

The author analyzes recent studies on the subject of recruitment and makes suggestions for improving recruitment programs.

————: "Post-Basic Baccalaureate Education for Nurses in Canada," *International Nursing Review*, 16: No. 2 (1969), 147-151.

Nineteen of the twenty-one university schools in Canada offer post-basic BS degree programs; RN's elect to study at one of these for two or three academic years after they've completed a basic diploma course. Since so few students enroll in the basic BS programs, it is unrealistic to discontinue the post-basic BS education for registered nurses.

Gordon, Marjory. "The Clinical Specialist as Change Agent," *Nursing Ottlook*, 17 (March, 1969), 37-39.

Views the clinical specialist as the responsible agent in planned change with expectation of improved patient care. She is concerned with closing the gap between knowledge and practice, using tools to evaluate needed behavior changes and analyzing results.

Gortner, Susan R. "Nursing Majors in 12 Western Universities: A Comparison of RN Students and Basic Senior Students," *Nursing Research*, 17 (March-April, 1968), 121-128.

Study of student characteristics, centering on the problem of discovering the differential attributes of two groups of BS students in nursing, RN students and Basic senior students. There is evidence to support and to discourage the continuance of separate programs for RN students. Some special handling of these students seems warranted because of their strong professional motivations, theoretical inclinations and post-baccalaureate plans.

Gow, Kathleen. "Resolution of a Revolution," *American Journal of Nursing*, 67 (March, 1967), 578-582.

Nursing schools are not immune to student rebellion, but in this hospital school (in Toronto), the conflict concerning communication between student and faculty was resolved.

Graham, Lois E. "A Faculty Research Development Project in a BS Program in Nursing," *Nursing Research*, 17 (July-August, 1968), 321-326.

Article describes a project to stimulate research capabilities in faculty members and students in universities conducting advanced nursing programs.

————: "Are We Motivating Students to go on For Graduate Education?" *Nursing Outlook*, 16 (August, 1968), 48-50.

The answer to this question is mostly negative, according to responses on a questionnaire from 266 basic students in 11 schools of nursing (three types of undergraduate programs).

Grayson, George A. "Small Hospitals Can Attract and Hold Qualified Nurses," *Hospitals*, 43 (April 16, 1969), 58-60.

  The author suggests that the attitude of hospital administrators plays a crucial role in the success of such recruiting efforts and describes several steps a small hospital might take to improve its recruitment programs.

Greenfield, Harry I. "Manpower Problems in the Allied Health Field," *Journal of the American Medical Association*, 206 (November 11, 1968), 1542-1544.

  Author discusses division of labor in health, cost-saving potential, and recommends the coordination and planning of health services on an areawide basis.

Griffith, Elsie I. "A Rational Approach to Patient Service Review," *Nursing Outlook*, 17 (April, 1969), 49-51.

  An effective review of patient service determines, among other things, the quality of care rendered and the proper use of appropriate resources — public health agencies are offered a method of patient review which is orderly, rational, continuous, and concerned with inter- and intra- agency services.

Gross, Paul A. and Robert A. Brown. "Contrasting Job Satisfaction Elements Shown for RN's and LPN's," *Hospitals*, 41 (February 16, 1967), 73, 76-79, 82, 87-92.

  Psychological tests show registered nurses and licensed practical nurses need different work assignments for job satisfaction.

Group, Thetis M. "If a Nurse is to Help in Ghettos," *American Journal of Nursing*, 69 (December, 1969), 2635-2636.

  According to the author, today's curriculum is inadequate to prepare nurses to work with anyone but the middle-class, and she suggests changes to be made.

Gunter, Laurie. "The Developing Nursing Student," *Nursing Research*, 18 (January-February, 1969), 60-64.

  Part I: A Study of Self-Actualizing Values. Findings of the study show the sophomore nursing student as developing toward self-actualization or emotional maturity. Findings are discussed in terms of their possible implications for nursing education.

Hacker, Carlotta L. "A New Category of Health Worker for Canada?" *The Canadian Nurse*, 35 (January, 1969), 38-43.

  The author quotes doctors and nurses about the subject of Physician Assistants' Associates, and Nurse Specialists. Many feel that nurses should be trained and take on duties such as the pediatric nurse practitioner.

Hale, Thomas. "Paramedical Crazy Quilt Needs More Than Just Patching to Mend Staffing Crisis," *Modern Hospital*, 110 (February, 1968), 82-87.

  The paramedical field must face and overcome three major problems — "dead ends", over-education and under-education — before hospitals can be run with maximum efficiency.

Hamil, Evelyn M. "The Changing Director of Nurses," *Nursing Outlook*, 17 (December, 1969), 64.

  Author sees the technical knowledge of nursing as an insignificant part of the preparation of a director of nursing service. It is rather the ability to plan, organize, dream and create, utilizing the skills and resources of others. She suggests preparation in health and public administration on a foundation of behavioral sciences.

Hamilton, C. B., M. K. Pratt and M. Groen. "The Nurses' Active Role in Assessment," *Nursing Clinics of North America*, 4 (June, 1969), 249-262.

  Nurses take responsibility for developing, evaluating and utilizing a patient care tool at Rancho Los Amigos.

Hamilton, Lee David. "A Nurses' Aide Program for Youthful Dropouts," *American Journal of Nursing*, 69 (March, 1969), 518-520.

At Clearfield, Utah, the only OEO Job Corps Center with an aide training program, young men are being helped to enter the health field and reach toward further education and training.

Hangartner, Carl A. "Re-examining the Hospital's Role in Nursing Education," *Hospital Progress*, (December, 1969), 64-66, 70.

Author describes relationship that should exist between the hospital and the college or university — stresses hospital role for in-service continuing and orientation — but the two are "educational partners".

Hanisch, Verna K. "Statewide Orientation Program to Public Health," *Nursing Outlook*, 17 (April, 1969), 52-54.

The state health department in New Jersey established a tuition-free, state-sponsored in-service training program for newly employed nurses in local community agencies with the ultimate objective of improving patient care.

Hannan, C. Phillip. "Planning and Implementing a Workable Unit Management System," *Hospital Progress*, (May, 1969), 120-136.

St. Joseph's Hospital in Chicago implemented this system because they didn't want nurses performing non-nursing functions.

Hanson, Rachel, Gene Minor and Elizabeth P. Wirick. "Tuning In and Tuning Out," *Nursing Outlook*, 16 (May, 1968), 40-42.

Loretto Heights College, school of nursing, in Colorado, had in its curriculum, *Communication*, but a new course dealing specifically with the dynamics of communication seems to have solved the communication problem between students and faculty.

Harrington, Helen Ann and E. Charlotte Theis. "Institutional Factors Perceived by BS Graduates as Influencing Their Performance as Staff Nurses," *Nursing Research*, 17 (May-June, 1968), 228-235.

Three hospitals were used: two typical hospitals and the Loeb Center. Results: Attitudes and expectations of administrative and supervisory personnel, work assignment and communication were seen by nurses as major factors influencing their ability to perform professional nursing functions. This influence was a deterrent in two "typical" hospitals but not at Loeb.

Harris, Virginia J. "This I Believe...About Practical Nursing Education," *Nursing Outlook*, 17 (June, 1969), 40-41.

Author maintains that we are underselling the practical nurse. She believes that the LPN has the right to the highest level of education of which she is capable.

Hartman, Jane. "Dietary Duties Bite Into Nurse's Schedule," *Modern Hospital*, 108 (January, 1967), 128-130.

In view of the nursing shortage, hospitals would do well to leave routine food service chores to the professional hands of the dietary worker.

Harty, Margaret. "Editorial: A Tragic Dichotomy," *Nursing Outlook*, 17 (July, 1969), 19.

The author urges nursing education and nursing service to cooperate in defining professional competence.

Harty, Margaret Brown. "Trends in Nursing Education," *American Journal of Nursing*, 68 (April, 1968), 767-772.

The movement of basic BS nursing programs from hospitals to universities has been slow but steady for 50 years. The author reviews some recent developments, cites figures and indicates some of the problems the profession faces and the kinds of decisions it must make.

Harvey, James D. "Toward More Effective Utilization of Health Manpower," *Hospitals*, 43 (January 1, 1969), 35-38, 96.

The author examines recent developments including personnel improvement through incentives, education and training, job definition, automation, self-help for patients, and better space planning and design.

Hauer, Rose Marie. "Perspective on Directing Hospital Nursing Service," *American Journal of Nursing*, 69 (December, 1969), 2626-2629.

Author believes nursing service director is an administrator not a practitioner, a policy-maker and planner, not an overseer of daily detail.

Haynes, M. Alfred and Victor H. Dates. "Educational Opportunities in the Health Professions for Negroes in the State of Maryland," *Journal of Medical Education*, 43 (October, 1968), 1075-1082.

Author contends that the number of Negroes in the health professions in Maryland relates to the availability of qualified candidates, the cost of higher education, and to discrimination in admission practices. Proposals are made to increase the opportunities for Negroes which will also help meet the increasing demands for health manpower.

Hedman, Lorraine L. and Elaine Mansfield. "Hospital to Hospital Via T. V.," *American Journal of Nursing*, 67 (April, 1967), 808-810.

Closed circuit TV between two psychiatric hospitals has opened new in-service education vistas for both. Nurses 112 miles apart see and hear each other in TV group sessions. They cooperate in making tapes for in-service education (Nebraska Psychiatric Institute and Norfolk State Hospital).

Heidgerken, Loretta. "Nursing as a Career: Is It Relevant?" *American Journal of Nursing*, 69 (June, 1969), 1217-1222.

Although more young persons are becoming nurses today, the percentage of high school graduates entering schools of nursing is not keeping pace with the growth of population. The reasons for a loss in the past 15 years of approximately three percent of high school graduates each year to other careers bear examination. The author covers: career choice theories, changing sex image, health careers, role models, image of nursing, etc.

Heidgerken, Loretta F. "This I Believe. . .About a Philosophy of Education," *Nursing Outlook*, 17 (April, 1969), 42-43.

A nurse educator, reminds us of our responsibility to distinguish clearly the differences in the purpose and nature of professional and technical education in nursing.

Heller, William M. "Data Processing in Drug Distribution Systems," *Hospitals*, 42 (December 1, 1968), 73-78.

Computer system offers faster processing of medication orders, with better quality control. Patient care is improved and nurses' time is saved.

Henderson, Virginia. "Excellence in Nursing," *American Journal of Nursing*, 69 (October, 1969), 2133-2137.

Excellence in nursing is initiated by careful choice and preparation of students, and development of measures for evaluation of practice. The author feels that students of the health professions should study together during their basic preparation.

Hershey, Nathan. "An Alternative to Mandatory Licensure of Health Professionals," *Hospital Progress*, (March, 1969), 71-74.

Mandatory licensure of health personnel limits the administrator's flexibility and is anachronistic. The author suggests a way out of the dilemma, while still maintaining control; he speaks about the physician's assistant and the nurse-midwife.

Hofmann, Paul B., William A. Gouveia and G. Octo Barnett. "Computers: Great Future, Perilous Present," *Modern Hospital*, 110 (July, 1968), 98-100, 148.

What computers can accomplish — and what they cannot. Authors remind us that a hospital information system should center on the patient, not on the department (i.e., accounting) needs.

Hohle, Beth H., Jane K. McInnis and Almyra C. Gates. "The Public Health Nurse as a Member of the Interdisciplinary Team," *Nursing Clinics of North America*, 4 (June, 1969), 311-319.

The recent enactment of legislation in the health field has resulted in new health workers to provide care outside the hospital. Where does the PHN, for so long the primary family contact, fit into the new structure?

Hornback, May S. and Helen R. Brunclik. "Party Line for Nurses," *Nursing Outlook*, 16 (May, 1968), 30-31.

The use of telectures is one more approach to continuing education for RN's. An experiment in 1966 was so successful that the University of Wisconsin Extension Nursing Department is now using a statewide educational telephone network and FM radio to supplement in-service education for nurses.

House, Roy C. "Work Standards Improve Care, Save Money," *Modern Hospital*, 108 (February, 1967), 91-94.

By establishing work standards, this hospital eliminated chaos in one department, improved efficiency in others and developed a new patient classification system. The engineers suggested discontinuing hiring of nurses but the hospital questioned this because of the nursing shortage.

Hutchins, Nettie. "Mediated Self-Instruction in Nursing Education," *The Journal of Nursing Education*, 7 (April, 1968), 3-8, 24-26.

The author proposes this method as a middle position, between student and teacher and also proposes a mediated learning center.

Hymovich, Debra P. and Marjorie P. Johns. "Whither Pharmacology in the Curriculum?" *Nursing Outlook*, 16 (August, 1968), 58-60.

With the many drug changes today, how much can the nurse be expected to know about pharmacology? With a pharmacodynamic approach to teaching, these students learn, without rote memorization, the usage and effects of drugs.

Iafolla, Mary Ann. "Guidance in Nursing Education," *Journal of Nursing Education*, 8 (January, 1969), 15-22.

The author states that a sound program of guidance in nursing education, when comprehensively organized and professionally conducted, should culminate in a substantial decrease in the school's attrition rate. She outlines, carefully, the possible duties of a qualified guidance counselor and stresses that this person should be employed full-time and be certified by the state.

Ingles, Thelma. "A New Health Worker," *American Journal of Nursing*, 68 (May, 1968), 1059-1061.

Author discusses the Physician's Assistant Training program at Duke University; asserts that they don't have to conflict with nurses.

———: "A Proposal for Health Care Education," *American Journal of Nursing*, 68 (October, 1968), 2135-2140.

A proposal for a new approach to the education for health workers in which persons interested in health care careers could proceed along several paths from a *core curriculum*. Comments pro and con follow the proposal (e.g., Montag-con). The author further asserts that a core curriculum, only one type of nurse, and a new worker, a clinical associate, may be one answer to the confusion, waste of time and divisiveness which exists in health care education.

Ingmire, Alice E. and Michael G. Blansfield. "Inservice Seminars Help Nurses Improve Patient Relationships," *Hospitals*, 41 (August 1, 1967), 68-75.

> An in-service education program for nurses is using behavioral science concepts to improve relations with patients and staff. Authors state that continuing education programs are vitally important in preparing hospital personnel to function in new and changing roles.

Irving, Susan. "Psychiatric Nursing Course for LPN's," *Nursing Outlook*, 15 (December, 1967), 44-45.

> In the first such course in the state of Washington, an advanced course in psychiatric nursing that carries 15 community college credits provides LPN's with an opportunity to increase their interpersonal skills and thus give more comprehensive patient care.

Jacobs, Donald J. "Position Control Plan Shows Rise in Cost of Nursing Service," *Hospitals*, 41 (June 1, 1967), 73-76.

> Woodlawn Hospital (Chicago) conducted a study of the use of nursing personnel. Results: utilization could be drastically improved through use of a nurse position control plan; nurse utilization was improved, the need for additional nursing personnel was reduced, the rapidly rising cost of nursing service was reduced and patients were provided with more care by RN's.

Jacox, Ada K. "Who Defines and Controls Nursing Practice?" *American Journal of Nursing*, 69 (May, 1969), 977-982.

> Are nurses going to use their collective power to focus on the improvement of nursing practice and patient care, or will they permit hospital administrators to use them as bureaucrats employed to meet the needs of hospital organization?

James, George. "The Professional Associations' Responsibilities in the Field of Health Manpower," *American Journal of Public Health*, 57 (April, 1967), 593-601.

> The author speaks of medicine but is really saying that accreditation and the setting of standards by professional associations are useful only as long as they remain effective weapons in the fight for better health care.

Jenny, Martha R. "A Development for Nursing," *Nursing Outlook*, 17 (February, 1969), 35-36.

> RMP's have great potential for nursing in the areas of prevention, treatment, and rehabilitation, particularly as they are related to the care of patients with heart disease, stroke and cancer. Author stresses the nurse working on studies, etc.

Johns, Marjorie P. "Changeover Time at Northeastern," *Nursing Outlook*, 17 (July, 1969), 40-42.

> Nursing students alternate work experiences and academic studies. Reaching the midpoint in a work-study program is significant because care courses are completed and students are now ready to embark on the upper division curriculum.

Johnson, Dorothy A. "Nursing Service," *Hospitals*, 42 (April 1, 1969), 115-120.

> Good review of 1967 nursing literature addresses itself to the problems of emerging professionalism (in most cases nurses are still not making completely independent decisions), the skills required for administrative vs. clinical practice, and is enthusiastic in support of clinical specialization.

Johnson, Dorothy E., Joan A. Wilcox and Harriet C. Moidel. "The Clinical Specialist As A Practitioner," *American Journal of Nursing*, 67 (November, 1967), 2298-2303.

> Authors focus on the contributions of the nurse specialist in the practitioner (rather than instructor or consultant) phase of her role. She assumes increased responsibility and accountability for the total care a patient receives and must have adequate authority to make nursing decisions and control nursing practice.

Johnson, Everett A. "Nursing Reorganization Strengthens Head Nurse Role, Provides Special Nursing Consultants," *Hospitals,* 42 (June 16, 1968), 85-90.

Author describes how the Methodist Hospital of Gary, Indiana, reorganized its nursing service to strengthen the position of head nurse and to provide three specialized nursing supervisors who act as consultants to the head nurses in problem solving and who support the hospital's associate director.

Johnson, Jean E., Donna Diers and Ann T. Slairnsky. "Research Projects for Teaching Methodology," *Nursing Outlook,* 16 (November, 1968), 27-29.

Students participating in ongoing research projects learned research methodology and at the same time acquired an enthusiasm for continuing research in nursing practice.

Jones, Phyllis, E. Editorial, *Canadian Nurse,* 63 (June, 1967), 25.

A suggestion that patient care could be enhanced if public health nurses were utilized as special assistants by medical practitioners. Whether they should be in the employ of the physician is questioned.

Josephus, Sr. Mary and Sr. Mary Venarda. "How Mercy Planned Its Communications," *Modern Hospital,* 109 (July, 1967), 87-89.

A Chicago hospital has deleted the traditional nurses station, replaced it with an "administrative communication center" and a series of equipment that will place information and supplies at each patient's bedside.

Juliana, Sister. "An Experience in Transition in Nursing Education," *Hospital Progress,* 48 (February, 1967), 67, 86-88.

St. Mary's Hospital in Evansville, Indiana, phased out its three year diploma program and now serves as a clinical field for students enrolled in the BS program of Evansville College.

Jupiter, Robert. "Patient Transport Service Saves Valuable Nursing Hours," *Hospitals,* 42 (March 16, 1968), 53-54.

A centralized transportation service is estimated to save 560 nursing hours weekly.

Kakosh, Marguerite E. "Profile of the College Graduate in Basic Nursing," *Nursing Outlook,* 15 (May, 1967), 64-65.

Article describes a graduate program at New York Medical College. The nursing profession is enriched by students who bring to the generic program a broad background of liberal arts.

Kelby, Nancy. "The Student Voice in Curriculum Planning — Threat or Promise?" *Nursing Outlook,* 17 (April, 1969), 59-61.

Nursing students are beginning to revolt against hierarchical authority and to present their demands. Faculty must face up to the change and decide whether it will come by evolution or revolution.

Keller, Nancy S. "Teaching by Concepts," *Nursing Outlook,* 17 (January, 1969), 32-34.

Describes a sophomore curriculum, constructed to reflect the basic purpose of the nursing school at the Medical College of Virginia: that of preparing a nurse and advocate for the patient whose basic skills are assessment, goal-setting, decision-making, and purposeful communication.

Kelly, Dorothy N. "Equating the Nurse's Economic Rewards with the Service Given," *American Journal of Nursing,* 67 (August, 1967), 1642-1645.

It is unprofessional not to equate nursing's economic rewards with realistic economic forces and achieve them by speaking out, united, to demand better salaries, better status and better patient care.

Kelly, Marjorie E. "Low-Cost Refresher Program Helps Inactive Nurses Make Comeback," *Hospitals*, 43 (January 16, 1969), 74-76.

Upon completion of a refresher course, nurses often return to hospitals with renewed confidence in their ability to do the job.

Kelly, Nancy Cardinal. "Nurses Must Love Hospital Administrators," *Nursing Outlook*, 16 (September, 1968), 28-31.

"Spying" on workers in other departments, counting virtually non-existent linens, taking surveys of high-flying mosquitoes and elusive roaches — these supervisory duties give proof to that controversial title.

Kenneth, Hester Y. "Medical and Nursing Students Learn Together," *Nursing Outlook*, 17 (November, 1969), 46-49.

At San Francisco Medical Center, joint clinical experiences are provided for medical and nursing students to provide interdisciplinary experiences for health science students. The program utilizes faculty from each of the University of California's health science professional schools.

———: "Students Learn to Use Consultants," *Nursing Outlook*, 15 (December, 1967), 39-41.

Lectures, discussions and a group demonstration in a course on community nursing help students learn principles underlying how and when to use consultation. Professional consultants have not been extensively or appropriately used in nursing; thus, this experiment.

Keyes, Clifford F. "A Four-Year Plan for Salary Increases," *Hospital Progress*, (January, 1967), 64-65, 76.

St. Joseph's Hospital in Tucson, raised salaries "across-the-board" in a four-year plan, by comparing its salary scale to local industry and business. Staff nurses should receive the pay of a public school teacher.

Keys, Marjorie L. and Jean F. Aeschliman. "Our Team Includes the Private Nurse Practitioner," *Nursing Outlook*, 15 (January, 1967), 32-33.

In an effort to close the gap between hospital staff and private nurse practitioners, an orientation and in-service program was planned, implemented and shared by both groups.

Killam, Lee. "In Good Faith," *American Journal of Nursing*, 67 (September, 1967), 1883-1885.

One answer for the young practitioner's need for practice and for economic security is a professional nurse residency and a salary which grows with the nurse's experience and improved performance.

King, Lambert and Lynnae Schwartz. "Student Activists See Health in New Ways," *Modern Hospital*, 110 (May, 1968), 118-120.

Some medical and nursing students are finding involvement in social issues a vital addition to their formal curricula.

Kinsinger, Robert. "A Core Curriculum for the Health Field," *Nursing Outlook*, 15 (February, 1967), 28-29.

A shift of instructional concentration in AD programs would help increase the quality of nursing instruction, decrease cost, and provide students with a better understanding of the health field.

Kirkpatrick, W.J.A. "The In and Out Nurse: Thoughts on the Role of the Psychiatric Nurse in the Community and the Preparation Required," *Canadian Journal of Psychiatric Nursing*, 9 (February, 1968), 6-9.

The skills required in community and institutional mental health are similar enough to permit nurses to move between the two settings and function as a coordinator of patient care. Preparation for, and practice of, this role are discussed.

Kissick, William L. "Effective Utilization: The Critical Factor in Health Manpower," *American Journal of Public Health*, 58 (January, 1968), 23-29.

Health manpower and its utilization are now priority concerns. Approaches to improve utilization, such as downward transfer of functions, education (core curriculum) and career mobility and the application of technology are discussed.

———: "How Imagination and Innovation Can Help Bridge Manpower Gaps," *Hospitals*, 41 (October 1, 1967), 76-83, 146.

Excellent review article on some possibilities for meeting health manpower needs includes discussion of recruitment, core curricula, and work analysis.

Klahm, James E. "Self-Concept and Change-Seeking Need of First-Year Student Nurses," *Journal of Nursing Education*, 8 (April, 1969), 11-16.

An important way to lower the dropout rate in nursing programs would appear to be the development of a more effective preadmission selection method. The method should be designed for students for admission to the program who have the highest potential for remaining in nursing.

Knudson, Eleanor Gray. "Deterrents to Developing Interest in Occupational Advancement Among Nurses," *The Journal of Nursing Education*, 7 (January, 1968), 27-31.

A study shows that nurses in a certain area, were not interested in advancement because they didn't want to leave patient care: author suggests changing the image of the administrative and supervisory nurses — nursing leadership is needed!

———: "Nurses and Occupational Advancement," *Nursing Outlook*, 17 (August, 1969), 29-31.

Study identifies nurses interested in leadership positions and the author makes recommendations on how to tap this potential resource.

Koch, Harriet B. "Television in Nursing Education," *The Journal of Nursing Education*, 7 (April, 1968), 37-43.

Instructional TV will replace a definite quantity of the written word; it will release many instructors from repetitious work and it will standardize a great deal of the educational process.

Kramer, Marlene. "Collegiate Graduate Nurses in Medical Center Hospitals: Mutual Challenge or Duel?" *Nursing Research*, 18 (May-June, 1969), 196-210.

The author's study showed that there was a positive relationship between low nurse role deprivation and the presence of innovative baccalaureate nurse roles and the presence of dual promotion ladders. Also, there is a trend towards renewed emphasis on the clinical and interdisciplinary aspects of nursing — greater opportunity for the practice of clinical nursing rather than absorption in managerial tasks.

———: "Team Teaching is More Than Team Planning," *Nursing Outlook*, 16 (July, 1968), 47-50.

Author describes briefly the composition and functioning of a teaching team in an integrated curriculum, illustrating team teaching in contrast to team planning and evaluation, and reports faculty and student reactions to the method.

Kriegel, Julia. "Are We Earning Our Salaries?" *Nursing Outlook*, 15 (December, 1967), 60-61.

Nurses often expect to be paid as professional people for work that is routine. The nurse needs to learn to evaluate the quality of her work, to delegate that which is routine and be given the opportunity and the knowledge to practice professionally.

Lambertsen, Eleanor C. "Defendants of College Nursing Programs Should Answer Critics," *Modern Hospital*, 108 (March, 1967), 156.

Not all hospital administrators are fighting the trend to collegiate education for nurses.

———: "Good Nursing Requires Good Management," *Modern Hospital*, 110 (November, 1968), 124.

The nature of the authority and responsibility of the director of nursing entails competence as a generalist in nursing practice. She is not a clinical practitioner but an administrator.

———: "Knowing Roles Aids Doctor-Nurse Accord," *Modern Hospital*, 112 (January, 1969), 75-77.

The author says that professionals collaborate best as colleagues who recognize each other's particular skills.

———: "Let's Stop Cold War Between Nurses and Administrators," *Modern Hospital*, 109 (September, 1967), 130.

Putting the nursing director on the management team can be a major step in eliminating administrative problems.

———: "Must Agree on Definitions of Nursing Functions to Avoid Wasting Manpower," *Modern Hospital*, 109 (July, 1967), 120.

Every effort must be made to support practices which delineate functions and determine the training necessary to perform them.

———: "New Knowledge Makes New Demands on Nursing," *Modern Hospital*, 112 (March, 1969), 138.

The author suggests guidelines for continuing education to keep nurses informed in an age of constant change.

———: "No School Can Prepare Nurses For All the Hospital Situations," *Modern Hospital*, 108 (February, 1967), 123.

Hospitals must take the responsibility for orienting new graduates to its particular needs.

———: "Nurse As Care Coordinator Must Be On 'Patient's Side'," *Modern Hospital*, 113 (July, 1969), 116.

Restorative, rehabilitative or therapeutic services of any health specialty are dependent upon constant reinforcement. Such reinforcement provided by nurses in their sustaining relationship with patient and family.

———: "Nurses Must Be Teachers and Must Know These Principles," *Modern Hospital*, 110 (February, 1968), 126.

Outlines the teaching-learning process necessary for increasing self-direction on part of patient and family.

———: "Nursing Research Should Emphasize Improving the Quality of Patient Care," *Modern Hospital*, 108 (April, 1967), 164.

Details abilities essential in the nurse researcher.

———: "Re-Organize Nursing to Re-Emphasize Care," *Modern Hospital*, 108 (January, 1967), 68-71, 138.

Proposal to reorganize nursing service department making director of nursing service, a skilled generalist in hospital affairs rather than a nurse skilled in clinical patient care.

———: "Shortages of other Specialists may be Hidden in Nurse Shortage," *Modern Hospital*, 113 (October, 1969), 136.

Society demands specialized health services but does not demand that they be delivered by specialists. When such specialists are not available, the role of the nurse has traditionally expanded to include the delivery of these services thus a shortage of nursing is perceived as a shortage of nurses.

———: "The Emerging Health Occupations," *Nursing Forum*, VII: No. 1 (1968), 87-97.
    Author writes on the implications for nursing of the emerging new occupations in the health field, cautioning that the more dominant health professionals — medicine — as they concentrate on a more distinctive core of services are trapping nursing in the phenomenon of the shifting areas of responsibility for supportive services.

———: "The Implications of New Techniques in Ward Management As They Affect Nursing," *International Nursing Review*, 16 (January, 1969), 4-15.
    Effective techniques of ward management are derived from administrative theory which, in turn, is derived from the disciplines of psychology and sociology. Quality of patient care services can be advanced by the application of principles of administration and introduction of work simplification techniques. The process demands an awareness that problems are reflections of organization of hospitals along dual lines — administrative and professional hierarchy.

———: "Today's Nurse Has Five Career Choices," *Modern Hospital*, 111 (October, 1968), 124.
    Nursing offers a variety of careers beyond patient therapy for those with postgraduate training — author briefly describes each.

———: "We're Not Using the Nurses We Have to Best Advantage," *Modern Hospital*, 110 (May, 1968) 146.
    The author suggests educational changes, since demands for nurses in all fields of practice exceed the supply, and hospitals must make effective use of the nurse power they have.

———: "When You Change Routines, Be Sure You Improve the Care," *Modern Hospital*, 109 (October, 1967), 140.
    A Brooklyn hospital switched the responsibility for food service on patient wards from the nurses to the dietary department — all except the pediatric ward!

———: "Why Head Nurse Often Favors Doctor Over Administrator," *Modern Hospital*, 110 (April, 1968), 134.
    To maintain good working relationships, the head nurse should have neither a predominantly organizational nor a predominantly professional orientation.

Lawrence, Virginia. "The Unit Manager at Massachusetts General Hospital," *Hospital Progress*, 50 (September, 1969), 22, 26, 30.
    Success of this unit coordinator program is attributed to careful selection and training of personnel and its policy of equal partnership between manager and head nurse.

Lee, Bob. "Houston: They Emphasize Their Nursing," *Modern Hospital*, 108 (March, 1967), 108-109.
    In-service training for nurses in cardiac care at St. Joseph's Hospital; want to establish a regional training center.

Lenahan, Mildred J. "Looking for Teacher Aids?" *Nursing Outlook*, 16 (October, 1968), 48-49.
    Article provides helpful suggestions on where and how to obtain literature once you have decided on what and why you want it.

Leonard, Robert C. "Developing Research in a Practice-Oriented Discipline," *American Journal of Nursing*, 67 (July, 1967), 1472-1475.
    The author discusses his observations of nurses and research students, particularly at the Masters' level at Yale University, and the problems of integrating research into a university school of nursing.

——— and James K. Skipper, Letter to Editor, *Nursing Research*, 18 (March-April, 1969), 173.

Practice-oriented clinical research can make fundamental contributions to general knowledge. It is this basic research which identifies a unique place for nursing among the academic disciplines. The roles of "researcher" and "nurse" cannot be separated.

Most successful way to integrate basic science and professional practice is through practice-oriented, basic, clinical research.

"Let's Examine...The Selection of a Proficiency Examination," *Nursing Outlook*, 17 (December, 1969), 36.

The article deals with how the faculty of an institution can assess the usefulness and suitability of a proficiency examination.

Levine, Eugene. "Nurse Manpower: Yesterday, Today and Tomorrow," *American Journal of Nursing*, 69 (February, 1969), 290-296.

The author tells why he thinks nursing in 1980 will be more challenging, rewarding and effective. He covers such topics as nursing manpower in the early 1950's, federal programs, planning agencies, nurse education, nurse demand, nurse practice settings, nurse role, nurse utilization, career ladders, etc.

Lewis, Charles E. "Local Action Groups Involve Communities in Kansas Program," *Hospitals*, 43 (July 1, 1968), 60-62.

A case study of the KRMP. The author describes projects now under way dealing with research, education, work evaluation, communications, and a library network.

——— and Barbara A. Resnik. "Nurse Clinics and Progressive Ambulatory Patient Care," *New England Journal of Medicine*, 277 (December 7, 1969), 1236-1241.

Report of Kansas study utilizing nurse clinics for primary care of patients with chronic medical problems.

Early concern re: whether this care is "nursing" or "medicine" was apparently academic. Patients see it as a primary source of the kind of care they wanted (and needed) at this particular phase of their illness. Essential to focus on patient rather than on needs and image of each professional discipline.

Lewis, Edith. "Four Nurses Who Wanted to Make a Difference," *American Journal of Nursing*, 69 (April, 1969), 777-782.

Four newly graduated RN's spend a year in a nursing care demonstration unit for chronically ill. Setting goals, serving as role models and instructing auxiliary personnel were seen as important professional nurse roles.

Lewis, Edith P. "The Cedars of Lebanon Story," *American Journal of Nursing*, 69 (November, 1969), 2385-2390.

The conditions under which a strike of nurses at Los Angeles "hospital of the stars" was settled may very well set a new and improved pattern for relationships between nurses and hospitals in Southern California.

Lindabury, Virginia A. "That's What We Want For Christmas," *The Canadian Nurse*, 63 (December, 1967), 27.

This editor wants better recruitment policies and the return of 22,000 inactive RN's to nursing practice.

Linden, Kathryn. "The Multimedia Approach to Teaching Nursing," *Nursing Outlook*, 17 (May, 1969), 36-40.

The director of the ANA-NLN Film Service offers a wealth of information about the cost, use, and value of films, videotapes, projectors, and other "hardware" used to help teach nursing.

Lipton, Nancy. "Nursing Education As A Challenge to the Professionalization of Nursing," *Nursing Forum*, VII: No. 2 (1968).

The author discusses trends of education through Goldmark and Brown, etc., and makes her own recommendations: 1. implement the recommendations of the ANA position paper; 2. recruitment programs; 3. enlarge the existing BS programs, rather than beginning new BS programs.

Lister, Doris Watford. "Clinical Exploration of Nursing Theory," *Nursing Outlook*, 15 (November, 1967), 58-62.

The article describes a course written by a faculty member and a group of graduate students, which uses research findings and attempts to establish a pattern of studying, identifying and refining the nursing process; they developed generalizations based on systematic observations and analysis.

Little, Dolores. "The Nurse Specialist," *American Journal of Nursing*, 67 (March, 1967), 552-556.

Description of University of Washington study designed to attempt to define the specialist role. Poses questions such as: should she be a part of nursing service, what should her educational background be, what caseload should she have? Included in the discussion are relationships with physicians and some problems encountered in implementing the theoretical role of the specialist.

Long, Linda. "Tomorrow's Nursing Education in Saskatchewan," *The Canadian Nurse*, 63 (April, 1967), 30-33.

One report (1966) recommends regionalization of schools of nursing so that the best use can be made of all resources (teacher, student, clinical, physical and financial).

Lucek, Dorothy. "Refresher Course — The First Step," *Nursing Outlook*, 16 (September, 1968), 23-25.

The Brooklyn Hospital offers the course, which is only one step of a three-step process toward reactivating RN's. The other steps are the creation of suitable working conditions and provisions for continued educational guidance.

Luginbuhl, W. H. and Edward C. Andrews, Jr. "A New Curriculum: Its Evaluation, Design and Implementation," *The Journal of Medical Education*, 42 (September, 1967), 826-832.

The University of Vermont College of Medicine has a new four-year curriculum, divided into three parts: 1. One and one-half years of basic science instruction; 2. One year devoted to the clinical sciences — these two parts provide *all* medical students with the minimum knowledge and skills essential for every physician; 3. One and one-half years of a "course major."

Lysaught, Jerome P. "Enhanced Capacity of Self-Instruction," *The Journal of Medical Education*, 44 (July, 1969), 580-584.

The author's ideas concerning medical education can be applied equally well to nursing education; ideas such as a core body of knowledge and the use of self-instruction as a valuable tool for education.

MacGregor, Frances C. "Nursing in Transition — Challenge for the Future," *International Nursing Review*, 14, No. 6 (November-December, 1967), 41-43.

The author, a professor of Social Science at New York-Cornell Hospital, stresses the need for: more and better behavioral science courses for all levels of nursing and medical students; special and advanced programs for students; making room for students who don't necessarily fit the traditional stereotype of a nursing student; recruit students interested in nursing research.

———: "Talent Salvage in Nursing," *Nursing Outlook*, 16 (August, 1968), 33-37.

A follow-up study of 19 baccalaureate graduates, who participated in a research-oriented honors program, reveals their scientific approach to nursing — as practitioners, teachers and researchers.

Magraw, Richard. "Multiple Entry Points and Advanced Standing: Implications for Enrollment and Teaching Levels," *Journal of Medical Education*, 44 (April, 1969), 266-269.

Author discusses the effects of multiple entry points and admission to advanced standing on medical school enrollment and teaching levels.

Mahar, Irene R. "Where There's A Will," *Nursing Outlook*, 17 (October, 1969), 55-57.

A faculty member describes various interdisciplinary learning experiences which she initiated for senior students in the public health nursing laboratory. She feels that joint educational experiences for students in the health disciplines will improve future working relationships and lead to better health services.

Makin, Mildred C. "Phasing Out A Diploma Program Need Not Be A 'Death Watch'," *Nursing Outlook*, 15 (October, 1967), 31-32.

At McLean Hospital in Waverly, Massachusetts, discontinuing the diploma program caused many anxieties. For some 85 years, it had been a source of study of male nurses and also nurses with more than the usual knowledge of psychiatric nursing principles.

Malkin, Evelyn: "A College Establishes A Generic Baccalaureate Nursing Program," *Nursing Outlook*, 15 (October, 1967), pp. 24-27.

The experiences of one hospital and a state college in establishing a generic BS nursing program and phasing out a diploma program proved that both problems and satisfactions can occur among the faculties, staffs, and students during such a transition.

Mancott, Anatol. "Let's Examine Prediction of Performance in Chemistry," *Nursing Outlook*, 17 (November, 1969), 55.

A study done at Queensborough Community College in 1968 indicates that it is essential to test incoming students (Lorge-Thorndike Intelligence Test, Verbal and Nonverbal Batteries, Level 5, Form A) so those who were shown deficient in nonverbal skills could have remedial work before registering for the general chemistry course.

Mandin, Jean. "A New Dimension in Nursing Education," *Hospital Progress*, 49 (February, 1968), 16, 26.

The responsibility for the education of nurses in Canada has passed from the Department of Public Health to the Department of Education. The author predicts that the arrangement will produce an influx of professional, prepared nurses.

Mannion, Shirley E. "Upgrading LPN's to RN's," *Journal of Practical Nursing*, 19 (September, 1969), 31-32, 47.

Description of Arizona program initiated in February, 1969 to prepare qualified LPN's to take RN licensing examinations. Selection of candidates and description of curriculum is discussed.

Mansfield, Elaine. "Care Plans to Stimulate Learning," *American Journal of Nursing*, 68 (December, 1968), 2592-2593.

The psychiatric nursing care plan described is used in inservice education to focus nurses' attention on individualized care; it is designed, not for service, but for in-service education.

Marram, Gwen D. "An Untapped Source of Registered Nurses," *Nursing Outlook*, 17 (July, 1969), 48-49.

A surprising number of foreign nurses could provide a sizeable nursing resource if there were statewide planning for consistency and coordination in courses designed to permit these nurses to overcome educational deficiencies.

Marshall, Melody J. and John C. Bruhn. "Refresher Courses and the Reactivation of Nurses," *Nursing Outlook*, 15 (January, 1967), 59-61.

The extent of professional disillusionment and detachment is undoubtedly a potent factor deterring inactive nurses from taking refresher courses and returning to active practice.

Marston, Robert Q. and Karl Yordy. "A Nation Starts A Program: Regional Medical Programs, 1965-1966," *Journal of Medical Education*, 42 (January, 1967), 17-27.

Article discusses the background, development, planning grant applications, and operational grants of RMPs.

Martin, Almeda. "Associate Degree Nursing. . . Are Changes Needed in the Practice Field for New Graduates?" *Journal of Nursing Education*, 8 (August, 1969), 7-12.

The author stresses the need for faculty to return to the clinical field to practice in order to upgrade their skills and simultaneously to assure nursing practitioners of their competence in "doing" as well as in teaching. The author also stresses the need for orientation programs for AD graduates.

Martin, Ruth M. "Teaching Family Planning — A Survey," *Nursing Outlook*, 15 (December, 1967), 32-35.

A survey of 72 nursing schools throughout the U. S. revealed that 68 taught family planning and related subjects, to some degree. This survey, according to the author, is among the first of its kind.

Mase, Darrel J. "The Growth and Development of the Allied Health Schools," *Journal of the American Medical Association*, 206 (November 11, 1968), 1548-1550.

The author describes the need for Allied Health Schools, the role of junior colleges, etc.

———: "The Role of the Medical Center in the Education of Health Related Personnel," *The Journal of Medical Education*, 42 (June, 1967), 489-493.

The author suggests that a health center for the education and training of those in the health professions makes possible a sharing of facilities, better utilization of limited teaching staffs, opportunities for interdisciplinary teaching and research, and improved patient care.

Mason, Beatrice K. "Staff Organization Improves Nurse-Physician Cooperation," *Hospitals*, 42 (June 16, 1968), 90.

At Tucson (Arizona) Medical Center's acute general hospital, the nursing staff organization is tailored to the physical arrangement of the center. Five line operational committees have direct responsibility for policies and procedures on their respective units (organizational chart included).

Masur, Jack. "All Hospitals Are Not Equal," *Hospitals*, 42 (July 1, 1968), 24a-24d.

Author writes about potential success of RMPs and past failures.

Mayberry, Minerva A. "Are Nurse Refresher Programs Worthwhile?" *Hospitals*, 41 (June 1, 1967), 95-100.

The New Jersey Hospital Association sponsored a program that has drawn back into hospital service 427 of the 680 inactive nurses who have completed the course.

McAdams, Dan. "The Licensure Dilemma," *Hospital Progress*, (July, 1969), 49-53.

Of the three alternatives to the solutions to the dilemma of compulsory state licensure of health professionals, the most feasible seems to be that of investing health care institutions with the responsibility for regulating the provision of services. Such a plan would use a private agency, such as the Joint Committee on Accreditation of Hospitals, as the base agency to establish bounds within which each institution could work to provide flexible job mixes.

McClellan, Marilyn. "Staff Development in Action," *American Journal of Nursing*, 68 (February, 1968), 298-300.

The credits and debits of a broad three-year program at the University of Rochester Medical Center designed to foster self-development. The author describes an extensive attempt to supplement and compliment the basic preparation of all nursing employees from supervisor to ward secretary, an effort embracing both classroom and clinical teaching and learning.

McCormack, Regina E. and Ronald L. Crawford. "Attitudes of Professional Nurses Toward Primary Care," *Nursing Research*, 18 (November-December, 1969), 542-544.

Report of a Virginia survey to determine receptivity toward an expanded role in primary patient care found that a majority of nurses favored this trend, would be willing to undertake preparatory programs and believed such a trend would reflect favorably on the profession's image and recruitment efforts.

McCreary, John F. "The Health Team Approach to Medical Education," *Journal of the American Medical Association*, 206 (November 11, 1968), 1554-1557.

The author describes a program being developed at the University of British Columbia which integrates medical and related health professions courses, students and teachers, especially nurses: A real interprofessional curriculum!

McGrath, Marion E. "Teaching Students to Teach," *Nursing Outlook*, 15 (September, 1967), 69-71.

Teaching patients should be a natural part of the nursing care. At the Mary Hitchcock Memorial Hospital in Hanover, New Hampshire, the faculty believe that students can be taught the skills of teaching patients in the freshman year.

McKinley, Jean E. "Inservice Education for Leadership," *Nursing Outlook*, 16 (September, 1968), 47-49.

Columbia Hospital for Women in Washington, D. C. developed a leadership program for nurses of widely varying ages and training to broaden their knowledge of basic principles and their application to nursing service; one 30-hour program which has continued.

McLaughlin, Herbert. "Systems Study Supports Triangular Shapes," *Modern Hospital*, 112 (May, 1969), 105-109.

Advanced technics for systems evaluation described here demonstrate values of a Salt Lake City hospital's triangular nursing units.

McNeil, Helen J. "How To Become Involved In Community Planning," *Nursing Outlook*, 17 (February, 1969), 44-47.

The nurse, as both a health professional and a consumer, has unique skills to contribute to community health planning. She is familiar with available agencies and facilities, has interviewing and teaching skills useful in surveying needs.

McNerney, Walter J. "Changing the Health Care System," *American Journal of Nursing*, 69 (November, 1969), 2428-2435.

The author believes that nurses, rather than playing handmaiden to the doctor, can be utilized, at times, as "primary care providers."

McNicholas, Ellen L. "International Nurse — Practitioner Committees," *International Nursing Review*, 16 (July, 1969), 279-286.

Is it not the time to consider organization of international committees of Nurse Practitioners in specialties? Epidemiological and etiological research would be benefited.

Melton, Marli Schenck. "Health Manpower and Negro Health: The Negro Physician," *The Journal of Medical Education*, 43 (July, 1968), 798-814.

Mentions proposal for a more complete integration of curriculum, job training and continuing education among the various health professionals; this would permit more entry into health careers which would not result in dead-ends.

"Mental Health Nursing in Canada — An Emerging Role," *International Nursing Review*, 16 (April, 1969), 161-165.

The majority of nurses working in mental health institutions in four Western Provinces are registered psychiatric nurses, who have received all training in mental hospitals. Canadian Nursing Association believes that specialization should follow, not be part of, basic program.

Metzger, Norman. "Sound Orientation Can Reduce Turnover," *Hospitals*, 41 (September 1, 1967), 62-64.

Author lists the objectives and discusses the implementation of such a program.

Mickelson, Barbara. "Breakthrough to Nursing — Students Pave the Way for Minority Groups," *International Nursing Review*, 15, No. 1 (January, 1968), 61-65.

The National Student Nurses' Association has declared that nursing must provide opportunities within the profession for people, without consideration of race, etc. In 1965, this organization launched a recruitment program among minority groups and this program has continued in the way of tutoring, adjustment help, etc.

Millard, Richard Jr. "Liberal and Professional Nursing Education," *Nursing Outlook*, 16 (July, 1968), 22-25.

The aim of liberal, professional education is to develop perceptive men and women who understand what they are doing and why, and have a grasp of the service, experimental, and learning possibilities for more effective practice of their profession — author supports education in a collegiate setting.

Miller, David L. "A Mythologist Looks at the Realities of Comprehensive Health Planning," *Nursing Outlook*, 17 (July, 1969), 24-27.

Author pleads for an integration of the health professions — comprehensive health planning.

Miller, George E. "Continuing Education for What?" *The Journal of Medical Education*, 42 (April, 1967), 320-326.

The author suggests that continuing education should mean continuing self-education, not continuing instruction. He also discusses EDUCOM.

Mittman, Ben and Beatrice Bumgarner. "What Happened in San Francisco," *American Journal of Nursing*, 67 (January, 1967), 80-84.

These two nurses involved in the negotiations in San Francisco (Bay Area Hospitals) describe the events which led to a salary settlement.

Moore, Sister Anne Benedict. "Utilization of Graduates of ADN Programs," *Nursing Outlook*, 15 (December, 1967), 50-52.

This study (questionnaire) of 16 hospital departments of nursing service in California, employing a total of 100 AD nursing graduates, revealed that, in 15, these nurses are being used in positions for which they have not been academically prepared.

"More Hospital Involvement Needed: Group Views Regional Medical Programs," *Hospitals*, 42 (July 1, 1968), 21-24a.

> This article describes part of the Invitational Conference on Hospital Involvement in Regional Medical Programs stressing that hospital involvement is less than satisfactory.

Morgan, Philip W. "New Jersey Students Explore Hospital Career Opportunities," *Hospitals*, 42 (December 16, 1968), 41-45.

> A cooperative program to introduce high school students to career opportunities in hospitals has produced rewarding results.

Moses, Dorothy V. and Carolyn S. Lake. "Geriatrics in the Baccalaureate Nursing Curriculum," *Nursing Outlook*, 16 (July, 1968), 41-43.

> A study was conducted in 1966; questionnaires were sent to NLN accredited baccalaureate nursing schools. The survey revealed that wide variations of type and extent of geriatric nursing content and clinical experiences occurred in curriculums. Conclusion: More geriatrics are needed in courses at all levels, including continuing education courses.

Mowbray, Jean K. and Raymond G. Taylor. "Validity of Interest Inventories for the Prediction of Success in a School of Nursing," *Nursing Research*, 16 (Winter, 1967), 78-81.

> The study took place at the Bryn Mawr Hospital School of Nursing in 1963 because the faculty felt a responsibility to identify the factors which influence the withdrawal of students from their program. One result was that the overriding determinant of adjustment to nursing school is the social service orientation.

Moxley, John H. "The Predicament in Health Manpower," *American Journal of Nursing*, 68 (July, 1968), 1486-1490.

> A staff member of the National Advisory Commission on Health Manpower reviews the report and discusses implications for nursing. He touches on licensing and relicensing, and continuing education.

Mueller, E. Jane and Howard B. Lyman. "The Prediction of Scores on the State Board Test Pool Examination," *Nursing Research*, 18 (May-June, 1969), 263-267.

> Purpose: to formulate regression equations which could be used to predict success or failure on the licensing examination of students in a given educational program; to identify potential failures on the examination early enough in their careers for appropriate school action.

Muldrow, Catherine. "Now It's Students of Nursing," *American Journal of Nursing*, 69 (June, 1969), 1252-1253.

> At Rutgers, a small revolt, triggered, the author believes, by a larger revolt of liberal arts students came to the school of nursing but was not "put down."

Munro, John. "A Challenge that Confronts Us," *The Canadian Nurse*, 65 (August, 1969), 40-43.

> The author thinks that overall hospital costs and physician's costs would be lessened if the nurse would expand her scope of practice — taking over former physician duties which she could do as well if not better.

Murdaugh, Jessica. "There is a Difference," *Nursing Outlook*, 16 (October, 1968), 45-47.

> How the medical social worker and public health nurse can relate and function in the patient's best interest is the subject of this well-written article. A useful classification of family problems is included so that the PHN can utilize the skills of social work colleagues more fully and appropriately.

Murphy, Jeanne S. "Springfield Hospital Proves Best Strategy is to Attack All Nursing Fronts at Once," *Modern Hospital*, 108 (January, 1967), 90-94.

Article explains how hospital attacked and solved the problems of too few nurses, job dissatisfaction, resignations, etc.

Murphy, Marion. "Why A Masters-Prepared Practitioner in Public Health Nursing?" *Nursing Outlook*, 15 (March, 1967), 33-37.

Part I: A review of public health nursing's origin and development provides the foundation on which to build a strong case for the masters-prepared clinical specialist, who, unlike other clinical specialists, in nursing, must function as a generalist.

————: "Why A Masters-Prepared Practitioner in Public Health Nursing?" *Nursing Outlook*, 15 (April, 1967), 56-60.

Part II: Discusses graduate education for public health nursing and describes the functions of a nurse so prepared.

Mussallem, Helen K. "Manpower Problems in Nursing," *The Canadian Nurse*, 63 (August, 1967), 25-28.

There is no shortage of nurses. There is, however, a shortage of available nursing hours. Manpower could be increased by better utilization, reduction of turnover, more realistic salaries and working conditions.

————: "The Changing Role of the Nurse," *American Journal of Nursing*, 69 (March, 1969), 514-517.

Executive director of Canadian Nurses' Association sees the nurse of 1980 as a family practitioner, free to move between community and hospital, utilizing the latest technological advances to provide health care.

Myers, Emily and Ella Pott. "An Internship For New Graduates," *American Journal of Nursing*, 68 (January, 1968), 96-98.

Six months of patient assignments on various services throughout the hospital narrows the gap for new graduates between classroom theory and realistic practice.

Nahm, Helen. "The RN and Baccalaureate Education," *Nursing Forum*, VI, No. 1 (1967), 28-44.

The author discusses the ideas and expectations, of diploma or AD RN's who completed a BS degree in nursing at the University of California school of nursing in San Francisco in 1966.

Nash, Robert M. "Negroes Can Ease the Shortage: Let Them," *Modern Hospital*, 108 (January, 1967), 84-85.

A federal official cites a new survey showing how racial barriers still keep Negroes out of nursing. USPHS survey shows the percent of non-white nursing students in 25 cities (1966).

National League for Nursing. "Action for Quality," *National League for Nursing Publications Catalog*, No. 23-1327 (1968).

Eleven papers and a summary of presentations at a Boston conference of the NLN Council of AD Programs, February 29-March 2, 1968. Almost every phase of AD nursing education is discussed, as well as the performance of AD graduates.

————: "An Approach to the Teaching of Psychiatric Nursing in Diploma and AD Programs," *National League for Nursing Publications Catalog*, No. 33-1288 (1967).

A workshop report.

————: "Characteristics of Baccalaureate Education in Nursing," *National League for Nursing Publications Catalog*, No. 15-1319 (1968).

————: "Characteristics of Graduate Education in Nursing," *National League for Nursing Publications Catalog*, No. 15-1318 (1968).

———: "Community Planning for Nursing," *National League for Nursing Publications* Catalog, No. 19-1355 (1969).

A nationwide survey by the NLN Research and Development Service of the agencies active in community planning for nursing and how they are undertaking this.

———: "Developing Nursing Programs in Institutions of Higher Education," *National League for Nursing Publications Catalog*, No. 15-1315 (1969).

Report of a conference held in October, 1967, for administrators and faculty of junior, community and senior colleges interested in developing new nursing education resources.

———: "Educational Preparation for Nursing — 1967," *Nursing Outlook*, 16 (September, 1968), 52-56.

An annual report on admissions, enrollments and graduations in all nursing programs; indicates an even greater nurse shortage for the future.

———: "Statements Regarding Practical Nursing and Practical Nursing Education," *National League for Nursing Publications Catalog*, No. 38-1333 (1968).

A revised edition contains the NLN philosophy relating to practical nursing, characteristics of education for practical nursing, abilities needed by instructors of practical nurses and continuing education for the LPN and the VPN.

———: "The Shifting Scene — Building for Strength," *National League for Nursing Publications Catalog*, No. 15-1252 (1967).

Report of a 1965 meeting, tracing recent history of developments in the health services and the challenges these pose to graduate and undergraduate education in nursing.

Nelson, Roger B. "Full-Time Nurses Should Nurse Full-Time," *Modern Hospital*, 108 (January, 1967), 66-67.

If hospitals are to meet the nursing shortage, they must make nursing more attractive by steps to allow nurses to return to professional tasks.

"New Facilities Expand Hartford Hospital's School of Nursing," *Hospitals*, 41 (September 16, 1967), 52-56.

Article describes the nursing educational programs available at Hartford Hospital — one leading to a nursing diploma and a cooperative program with Mt. Holyoke College, leading to a diploma plus a baccalaureate.

New York State Nurses' Association and the Hospital Association of New York State. *American Journal of Nursing*, 67 (June, 1967), 1211-1214.

Deals with the transition in nursing education including institutions, continuing education, faculty, etc.

"Nova Scotia Nurses' Association Agree to 2-Year Program," *Canadian Hospital*, 44 (July, 1967), 60.

This association accepted an executive recommendation to reduce hospital training programs in nursing to two years by 1970.

"Nurses and Ambulatory Care," *The New England Journal of Medicine*, 277 (December 7, 1967), 1264-1265.

In the cost-effectiveness analysis, the nurse is cheaper than the doctor — the jobs of treatment can be exchanged when they are most suitable to the nurse and doctor — and the patient too.

"Nurses Are Making It Happen," *American Journal of Nursing*, 67 (February, 1967), 284-289.

Nurses are on the march for a better living for themselves and better care for their patients. This article describes interviews concerning conditions all over the country.

"Nursing Education Will Be College-Based," *Canadian Hospital*, 45 (June, 1968), 57, 60.

The RNAO held a symposium and panelists agreed that diploma programs would phase out and that carefully developed programs in the community colleges are the answer to the problems of present and future nursing education.

O'Brien, Margaret J. "A Nurse in School — Why?" *Nursing Clinics of North America*, 4 (June, 1969), 343-349.

When school nurses are relieved of routine and clerical tasks by utilization of auxiliary workers, there will be more opportunity for her to participate in counseling, interpret health needs of children to educators, and direct attention to problem of common health such as drug addiction, teen-age pregnancy and adolescent suicide.

——: "Team Nursing in School Health," *Nursing Outlook*, 17 (July, 1969), 28-30.

Selected schools in New York City utilized a team (public health nurse, staff nurses, public health assistants and the school physician) approach and a health audit to increase time spent by the public health nurse in professional work.

Ogden, Ann. "'Evanston Hospital High' Opens Opportunities for Employees," *Hospitals*, 43 (September 16, 1969), 58-60.

A classroom program sponsored by the hospital auxiliary provided an opportunity for employees to prepare for taking an educational development test leading to a high school equivalency certificate. In one case, a nurse aide, out of school for 25 years, received the certificate and plans to study for a nursing degree on an auxiliary scholarship.

Olson, David E. "Automated Nurses' Notes — First Step in a Computerized Record System," *Hospitals*, 41 (June 16, 1967), 68-78.

Check list of observations make nurses records more complete and take less nursing time to complete.

Olson, Edith V. "Needed: A Shake-Up in the Status Quo," *American Journal of Nursing*, 68 (July, 1968), 1491-1495.

It is time for a re-examination and review. The author suggests six new directions for nursing to take in solving old complaints, including continual re-examination of our beliefs about the educational preparation for professional and technical nurses and of our philosophy about refresher and continuing education.

O'Malley, Claire D. "Application of Systems Engineering in Nursing," *American Journal of Nursing*, 69 (October, 1969), 2155.

A California hospital uses systems engineering techniques to measure quantity and monitor quality of nursing care.

"On One Computer System Is Memory for Patient Care Data," *Modern Hospital*, 113 (July, 1969), 70-72.

Part of data processing system is automated nursing notes. Increases available nursing time and makes information immediately available.

Oram, Phyllis G. and Wilda R. Routhier. "Research as In-Service Education," *Nursing Outlook*, 16 (September, 1968), 20-22.

Realistically involving nursing personnel in a nursing research project will ultimately result in profitable in-service education and improved attitudes toward research.

Ortelt, Judith A. and Carole E. Glickman. "An Undergraduate Honors Program in Nursing," *Nursing Outlook*, 15 (July, 1967), 67-68.

Academically promising freshmen are encouraged to participate in an honors program for junior and senior nursing students at the University of Hawaii.

Osgood, Gretchen A. "Dimensions of Involvement," *Nursing Outlook*, 17 (September, 1969), 53-55.

Author discusses the funds and programs available to identify the disadvantaged with untapped potential and prepare them for a nursing career.

O'Shea, Helen Spustek. "A Guide to Evaluation of Clinical Performance," *American Journal of Nursing*, 67 (September, 1967), 1877-1879.

Characteristics essential for competence in bedside nursing and criteria for measurement were identified and are being used by the faculty in an AD program at Baltimore Junior College.

Ozimek, Dorothy. "The Preparation of a Generalist," *Nursing Outlook*, 16 (December, 1968), 28-29.

The focus of baccalaureate nursing education should be preparation of the generalist nurse. This preparation encompasses general education in anatomy, microbiology, etc. and professional education which is concerned with synthesizing and applying skills to problems in professional realm. The preparation of the nurse specialist should be the focus of graduate education.

Palmer, Helen. "Nurses for Nursing," *The Canadian Nurse*, 65 (May, 1969), 36-39.

In a Toronto hospital, introduction of ward manager system frees nurses of non-nursing functions.

Palmer, J. D. Keith, James P. O'Leary, Jr., and Harold M. Sterling. "Interfaculty Research-Training Crossover: An Experiment in Medical Education," *The Journal of Medical Education*, 42 (December, 1967), 1096-1100.

This technique could be incorporated into allied health professional education as a complement to a core curriculum. This format is particularly effective in dissolving interdisciplinary barriers.

Pankratz, Loren D. and Deanna M. Pankratz. "Determinants in Choosing a Nursing Career," *Nursing Research*, 16 (Spring, 1967), 169-172.

Ten statements about reasons for entering nursing were ranked by 166 nursing students and 144 RN's. Other influences such as age when nursing was first considered, age when final decision to enter nursing was made, significant individuals who influenced this decision, and satisfaction with result. If the concept of nursing were broadened, more individuals might find that their own needs could correspond to their image of nursing.

Pape, Ruth H. "Higher Education for the Nurse Practitioner," *Nursing Outlook*, 15 (February, 1967), 48-52.

An attempt to show how students in graduate programs reported their education experience and how they used it, or hope to use it, when they went back to the work world.

Parse, Rosemarie Rizzo. "The Advantages of the Associate Degree Nursing Program," The Journal of Nursing Education, 6 (August, 1967), 15-21, 24-25.

The author stresses the need for technical nurses which the AD program can best produce.

Pavalko, Ronald M. "Recruitment to Nursing: Some Research Findings," *Nursing Research*, 18 (January-February, 1969), 72-76.

Marriage results in a high degree of attrition from nursing.

Pellegrino, Edmund D. "Rationale for Nursing Education in the University," *American Journal of Nursing*, 68 (May, 1968), 1006-1009.

What can the university offer nursing and what can nursing offer the university? The future of nursing as a profession and its ultimate effectiveness as a social instrument are contingent upon the degree to which it establishes contact with the many university disciplines requisite to its growth.

Percy, Charles. "The View from Outside," *Modern Hospital*, 113 (December, 1969), 80.
    Senator Percy places priority on three objectives: 1) increasing the supply of health personnel; 2) overhaul of existing medical care operations; and 3) increasing the breadth of participation in existing programs.

Perlman, Lawrence V., et. al. "Public Health Nurses and the Prevention of Recurrences of Congestive Heart Failure," *Geriatrics*, 24 (September, 1969), 82-89.
    Five case studies illustrate the decrease in acute exacerbations of congestive failure when PHN role is expanded in area of counseling and referral.

Perry, Lucy, Marchusa Huff, Leona Adam and Emma Flinner. "An Experience in Preparing Programmed Instructional Material in Nursing," *Journal of Nursing Education*, 8 (January, 1969), 27-32.
    The authors describe a programmed instruction experiment at Indiana University School of Nursing. If students can learn better in less time than by other methods, the time must be spent in preparing programmed materials, the authors contend.

Peterson, Sharon. "The Psychiatric Nurse Specialist in a General Hospital," *Nursing Outlook*, 17 (February, 1969), 56-58.
    Psychiatric Nurse Specialist moves outside the psychiatric unit to achieve quality nursing care by: direct work with patient, consultations with staff nurses, consultation to head nurse committee, and teaching in specialty units. Conducts sensitivity training and sessions in interviewing and counseling techniques.

Plaisted, Lena M. "The Clinical Specialist in Rehabilitation Nursing," *American Journal of Nursing*, 69 (March, 1969), 562-564.
    The director of the Boston University graduate program in rehabilitation nursing describes the role of the clinical specialist as perceived by some graduates of the program.

Platou, Carl N. and W. Dennis Pederson. "Can More Part-Time Nurses Be Recruited?" *Hospitals*, 41 (May 16, 1967), 77-82.
    A survey of 708 unemployed RN's in a Minnesota County proves encouraging only if hospitals can make changes such as flexible schedules (hours when the children are at school), better salaries, and more appreciation.

Popiel, Elda S. "The Director of Continuing Education in Perspective," *Nursing Forum*, VIII, No. 1 (1969), 86-93.
    Author touches on identification of learning needs, curriculum and teaching methods, staff selection, public relations, evaluation and the roles of the Director.

———: "The Many Facets of Continuing Education in Nursing," *Journal of Nursing Education*, 8 (January, 1969), 3-13.
    The author describes continuing education and stresses self-development, in-service education, staff development, job orientation, refresher training.

Price, Elmina. "Data Processing — Present and Potential," *American Journal of Nursing*, 67 (December, 1967), 2558-2564.
    A review of the literature on automation in the health field that sorts fact from fancy. Implications for the patient and for the nurse are discussed. Brief descriptions of various kinds of computers are included.

Psathas, George and Jon Plapp. "Assessing the Effects of a Nursing Program: A Problem of Design," *Nursing Research*, 17 (July-August, 1968), 336-342.
    Study reports the application of the research design, the Recurrent Institutional Cycle Design, to sets of data regarding changes in personality needs, as measured by the Edwards Personal Preference Schedule — Subject: Nursing students in a three-year diploma program. The study focuses on the problems of designs in the study of institutional or training effects on personality.

Pueschel, Shirley J. "A Demographic Analysis of the Educational Structure of American Nursing," *Nursing Research*, 18 (May-June, 1969), 211-216.

Purposes of the study: To explore demographically the relationships of the educational attainment of American nursing with that of women in the other professional and technical groups and with women in the clerical occupations; the question of the expected time span involved in completing the structural change in nursing education will be approached through the demographic technique of the lifetable.

Puleo, Sister Mary Pius. "Comparison of On-The-Job and At-Home Use of Programmed Instruction and the Lecture Method in an In-Service Education Program," *Nursing Research*, 17 (July-August, 1968), 356-360.

Study done on staff nurses in a large general hospital: Programmed instruction for study at home proved to be superior to either study by means of programmed instruction on the job or the lecture method in in-service education.

Ragland, John Burt and K. Richard Knoll. "Pharmacists and Nurses Benefit From an IV Additive Program," *Hospitals*, 42 (August 16, 1968), 136-140.

Authors describe steps involved in organizing and maintaining program and discuss benefits derived — one of which is increased availability of nursing time for patient care.

Ramey, James W. "Teaching Medical Students by Videotape Simulation," *The Journal of Medical Education*, 43 (January, 1968), 55-59.

The author suggests this method be used in developing insight into the manner in which a health care team functions, and the interaction of the various team members in the hospital setting.

Ramphal, Marjorie. "Clinical Nursing Supervision," *American Journal of Nursing*, 68 (September, 1968), 1900-1902.

The clinical supervisor may be the head nurse, the supervisor or the team leader. *She* must be that nurse who has a case load which permits her to participate in patient care and thereby choose the techniques required to achieve the aim of the nursing care plan. Is it feasible for the traditional head nurse *functions* to be delegated to an LPN?

———: "Needed: A Career Ladder in Nursing," *American Journal of Nursing*, 68 (June, 1968), 1234-37.

This author suggests that the feasibility of special programs to permit some nurses to progress from technical nursing to professional nursing and, for the present from practical nursing to technical nursing, should be determined through research and experimentation and not deterred because of devotion to a caste system.

———: "This I Believe . . . About Excellence in Technical Nursing," *Nursing Outlook*, 16 (March, 1968), 36-38.

The measure of excellence in a technical nursing program does not lie in its resemblance to the professional nurse program. The author outlines what technical practice is, and what it is not and emphasizes that the development of techniques through research, the teaching of technique and the prescription of a technique for a given patient in a given setting are all the responsibility of the professional nurse.

Rankin, John W. "Four Carolina Hospitals Go On Line With Computer," *Modern Hospital*, III (October, 1968), 86-89.

Computer operation is expected to cut hospital stay by one day and reduce by 50 percent the time professional staff spends on paper-work. Doctors' orders, medication, radiology, dietary and nursing administration (staffing, nurses roles, etc.) will be part of the automated system.

Raphael, Sister Mary. "The Development and Activities of a Joint Physician-Nurse Liaison Committee," *Hospital Progress*, 49 (August, 1968), 80-83.

    After the national nurse-physician conference in 1965, a joint committee was formed in Idaho and made statements concerning joint practice problems.

Ravin, Robert, John Gilbert and John A. Comisky. "Two-Year Appraisal of a Centralized IV Additive Service," *Hospitals*, 41 (January 16, 1967), 88-92, 131.

    The function of compounding drugs (IV solutions) is returned to the pharmacist with saving in time and money, increased patient safety and good nurse-pharmacist acceptance.

Reader, George G. and Doris R. Schwartz. "Joint Planning for Patient Care," *Journal of the American Medical Association*, 201 (August 7, 1967), 364-367.

    This paper reviews the process of joint planning for care and predicts a beginning between physician and nurse which will spread to other disciplines.

Reed, Fay Carol. "Baccalaureate Education and Professional Practice," *Nursing Outlook*, 15 (January, 1967), 50-52.

    Baccalaureate program graduates can make their greatest contribution to patient care, provided the differences between them and graduates of other basic programs are recognized.

Reese, Eva M. "Public Health Nursing and Comprehensive Health Care," *Nursing Outlook*, 16 (January, 1968), 48-52.

    The author calls for the preparation of the specialist in general public health nursing at the masters level. Distributive nursing is "where the action is."

Regan, Patrick A. "Measuring the Effectiveness of a Unit Management Program," *Hospital Progress*, (December, 1969), 28-33.

    This plan at Methodist Hospital in Indianapolis, Indiana has increased the time which nurses can devote to direct patient care, but with a significant increase in payroll expense.

"Regional Medical Programs: The View From the Hospital," *Hospitals*, 42 (July 1, 1968), 63-64.

    Two respected health professionals, James T. Howell, M.D. and Dr. Eugene Sibery, agree on the hospital's position as focal point of RMP effectiveness.

Reinkemeyer, Sister Agnes M. "It Won't Be Hospital Nursing," *American Journal of Nursing*, 68 (September, 1968), 1936-1940.

    Do BS graduates shun hospital practice? Why? Findings from a study in Great Britain have some disturbing implications for nursing education and practice in the U.S. The root cause may be: valuation of the BS degree for its prestige significance rather than for the competencies it represents.

Reinkemeyer, Sister Mary Hubert. "An Inherited Pathology," *Nursing Outlook*, 15 (November, 1967), 51-53.

    Nurses' hostility toward university-based programs and university-educated nurses has a long history, and only nurses can modify, if not eliminate, this acquired negative attitude. This article is based on a study conducted by the author in England in 1965.

Remillet, June Gordon. "The 8 mm Film in Student and Patient Education," *The Journal of Nursing Education*, 7 (April, 1968), 27-35.

    This method of teaching has the advantage of self-study or self-pacing and of strengthening learning by repetition as individually needed. Also is useful for group teaching.

"Report of the Health Manpower Commission," *Journal of the American Medical Association*, 203 (February 12, 1968), 499-506.

The Recommendations of the Commission are presented here with accompanying comments from the AMA Committee. The Committee favors a higher professional role for nurses, especially in direct patient care; Commission favors relicensure, peer review, etc.

Reres, Mary E. "An Effective Review Course for Psychiatric Nurses," *Nursing Outlook*, 17 (May, 1969), 66-67.

A nursing instructor in a collegiate school, teaching psychiatric nursing theory in an 8-week summer course, demonstrated the usefulness of university faculty as resource persons in a state hospital.

"Research Made This Hospital Go Round — And Square," *Modern Hospital*, 109 (December, 1967), 98-101.

The new Rochester Methodist Hospital is elaborately equipped for patient care and deliberately designed for administrative research on such questions as what shape is best for nursing units.

Richards, Jean F. "Integrating a Clinical Specialist into a Hospital Nursing Service," *Nursing Outlook*, 17 (March, 1969), 23-25.

The utilization of the clinical nurse specialist can be enhanced if the director of nursing service is aware of the sensitivities and attitudes of present staff, makes realistic commitments to implement this position, recognizes the anticipated contributions of this skilled practitioner, by both proper placement in organization and by adequate salary.

Richardson, William C. and Duncan Neuhauser. "Does the Public Know What It Wants?" *Modern Hospital*, 110 (May, 1968), 115-117, 172.

Policy decisions would be more coherent if policy makers would first decide just what they think of human nature.

Rihm, Sister Alma. "From a Diploma to an Associate Degree Program in Nursing," *Nursing Outlook*, 17 (January, 1969), 25-26.

Transition from a diploma to a new AD program is facilitated when the existent faculty structure can be used for planning and the faculty members can move with ease into the university setting. A diploma program was phased out and a new AD program established at the University of Albuquerque.

Roberts, Doris E., et. al. "Epidemiologic Analysis in School Populations as a Basis for Change in School Nursing Practice," *American Journal of Public Health*, 59 (December, 1969), 2157-2166.

Methods and preliminary findings in the first phase of a longitudinal study of a school population are presented. Absence and attendance patterns were studied, and a statistical model was developed which can be used in evaluating effects of change in nursing programs on the functional state of students.

Robertson, Leon S., John Kosa, Joel J. Alpert and Margaret C. Heagarty. "Anticipated Acceptance of Neighborhood Health Clinics by the Urban Poor," *Journal of the American Medical Association*, 205 (September 16, 1968), 815-818.

A study concluded that only to the extent that neighborhood clinics provide personalized, comprehensive care, can we expect them to replace the present uncoordinated, fragmented pattern of health care prevalent in their target populations.

Robinson, S. C. "A Doctor Looks at Nursing Education," *The Canadian Nurse*, 64 (July, 1968), 38-40.

The author contends that all nurses should have core knowledge and skills, regardless of what they will do. The core experience should take no longer than two years, and then the student can proceed into further training, by a series of elective programs. The elective third year should be directed toward a career goal.

Robischon, Paulette and Evelyn G. Sobel. "It's the Principle, Not the Setting," *Nursing Outlook*, 15 (May, 1967), 36-39.

Educational philosophy and empirical necessity motivated this faculty to experiment in the use of an ambulatory care unit for laboratory study in community nursing.

Rogers, Kenneth D., Mary Mally and Florence L. Marcus. "A General Medical Practice Using Nonphysician Personnel," *Journal of the American Medical Association*, 206 (November 18, 1968), 1753-1757.

Demonstration project in Pittsburgh utilized PHN, office nurse, social worker and technician to care for population of 2500. Some traditional-physician care was delegated to nurses without patient expressed dissatisfaction and with 50 percent increase in available physician time. The project has since been duplicated twice in the Pittsburgh area.

Rosinski, Edwin F. "The Community Hospital as a Center for Training and Education," *Journal of the American Medical Association*, 206 (November 25, 1968), 1955-1957.

Community hospitals should work in partnership with community colleges to develop innovative training programs producing a vast array of health personnel.

Ross, Carmen F. "In Support of Practical Nursing Education," *Nursing Outlook*, 16 (June, 1968), 36-37.

Author refers to the ANA Position Paper and gives arguments for the continuation of LPN programs.

Rottkamp, Barbara C. "Attrition Rates in Basic Baccalaureate Nursing Programs," *Nursing Outlook*, 16 (June, 1968), 44-47.

A review of the studies of nursing student attrition in this country reveals that careful study of facets of the problem and curative action could reduce the number of students who fall by the way.

Rowe, Harold R. and Hessel H. Flitter. "Junior Colleges Hold Their Nursing Students," *Nursing Outlook*, 15 (February, 1967), 35-37.

An overview of recent studies on AD programs in nursing indicates a low rate of student attrition in comparison to the rate for students enrolled in most other programs offered by junior colleges.

Ruiz, Rene A., Hester I. Thurston and Neila A. Poshek. "Intellectual Factors, Biographical Information, and Personality Variables as Related to Performance on the Professional Nurse Licensure Examination," *Nursing Research*, 16 (Winter, 1967), 74-78.

The study included BS and diploma students from Topeka, Kansas. BS graduates did slightly, but significantly better.

Rutstein, David D. "Can *Non* Doctors End the Doctor Shortage?" *Medical Economics*, (June 24, 1968), 155-166.

Nurses should be doing more of the tasks formerly done by the physicians — they should work at their highest capability levels.

Ryder, Claire F., Pauline G. Stitt, and William F. Elkin. "Home Health Services — Past, Present, Future," *American Journal Of Public Health*, 59 (September, 1969), 1720-1729.

Authors discuss trends in home health services, describe new directions and explore future developments.

Sable, David E. "Personalization On The Coronary Care Unit," *American Journal of Nursing*, 69 (July, 1969), 1439-1442.

When nurse is open and interacts with patients as a 'person' rather than as a professional there is less denial, hopelessness and anxiety and fewer perceptual aberrations.

Sanford, Nancy. "Students and Studies," *American Journal of Nursing*, 68 (April, 1968), 805-806.

Practice in conducting small studies helps students gain confidence in their ability to solve nursing problems and arouses their interest in nursing research.

Schaan, Sister Mary Catherine. "The Nurse: A Thoughtful Generalist-Specialist," *The Journal of Nursing Education*, 6 (November, 1967), 3-6.

The author quotes Earl McGrath and Charles Russell, in arguing for a BS program in nursing.

Schaefer, Morris. "Current Issues in Health Organization," *American Journal of Public Health*, 58 (July, 1968), 1192-1199.

Health Administration by its very nature is enmeshed in political activity. This fact has been denied by health professionals. Current problems and issues in organization demand a reorientation of attitude and ideology in public health administration.

Schechter, Daniel S. "Innovation in Training and Education," *Hospitals*, 41 (June 1, 1967), 55-58.

The author describes the use of methods such as closed-circuit TV and programmed instruction to improve the professional and technical skills of smaller hospital personnel.

Scheinfeldt, Jean. "Opening Doors Wider in Nursing," *American Journal of Nursing*, 67 (July, 1967), 1461-1464.

A description of ODWIN: If minority group members are to be both encouraged and assisted to pursue nursing careers, they need informed guidance early in high school, demonstration that nursing is truly non-discriminatory, and often, supplemental education to overcome the handicaps of inadequate early schooling.

Schlotfeldt, Rozella M. and Jannetta MacPhail. "An Experiment in Nursing Rationale and Characteristics," *American Journal of Nursing*, 69 (May, 1969), 1018-1023.

Study in progress at Case Western Reserve which tests the hypothesis that there is need for academic leadership in delivery of, and education for, nursing care.

——— and ———: "Introducing Planned Change," *American Journal of Nursing*, 69 (June, 1969), 1247-1251.

Second of three-part series details steps taken to implement change in nursing roles. Success depends on careful planning and timing, administrative sanctions and adequate articulation of the system to permit incumbents to meet the changed expectations.

——— and ———: "Experiment in Nursing: Implementing Planned Change," *American Journal of Nursing*, 69 (July, 1969), 1475-1480.

This paper discusses changes in roles in nursing education and nursing care and the learning and research climates in a complex health science center. The authors stress the idea that those faculty who guide the learning of students in the hospital are expected to engage in clinical practice.

—— and Mildred Montag: "Preparation of Nurses for Faculty Positions," *Nursing Outlook*, 15 (January, 1967), 26-31.

In a two part article, Dr. Schlotfeldt maintains that the need to develop special programs to prepare nurse teachers for each of the currently existing types of nursing programs "cannot be defended"; Dr. Montag's answer is "yes" to the question, "Should we prepare teachers (of nursing) specifically for the kinds of nursing programs we envision?"

Schmidt, Alexander M. and Robert Q. Marston. "Regional Medical Programs: A View From the Federal Level," *Journal of Medical Education*, 43 (July, 1968), 828-834.

Author discusses the progress, expectations, limitations, and role of quality of regional medical programs and also discusses some other federal programs.

Schmidt, Etta B. "More Schools, More LPN's, More Duties," *Modern Hospital*, 108 (January, 1967), 82-83.

The author asserts that more LPN's will be needed, especially since bedside nurses are needed and hospital schools are dwindling and AD courses don't teach bedside nursing!

Schmidt, Mildred S. and William Lyons. "Credit For What You Know," *American Journal of Nursing*, 69 (January, 1969), 101-104.

New York State has begun administering examinations in three clinical areas. It is hoped that candidates who are successful will receive college credit and will not have to repeat work in which they have demonstrated proficiency.

Schmitt, Edith. "Transition From Student to Graduate," *American Journal of Nursing*, 67 (December, 1967), 2573-2575.

To give senior students in a BS program a taste of the working situation that they will encounter, faculty members established a course during which students function as staff nurses for 17 days and concentrate in the academic hours of the course on the activities of team leadership.

Schutt, Barbara. "And Now Practical Doctors?" *American Journal of Nursing*, 67 (July, 1967), 1411.

The editor discusses the present multiplicity of professional health workers and how nursing can be influenced.

———: "Community-Based Education," *American Journal of Nursing*, 67 (November, 1967), 2297.

The author approves the great growth in AD programs and feels that in-service education is definitely needed.

Scott, Jessie M. "Three Years With the Nurse Training Act," *American Journal of Nursing*, 67 (October, 1967), 2107-2109.

Under this federal legislation, over one million dollars has been disbursed in assistance to students, and grants to nursing schools for construction and projects to improve educational programs.

Scott, Joe L. "Educational Child Care," *Hospitals*, 43 (November 16, 1969), 51-54.

A hospital's day care center lets employees get back to work. Nursing service has used the center more than any other department.

Senf, Harriet R. "The Oral Examination for Nursing Students," *Nursing Outlook*, 15 (September, 1967), 58-59.

Four instructors decided to try oral testing and now support it as a useful method of evaluation.

Sharp, Lawrence J. and Mary S. Tschuding. "Nursing Faculty Research Development: Report of an Experience," *Nursing Research*, 16 (Spring, 1967), 161-166.

 From 1959-1964, the University of Washington School of Nursing faculty was engaged in an extensive program of research development. The project was designed to increase faculty participation in nursing research and to assist in the advancement of nursing knowledge.

Shriver, Beatrice M., Franklin N. Arnhoff and Esther A. Garrison. "Follow-Up on Mental Health Trainees," *American Journal of Nursing*, 67 (December, 1967), 2569-2572.

 The article reports a survey, by the National Institute of Mental Health, of a group of psychiatric and mental health nurses who received federal stipends to study under the institute's program and what has happened to these nurses.

Shupe, Donald R. "On The Use of Chi-Square in Nursing Research," *Nursing Research*, 16 (Summer, 1967), 279-282.

 Article developed from a USPHS grant to study the development of faculty competence in research. The author points out the common misuses of X_2 in nursing literature.

Siegel, Fanny F. "Should Supervisors and Head Nurses Teach Nursing Aides?" *Nursing Outlook*, 16 (June, 1968), 24-26.

 As one step in the overall in-service program, the basic training of nursing aides helps the aide learn to assist the nurse, the head nurse to gain experience in demonstrating standards of performance, and the supervisor to develop interpersonal relations skills.

Sieverts, Steven. "Coordinating Institutional Plans to Form a Comprehensive Regional Plan," *Hospitals*, 41 (November 16, 1967), 58-62.

 Areawide planning agency in Pennsylvania uses hospital-by-hospital approach in developing an orderly, no-service-gap plan for health care.

———: "P. L. 89-749 Poses Three Critical Issues for Health Planners," *Modern Hospital*, 111 (July, 1968), 88-90.

 Emphasis on the word "comprehensive" requires a broad view of the whole health picture and permits problems to be solved one at a time.

Silver, Henry and Loretta Ford. "The Pediatric Nurse Practitioner at Colorado," *American Journal of Nursing*, 67 (June, 1967), 1443-1444.

 The article describes the training for this extended role.

———, ——— and Lewis R. Day. "The Pediatric Nurse Practitioner Program," *Journal of the American Medical Association*, (April 22, 1968), 88-92.

 Discussion of pediatric nurse practitioner program in Denver with major emphasis on nurse role.

Simpson, M. June. "The Medium for the Message in Maternal-Child Nursing," *American Journal of Nursing*, 67 (November, 1967), 2343-2344.

 TV makes it possible for students in this AD program to have clinical obstetric and pediatric experience in their classrooms.

Sjoberg, Kay. "Unit Assignment — A New Concept," *The Canadian Nurse*, 65 (July, 1969), 29-31.

 A 47-bed research ward is divided into units, (three bed intensive care, five-bed above average care, etc.) each of which can be handled by one RN with adequate assistance and supplies. Service staff is available for non-nursing duties. System allows individual nursing innovations.

Skaggs, Kenneth G. "Allied Health Programs in the Junior Colleges," *Journal of the American Medical Association*, 206 (November 11, 1968), 1551-1553.

 The author discusses the junior college as the institution to educate "support" personnel, including AD nursing programs.

Skipper, Jr., James K., Powhatan J. Wooldridge and Robert C. Leonard. "The Use and Misuse of Behavioral Science in Nursing Education," *Journal of Nursing Education*, 8 (January, 1969), 23-26.

The authors argue for a reorientation and enhanced understanding of the potential uses of present courses in the nursing curriculum, not so much for an extension of behavioral science content.

Slater, Carl. "Student Participation in Curriculum Planning and Evaluation," *Journal of Medical Education*, 44 (August, 1969), 675-678.

The author concludes that students should be formal participants in the decision-making related to curriculum planning in all medical schools.

Slater, Robert J. and Elizabeth Reichert. "Editorial: Quality in Health Care," *Journal of Medical Education*, 43 (August, 1968), 931-932.

The members of the National Health Council agreed that licensure should be maintained in the health professions but that periodic review and recertification would assure better quality of ongoing performance. Participants felt that experience with nationally standardized certification by peer professional organizations has proved promising.

Smith, Eleanor F. "Nursing Service Administration is Nursing, Too," *Nursing Outlook*, 16 (September, 1968), 19.

In placing emphasis on clinical specialty and "freeing the nurse to nurse" we must remember that there remain administrative functions that can only be done by nurses and such nurses have not "deserted" the profession.

Smith, James L. "The Computer: Its Impact on the Physician, the Nurse, and the Administrator," *Hospitals*, 43 (September 16, 1969), 61-65.

The author contends that careful examination of present uses and of developmental trends in computer hardware and software make it possible to assay some predictions about the effects of a computer-based total hospital information system on the roles of health care personnel.

Smith, Jean H. and Helen A. Slaven. "A Hospital Assesses and Alters Its Role in Nursing Education," *Nursing Outlook*, 15 (October, 1967), 28-30.

The closing of a diploma nursing school after 60 years of enviable reputation caused great concern to its sponsors, faculty and students. Only through very careful planning and close communication was it accomplished without serious difficulty.

Smith, Jeanne E. "Personality Structure in Beginning Nursing Students: A Factor Analytic Study," *Nursing Research*, 17 (March-April, 1968), 140-144.

Two Personality Inventories measuring 21 variables were given to 546 freshmen nursing students from 10 hospital-based schools around Baltimore. Each factor describes a dimension of the personality which is probably involved in some way with the motivational drives which result in the choice of nursing as a career.

Smyth, Sister Mary Paul and Sister Nathalie Elder. "Nursing Education Curriculums, 1968: Direction or Drift," *Nursing Outlook*, 16 (December, 1968), 41-43.

A survey of NLN approved BS curriculums was conducted during the summer of 1967; it raised the question: "Are our BS nursing curriculums really educating generalists for professional practice, or are we preparing a hybred for specialized technical practice?"

Somers, Anne R. "Meeting Health Manpower Requirements Through Increased Productivity," *Hospitals*, 42 (March 16, 1968), 43-48, 116.

Excellent review article of the background of manpower problems, including improper utilization of nursing skills.

Sorensen, Gladys. "An Honors Program in Nursing," *Nursing Outlook*, 16 (May, 1968), 59-61.

Intellectually superior students are given an opportunity to broaden and deepen their interest in the profession through special lectures and seminars, independent study and research, at the University of Arizona College of Nursing.

Spencer, Carlee S. and Frank M. Mele. "A Community Approach to Nursing Manpower," *Nursing Outlook*, 17 (February, 1969), 28-30.

A local, voluntary body, armed with accurate information, can directly influence both the number and quality of nursing care personnel available in a given community. The author urges that three groups need representation in the proposed body: the trainers and educators of nursing personnel, the users and consumers of nursing service, and nursing personnel themselves!

"Square Nursing Units Joined in Radical Design," *Modern Hospital*, 110 (April, 1968), 90-93.

Lincoln (Nebraska) General's rebuilding program included functional planning, generous spacing, and unconventional nursing units.

Stacey, James. "RN's Tell Why They Took Off Their Caps," *Modern Hospital*, 108 (January, 1967), 76-77.

Inflexible schedules, burdensome chores, and lack of recognition — these and other disadvantages caused these former practitioners to surrender.

"States Plan for Transition in Nursing Education," *American Journal of Nursing*, 67 (June, 1967), 1215-1216.

Summary of responses to an *AJN* query on the present activity for future education from 21 state nurse associations.

Stearly, Susan, Ann Noordenbos and Voula Crouch. "Pediatric Nurse Practitioner," *American Journal of Nursing*, 67 (October, 1967), 2083-2087.

The background and specialized preparation of the PNP is discussed. Her practice includes all child care, management of minor illnesses and occasional first aid.

Steed, Margaret E. "Trends in Diploma Nursing Education," *The Canadian Nurse*, 64 (February, 1968), 40-41.

Present programs should not be phased out until alternate plans and programs can ensure an increase in the number of graduates to meet the increased demand for stated needs.

Stein, Leonard I. "The Doctor-Nurse Game," *American Journal of Nursing*, 68 (January, 1968), 101-105.

Nurses and doctors successfully perform a type of interaction which, though efficient, creates serious obstacles and is basically a transactional neurosis, says this psychiatrist.

Stein, Rita F. "An Exploratory Study in the Development and Use of Automated Nursing Reports," *Nursing Research*, 18 (January-February, 1969), 14-21.

In the interest of more efficient patient care, observation and communication, and productive potential for clinical research, an automated (checklist) nursing report (note) was devised. Tended to give more information than narrative reports.

Steinberg, Sheldon S., Eunice O. Shatz, and Jacob R. Fishman. "New Careers: A Major Solution to the Environmental Health Problem," *American Journal of Public Health*, 59 (July, 1969), 1118-1123.

Authors see the solution to the "shortage" of health manpower in the public health field as the utilization of people indigenous to the poverty areas in new health careers. There must be career ladders for mobility beyond entry level.

Stevens, Leonard and Sister Theophone Umscheid. "Psychiatric Nursing As A First Course For Students," *American Journal of Nursing*, 68 (August, 1968), 1720-1724.

> Psychiatric nursing as a first course provides students with knowledge and skill they can apply throughout the rest of their program.

Stewart, Diane Y. "Nursing Organization — Circa 1969," *The Canadian Nurse*, 65 (February, 1969), 59-61.

> In a new hospital in Ontario, the "nurse supervisor" is now the "nursing administrator" and the "head nurse" is now the "nursing coordinator." The former is a specialist in her clinical area as well as an administrator; the latter is also a specialist in her clinical area and is responsible for the nursing activities on her unit.

Stobo, Elizabeth C. "Trends in the Preparation and Qualifications of the School Nurse," *American Journal of Public Health*, 59 (April, 1969), 669-672.

> A trend for graduate level education for professional nurses to work in schools is discussed. What is involved in such preparation forms various discipines and the need for their synthesis into a meaningful curriculum is presented and emphasized.

Stokes, Joseph. "More Physicians, More Highly Trained Nurses or a New Health Worker?" *American Journal of Nursing*, 67 (July, 1967), 1441-1442.

> The author asks whether the clinical role of the nurse should be extended to fill the doctor gap or should doctors' assistants be trained?

Stone, Joseph, Elizabeth Patterson and Leon Felsom. "The Effectiveness of Home Care for General Hospital Patients," *Journal of the American Medical Association*, 205 (July 15, 1968), 145-148.

> Report of study in Wisconsin in which it was found that when home care is of high quality, there is no significant difference in the results of that care vs. hospital care; patients express satisfaction and costs are cut by 75%.

Summers, Jack L. "Nurse and Pharmacist — Partners," *The Canadian Nurse*, 63 (February, 1967), 40-44.

> New organization of administering and dispensing medications on part of nurses and pharmacists would reduce widespread medication errors and relieve shortage of nursing time.

Summers, Virginia M. "An Occupational Health Nursing Study," *Nursing Outlook*, 15 (July, 1967), 64-65.

> Since baccalaureate programs in nursing prepare nurses to function in first-level positions in any setting, it is essential that content in occupational health nursing be identified and included in the curriculum. This study was conducted at Boston College, from 1964-1965.

"Summit: Regional Nurse Training Center," *Modern Hospital*, 108 (March, 1967), 110.

> Overlook Hospital in Summit, New Jersey, prepares cardiac nurses from surrounding hospitals.

Sweeney, Sharyn. "Health Programs and the Nixon Administration: Revision, Revamping of Existing Programs Expected in Wake of Great Society's Legislative Thrust," *Hospitals*, 43 (May 1, 1969), 24a-24h.

> Author discusses regional medical programs and comprehensive health planning and "radical" redirection for Hill Burton.

Taylor, Joe K. and Frances S. Richter. "What Motivates Students Into Nursing?" *Hospitals*, 43 (January 1, 1969), 59-61.

> A survey of freshmen from six nursing schools in Atlanta, Georgia explains why and when they selected nursing as a career.

"Teammates are Equal Partners," *The Canadian Nurse*, 64 (September, 1968), 36-41.
  Nurses complain that doctors do not recognize nurses as equal partners. Are nurses as guilty in relating to other health professionals? Interviews with medical social workers, occupational therapists, and dietitians outline roles and functions of each in the health care team.

"That's What We Want for Christmas," *The Canadian Nurse*, 63 (December, 1967), 27.
  This editorial suggests an orderly transition of nursing programs from hospitals to educational institutions — but it shouldn't take another half century!

"The Connecticut Mental Health Center," *Journal of Practical Nursing*, 19 (June, 1969), 24.
  Community mental health needs in New Haven area are being met by a program which involves in and out patient services, a crisis intervention unit. Interdisciplinary teams are used and the patient is treated in his own setting.

"The Delicate Business of Delegating More," *Medical Economics*, (September 30, 1968), 76-79.
  A productivity survey by this magazine showed that the trend towards increased delegation of clinical duties to qualified paramedical personnel is running strong.

"The Nurse and the Multiphasic Exam," *Nursing Outlook*, 16 (September, 1968), 41.
  In a Kaiser Clinic the nurses' main functions were in prevention of illness and provision of psychological support needed by patients undergoing strange tests.

"The Nurse Researcher and the Nursing Profession," *International Nursing Review*, 14 (November-December, 1967), 33-35.
  Emphasizes the need for combining both formal education and practice experience to produce meaningful nursing research.

"The Nursing Education Controversy: AHA Acts to Support Hospital Schools," *Hospitals*, 41 (June 1, 1967), 22a-22c.
  Article summarizes the various reactions to the ANA Position Paper.

"The Sick Poor," *American Journal of Nursing*, 69 (November, 1969), 2423-2454.
  Nurses, physicians, administrators, and behavioral scientists examine and explore the nature and extent of the nation's health care problems: causes, effects, and possible directions for change.

"The Surgeon General Looks at Nursing," *American Journal of Nursing*, 67 (January, 1967), 64-67.
  Dr. William Stewart discusses problems such as shortage of nurses, economics and education.

Theis, Charlotte and Helen Harrington. "Three Factors That Affect Practice — Communications, Assignments, Attitudes," *American Journal of Nursing*, 68 (July, 1968), 1478-1482.
  Whether or not the staff nurse functions to her highest capability is affected by all three. Loeb Center in New York has manipulated these variables to improve practice.

Thomas, Lauraine A. "A Rationale for Nursing Administration," *American Journal of Nursing*, 69 (April, 1969), 774-776.
  Nursing by administrative directive is not only frustrating but erodes the nurse's professional values. Only as the nurse is free to make her own nursing assessments and plan her care accordingly, will she develop her clinical expertise and the patient benefit from her skills.

Thomas, Lewis. "Needed: New Concepts in Medical Manpower," *Hospital Practice*, (March, 1969), 37-41.
  Author suggests alternative solutions to the manpower crisis including the setting up of paramedical institutes.

Thompson, Adrian J. "Small Hospitals Can Develop Effective Employee Training Programs," *Hospitals*, 42 (September 16, 1968), 67-70.

Small hospitals can conduct, and will benefit from, training programs to upgrade employees' knowledge and capabilities (including nurses).

Thompson, Doreen. "Hospital Makes Movie to Train Housekeeping Staff," *Modern Hospital*, 113 (December, 1969), 64.

A movie (budget $47) teaches isolation cleaning to 67 housekeeping personnel, many of whom have primary language other than English.

Thompson, John D., et. al. "Age a Factor in Amount of Nursing Care Given, AHA Study Shows," *Hospitals*, 43 (March 1, 1968), 33-38.

In AHA conducted study in nine areas of the country, the over-65 age group on medical surgical units requires more nursing care hours (at least 30 minutes/patient/day) than those under 65.

Thoren, Beverly, Dorothy Paulson Smith and Leroy Gould. "Attitude Study, Training Helps Employees Adapt to Use of Computers," *Hospitals*, 43 (March 1, 1969), 61-64.

Factors to be considered in planning technical innovations in hospitals. Decision-making powers tend to be decreased in middle-management areas and this group may not be enthusiastic.

Thurlow, Ralph M. "How People React to a Paramedic," *Medical Economics*, (August 18, 1969), 187.

Author reports of a survey done by Dr. Henry Silver concerning the pediatric nurse practitioner: 96 percent of the respondents are satisfied with the nurse practitioner's services.

Thurston, John R., Helen L. Brunclik and John F. Feldhusen. "Personality and the Prediction of Success in Nursing Education," *Nursing Research*, 18 (May-June, 1969), 258-262.

The purpose was to further refine and validate techniques which could eventually contribute to the accuracy of prediction of student success in nursing schools, and to an understanding of factors associated with nursing student performance.

———, ——— and ———: "The Relationship of Personality to Achievement in Nursing Education — Phase II," *Nursing Research*, 17 (May-June, 1968), 265-268.

Significant differences found on some scores and no significant differences found on others.

Tillotson, Olen L. "The Long Road Ahead," *The Canadian Nurse*, 64 (October, 1968), 52-54.

The rehabilitation nurse is a prime source of support for a patient involved in the long, often discouraging, return to self-care and employment. Due to her continuity of contact with the patient, she is also a resource person for the vocational rehabilitation counselor in determining timing and realistic goals for retraining.

Topf, Margaret and Ruth Gordon Byers. "Role Fusion on the Community Mental Health Multidisciplinary Team," *Nursing Research*, 18 (May-June, 1969), 270-274.

Role fusion is defined as a similarity of tasks performed and expected in two or more positions. Study shows significant sharing of tasks between psychiatrist, psychologist, social worker and nurse in individual therapy, group therapy supervision, education, consultation planning, evaluation, and research.

Towner, Alfred M. "No More Supervisors?" *Nursing Outlook*, 16 (February, 1968), 56-58.

Seven supervisory positions were eliminated at a saving of $39,000 in yearly salaries which was assigned to direct patient care via clinical specialists. The head nurse role is expanded to that of total responsibility for patient care 24 hours a day.

Trites, David K. and Neal W. Schwarton. "Nursing or Clerking?" *Nursing Outlook*, 15 (January, 1967), 55-56.

   A nurse could spend more time in patient care if she were relieved of many clerical activities related to physicians' medication orders, so concludes a report from 270 hospitals.

———, Frank D. Galbraith, Jr., John F. Leckwart, and Madelyne Sturdavant. "Radial Nursing Units Prove Best in Controlled Study," *Modern Hospital*, 112 (April, 1969), 94-99.

   Nearly two million items of data were analyzed by computer in this study — a comparison of radial, single corridor, and double corridor nursing units. Staff and patients preferred the radial design; also, the radial unit proved to be more efficient in terms of the amount of time nurses spent in traveling and direct care: Rochester (Minnesota) Methodist Hospital.

Uprichard, Muriel. "Ferment in Nursing," *International Nursing Review*, 16:3, 222-232.

   Nursing's heritage determines to some extent the difficulties it must conquer in search of professional status and development of a scientific knowledge base for practice.

U. S. Department of Health, Education, and Welfare. "Federal Funds for Nursing Education," *American Journal of Nursing*, 68 (February, 1968), 312-315.

   Excerpts from the official report submitted by the committee appointed by the Secretary of HEW to evaluate the programs initiated under the 1964 Nurse Training Act. Recommendations for the continuation and expansion of these programs are presented.

VanFossen, Marian A. "This I Believe...About Public Health Education in the Baccalaureate Nursing Program," *Nursing Outlook*, 16 (July, 1968), 38-40.

   When those in charge of collegiate programs in nursing care are willing to provide qualified instructors to teach in the community, they should be permitted to assume full responsibility, within the agency setting, for the education of their students.

Vaz, Dolores. "High School Senior Boys' Attitudes Toward Nursing As A Career," *Nursing Research*, 17 (November-December, 1968), 533-538.

   In this study (Rhode Island and Massachusetts), the sample overwhelmingly ranked nursing lowest on masculinity — involving all three hypotheses.

VerSteeg, Donna F. "The Fictional Nurse...Is She For Real?" *Nursing Outlook*, 16 (August, 1968), 20-23.

   A report of a small study compares the image of nurses and nursing projected by popular fiction to real nurses and nursing as reported in the literature.

Voss, Charlotte E. "A Cooperative Education Program in Nursing," *Nursing Outlook*, 17 (July, 1969), 38-40.

   A description of the work-study plan for AD and BS degree students at Northeastern University in Boston.

Walker, Dorothy J. "The Structural Dysfunction of Nursing," *Hospital Progress,* 50 (April, 1969), 90-94.

   Nursing has adopted the work distribution model from industry. Dysfunction occurs when the nurse must choose either quantity or quality of care. Crux of problem is the laminated nature of the structure of organization without clear lines of responsibility for administration.

—— and Bernadette P. Hungler. "A Proposed Approach to the Education of Nurses," *Nursing Outlook,* 16 (August, 1968), 24-26.

   High school graduates would be admitted to only one kind of university program in nursing, would continue without interruption, and be graduated seven years later with a truly professional degree — doctor of nursing.

Wallace, J. Douglas. "Developing an Effective Utilization Review Program," *Hospitals,* 41 (November 16, 1967), 70-73.

   Utilization review programs should be implemented by a coordinated team of persons representing all hospital departments, including nursing.

Wayne, Dora. "School Nursing and Team Teaching," *Nursing Outlook,* 17 (July, 1969), 37.

   School nurse joined three teachers in preparing a study unit for 6th graders.

Wedgery, Albert W. "Post-Basic Courses. . .A Major Nursing Need," *Canadian Hospital,* 45 (January, 1968), 45-46.

   The president of the Registered Nurses' Association of Ontario voices grave concern over the apparent lack of post-basic courses for nurses presently employed and outlines his plan of action.

Weil, Thomas P. "80 Basic Applications for ADP Equipment," *Hospitals,* 41 (May 1, 1967), 81-89.

   Interesting listing of possibilities for using coordinated data processing in hospitals, which would improve care at the same time it reduces personnel time requirements.

—— and Henry M. Parrish. "Development of a Coordinated Approach for the Training of Allied Health Personnel," *Journal of Medical Education,* 42 (July, 1967), 651-659.

   Authors propose a core curriculum for a major portion of the first two years of all of the allied health programs — for an interdisciplinary approach and for easier transfer from one discipline to another.

Weinert, RosaLee. "Refresher Course Program in Ohio," *American Journal of Nursing,* 68 (October, 1968), 2185-2189.

   Approximately 100 RN's a year are helped to make the transition from inactive status to active practice by Ohio's continuing program of refresher courses (a cooperative effort by the ONA, OLN, Ohio Department of Health, etc.) — financed under the Manpower, Development and Training Act.

Wemett, Mary F. "Study of the Use of Films as Self-Instructional Tools," *Nursing Research,* 16 (Winter, 1967), 83.

   Article describes a study done at the University of Rochester Department of Nursing. Study supports the premise that students can learn as effectively by using the self-instructional device and, teachers' and students' time were saved.

Wesbury, Stuart A. and Michael R. Schwartz. "Three-Step Program Lets Nurses Get Back to Nursing," *Modern Hospital,* 110 (January, 1968), 85-87.

   A nurse is responsible for all aspects of nursing service, a unit manager for all aspects of supportive services — 24 hours a day!

"What Happens to the Libraries of Nursing Schools in Transition?" *Nursing Outlook*, 17 (April, 1969), 40-41.

> The results of a small survey, by letter, answers some important questions regarding nursing school libraries involved in the process of educational transition.

"What's in a Name," *The Canadian Nurse*, 64 (April, 1968), 29.

> Clinical nurse specialists' responsibilities in analysis, planning, evaluating patient care, and collaborating with other health professionals.

White, Kerr L. "Personal Incentives, Professional Standards, and Public Accountability for Health Care," *Hospitals*, 42 (July 16, 1968), 74-78.

> The author discusses shortcomings of the prevailing "systems" of health care (Regional Medical Programs and the Comprehensive Health Services Act) and proposes that hospitals, physicians, medical groups and medical centers unite as "fourth parties" — organized under the auspices of public, private and voluntary agencies for the purpose of improving and maintaining the standards, the efficiency and the scope of health care services.

"Why A Hospital Council Urged $27 Million Pay Hike," *Modern Hospital*, 110 (March, 1968), 68-70.

> The hospital council of Western Pennsylvania, using the Hay (a consulting firm) method of point values, was able to make a direct comparison of dissimilar jobs, thus establishing new salary levels: e.g. a general duty nurse should be paid the same salary as a programmer.

Wilbur, Dwight L. "Quality and Availability of Health Care Under Regional Medical Programs," *Journal of the American Medical Association*, 203 (March 11, 1968), 945-949.

> The author writes from the perspective of the development of personal health service.

———: "Total Manpower Needs and Resources — Medicine and Nursing," *Nursing Outlook*, 17 (December, 1969), 32.

> Former AMA president admonishes nurses and physicians to consider that their primary responsibility is to advocate and promote health. He discusses three alternatives for meeting increasing health care demands, the composition of the health care team, and some of the differences between the professions that cause problems in communication.

Wilson, Vernon E. "Academic and Public Agencies Work Together in Missouri Program," *Hospitals*, 42 (July 1, 1968), 56-59.

> A case study of the MRMP. The author says that RMP's can provide the impetus for cooperation between all the academic disciplines and health-oriented agencies in the effort to aid physicians in delivering the highest quality medical care, directly to the patient in his own community, if possible, and at the lowest possible cost.

Wise, Harold B., et. al. "The Family Health Worker," *American Journal of Public Health*, 58 (October, 1968), 1828-1835.

> Report of the New York program to train and employ a new health care worker. Outlines criteria for selection, job description and training. PHN in this program is responsible for preventive care of families, and coordinates health and social care.

Wolin, Richard and Vesta Phelps. "The Psychiatric Nursing Seminar," *The Journal of Nursing Education*, 7 (November, 1968), 31-33.

> At the University of Buffalo, junior level nursing students receive didactic instruction by psychiatrists. The group seminar includes students, a nurse-clinician and a psychiatrist. This teaching method is supplemented by lectures, patient experience and supervision by nursing instructors.

Woolley, Alma S. "The 'Now' Generation in Nursing," *Nursing Outlook*, 16 (March, 1968), 26-28.

> A comparison of BS programs and nursing students today with those of the '40's and '50's by an instructor who graduated from a BS program in the past and teaches in one at the present.

Woolsey, Jr., Frank M. "Albany Program Emphasizes Community Strengths, Relationships," *Hospitals* 42 (July 1, 1968), 52-55.

> A case study of the Albany RMP. Article discusses the successes and problems of the ARMP.

Wylie, Norma A. "Hospital Design is a Nursing Affair," *The Canadian Nurse*, 65 (October, 1969), 42-44.

> At this hospital, a nurse is a permanent member of the planning team, working closely with the architect and medical staff in overall planning and design of the new Health Sciences Centre.

Yankauer, Alfred, John P. Connelly and Jacob J. Feldman. "Task Performance and Task Delegation in Pediatric Office Practice," *American Journal of Public Health*, 59 (July, 1969), 1104-1107.

> This is a report of a survey of pediatricians to determine the use of allied health workers, the desire to use them, the way in which specific tasks are delegated, and factors influencing this division of labor. The implications of the findings for public health are also discussed.

Yerby, Alonzo. "Improving Care for the Disadvantaged," *American Journal of Nursing*, 68 (May, 1968), 1043-1047.

> The author outlines the components necessary in a health care system for urban communities. He stresses regional planning.

Yingling, Mildred and Ann Jumper. "Relieving Visiting Nurses of Fee Assessment," *American Journal of Nursing*, 68 (August, 1968), 1702-1704.

> Fee assessment and interpretation of Medicare benefits is done by a clerk for the Denver VNA, with savings in nurse time and in money, more accurate billing and fewer patient questions concerning finances.

Young, Lucie S. "Nursing's Challenge," *Nursing Outlook*, 17 (May, 1969), 62-65.

> Author stresses need for the nurse to be on committees within a hospital concerning patient care, architecture, etc. Also wants horizontal advancement and financial rewards.

Zimmerman, James P. "Initiating a Unit Management System," *Hospital Progress*, 49 (February, 1968), 64-66, 72.

> Utilizing a unit manager system permits the nurse to spend more time with patients. However, the author cautions that each new unit management system must meet the particular hospital's needs and each must have provision for ongoing review and change.

APPENDIX H

SITE VISIT ACTIVITIES CONDUCTED BY THE STUDY STAFF

S hortly after the study began, we submitted our initial general research proposal to a panel of consultants. This group represented medicine, nursing, health administration, economics, sociology, education, and industry. One major constructive suggestion resulting from this meeting was that more emphasis should be given to the *future* aspects of health care, nursing practice, and nursing education. A further suggestion was that one way to approach this future orientation would be to undertake a series of visits to locations where new and different practices were ongoing that involved nursing personnel.

With these suggestions at hand, and with a beginning list of possible site visits contributed by the consultants, the staff undertook an extensive literature search, one aspect of which was to identify locations where innovations in the practice or education of nurses were either currently operating or else in the advanced planning stage. Over 100 locations were identified as a result of this activity and these were submitted to the Commissioners and the nursing and health professions advisory panels for their review. Additions and deletions to the list were made by these groups.

The final result was that 143 sites were identified where innovation in nursing practice or education was occurring. Some duplication of activities was determined to exist between sites and, further, in some cases, the literature on the innovation was quite extensive and a visit was not required. Therefore, we finally arrived at a

list of 100 programs and activities, located in over 85 physical sites, which were
planned for visitation.

As each of these 100 locations was contracted, additional screening resulted
in more deletions. However, referrals resulted in some additional locations for
visiting. The final tally of our field work is shown below.

Total Sites Identified by Study Staff		143
Sites Dropped (Duplication of Activities)	22	
Sites Dropped (Covered Sufficiently in Literature)	21	
Total Sites Planned for Visitation		100
Sites Dropped (After Further Screening)	23	
Sites Added (From Referrals)	9	
Total Number of Sites Visited		86
Total Number of Programs or Projects Discussed and Observed		103
Sites Covered by Research Reports and Sufficient Literature		42
Grand Total of Field Reports		145

The staff developed an interview guide to use during these visits, a copy of
which can be found in Appendix R. The entire staff spent a week in Boston in
February 1969 during which the interview guide and staff interviewing techniques
were tested and evaluated. The Boston metropolitan area was particularly good for
field testing our instruments and methods since it provided us with 10 innovative
locations in a relatively small geographical area. As a result of that field testing,
several refinements were made in the interview guide and in the staff's approach to
interviewing which helped us immeasurably in subsequent interviews.

The major subjects covered at each site interview were: a history and
description of the program and how it differed from past practice; the personnel
involved and their function in the innovation; methods of funding and administration; evaluation procedures; and future developments expected. After returning
from a field visit each interview was written up with the subjects listed above being
highlighted. In almost every instance two staff members conducted the interview so
that the final summary of the visit was more thorough and accurate. The summaries
of these visits served as resource material to the staff during the writing of the final
report, and the development of recommendations.

Even more valuable, however, was the first-hand knowledge and experience
gained from interviewing nearly 1,000 individuals during the course of these visits.
It is impossible to measure just how much of this field work is reflected in the
final report, but there is no question that it is a significant amount. The insight into
the health care field, its problems, frustrations and accomplishments cannot
possibly be acquired through literature or hearsay. For this reason alone, these visits
were an integral part of our study.

Table H-1 is a summary listing of sites, programs, and primary contact
persons included in the field visits.

TABLE H-1. SITE VISIT DATA

Location	Site	Site Visits (Program(s) or Project(s) (Discussed and/or Observed)	Primary Personal Contact(s)
California			
Downey	Rancho Los Amigos Hospital	Liaison Nurse Project	Mrs. Barbara Madden, Director of Nursing
Los Angeles	Los Angeles City College Department of Nursing	Associate Degree Program	Mrs. Fay O. Wilson, Chairman, Department of Nursing
Oakland	Oakland Public Schools	Strengthening School Nursing Service to Improve Health Care in Economically Deprived Neighborhoods	Dr. Doris S. Bryan, Supervisor of Nursing Services
Palo Alto	Stanford University School of Nursing	Reorganization of Basic Nursing Education and Setting Up a Graduate Program	Miss Grace E. Ringressy, Director, School of Nursing Dr. John L. Wilson, Associate Dean, Stanford University School of Medicine
San Francisco	University of California School of Nursing	Major Curriculum Revision, and Initial Stages of Developing a Doctoral Program	Dr. Helen Nahm, Dean, School of Nursing
	University of California H. C. Moffitt Hospital-Medical Center	Experimental Surgical Floor Involving Clinical Nurse Specialist and Unit Manager	Mr. Harold Hixon, Hospital Administrator Miss Irma Nickerson, Director Nursing Service

TABLE H-1. SITE VISIT DATA

San Pablo	Contra Costa Community College	One of the Oldest A.D. Nursing Programs in California. Not Accredited by NLN	Mrs. Bernice H. Hunn, Director Division of Health Sciences
Colorado			
Boulder	Western Interstate Commission for Higher Education	Current Issues in Nursing	Miss Jo Eleanor Elliott, Director of Nursing Programs
Denver	Saint Luke's Hospital School of Nursing	Highly Regarded Diploma Program	Miss Lillian DeYoung, Director School of Nursing
	City and County of Denver Department of Health and Hospitals	Psychiatric Nurse in the Hospital Setting, and Public Health Nurses and Pediatric Nurse	Dr. John Sbarbaro, Medical Coordinator, Neighborhood Health Program
			Miss Mildred Yingling, Associate Director, Denver Visiting Nurse Service
	University of Colorado Medical Center	Pediatric Nurse Practitioner Program	Dr. Loretta Ford, Head of Graduate Program in Community Health
			Dr. Henry K. Silver, Professor of Pediatrics

TABLE H-1. SITE VISIT DATA

Denver (continued)	University of Colorado School of Nursing	The Rural Community Health Nurse	Mrs. Elda Popiel, Assistant Dean of Continuing Education
	Fort Logan Mental Health Center	Nurses in the Multi-Disciplinary Mental Health Team	Dr. Donald Schiff, Director Staff Development Unit
			Dr. John Aycrigg, Associate Director
			Mrs. Helen Huber, Chief Nurse
Washington, D.C.	U.S. Department of Labor	Data Collection and Studies of Health Manpower	Mr. John R. Elliott, Special Assistant, Office of the Associate Manpower Administrator
	Office of the Surgeon General, Department of the Army	Training of Enlisted Men for Medical Specialties	Lt. Colonel Reginald Loyd
	Veterans Administration	General Discussion Regarding Trends in Health Care	Dr. Harold M. Schoolman, Director of Education Service
	U.S. Office of Education, Health Occupation Education	General Background Information	Miss Helen K. Powers, Chief

TABLE H-1. SITE VISIT DATA

Washington D.C. (continued)	Veterans Administration Department of Nursing Service	Professional Standards of VA as Related to Levels of Nursing Practice	Mrs. Beatrice James, Nursing
	U.S. Office of Education	Recognition of Accrediting Agencies for Determining Eligibility for Federal Funds	Mr. John Proffitt, Director Accreditation and Institutional Eligibility Unit
			Mrs. Marcia Winder, Program Assistant
	American Association of Junior Colleges	Nursing Education in the Junior College	Dr. Kenneth G. Skaggs, Coordinator of Occupational Education Project
	Veterans Administration Management Systems Service	Ward Nursing, Staffing Criteria, and Quality Care Evaluation	Miss Verna Grovert, Senior Nurse Coordinator
	Veterans Administration Hospital	Highly Automated Hospital	Miss Kathleen McNamara, Automated Hospital Information System
Florida			
Gainesville	University of Florida College of Health Related Professions	Nursing Students Participation in the Courses of the College	Dr. Patricia Laurencelle, Liaison Between the Educational Departments of the College of Health Related Professions and the University

TABLE H-1. SITE VISIT DATA

Gainesville (continued)	University of Florida College of Nursing	Psychological Assistant Program, and the Technical and Professional Role in Nursing	Dr. Mary H. McCaulley, Assistant Professor, Department of Clinical Psychology
			Miss Marion E. McKenna, Teaching Associate and Project Director, Kellogg Project
Georgia			
Atlanta	Southern Regional Education Board	Current Issues in Nursing Program of the Nursing Education Project	Miss Helen C. Belcher, Director Nursing Education Project
	Veterans Administration Hospital	Friesen Design Hospital	Dr. John G. Hood, Director Dr. Julian Jarman, Chief of Staff
			Miss Nell Thomasson, Chief Nurse
Illinois			
Chicago	Charles F. Read Mental Health Center	Nursing Role in Crisis Clinic	Dr. Helen Sunukjian, Chief, Crisis Intervention Program
Evanston	Evanston Hospital	Triad System and the Administration of Nursing Services	Mr. John Danielson, Executive Vice President
			Miss Dorothy Johnson, Chairman, Department of Nursing

TABLE H-1. SITE VISIT DATA

Kansas

Kansas City	University of Kansas Medical Center	Nurse Clinician Program, and Development of the Nursing Clinic for Ambulatory Patient Care	Dr. Martha Pitel, Chairman

Maryland

Bethesda	Bureau of Health Professions Education and Manpower Training, Division of Nursing	Studies on Manpower Requirements in Nursing, and Studies on Costs of Nursing Education	Dr. Eugene Levine, Chief, Manpower Analysis and Resources Branch Mr. Stanley Siegel, Assistant Chief

Massachusetts

Boston	Boston University School of Nursing	Two Doctoral Programs in Nursing: 1) Nurse-Scientist, R.N. with Masters Obtain Ph.D. in Such Disciplines as Sociology and Psychology 2) Nursing Science, Ph.D. in Psychiatry	Dr. Irene Palmer, Dean
	The Children's Hospital Medical Center	Clinical Scheduling by Computer, and Hotel with a Nursing Station	Dr. Leonard W. Cronkhite, Jr., General Director
	Northeastern University College of Nursing	Nursing Education in a Cooperative Work Study Program	Mrs. Juanita O. Long, Acting Dean, College of Nursing

TABLE H-1. SITE VISIT DATA

Boston (continued)	Massachusetts General Hospital	Pediatric Nurse Practitioner, Unit Nurse Teacher, Nursing Internship Program	Dr. John Knowles, General Director Miss Mary MacDonald, Director of Nursing Dr. John Newman, Associate Hospital Administrator Miss Natalie Petzold, Director, School of Nursing
	Hospital Planning for Greater Boston, Inc.	Manpower Planning with Emphasis on Identifying Needs	Mr. John Donaher, Director
	Boston Department of Health and Hospitals, Nursing Advisory Committee	Coordination and Effective Utilization of Public Health Nursing Services	Miss Catherine M. Sullivan, Assistant Deputy Commissioner for Nursing
Cambridge	Cambridge Hospital	Planning Stage for a New Hospital School of Nursing and Its Affiliation with an Educational Facility	Dr. James B. Hartgering, Commissioner of Health, Hospitals, and Welfare for the City of Cambridge
	MIT-Harvard Joint Center for Urban Studies	Community Health Information System	Mrs. Katharine G. Bauer Research Associate
Charlestown	Bunker Hill Health Center	Community Health Center Providing Comprehensive Health Care, under Sponsorship of Massachusetts General Hospital	Miss Ruth M. Farrisey, Executive Officer of Clinics and Assistant Director of Nursing Service, Massachusetts General Hospital

TABLE H-1. SITE VISIT DATA

Location	Institution	Description	Contact
Chestnut Hill	Boston College, College of Nursing	1966-68 Nursing Home Study Funded by PHS	Miss Mary Shaughnessy, Associate Professor of Nursing
Dorchester	Columbia Point Health Center	First Neighborhood Health Center Funded under OEO (Dec. '65). Operated by Tufts University	Mrs. Joan Davidson, Assistant Director of Nursing
Greenfield	Franklin County Public Hospital	Extensive Automation of Patient Care Activities	Mr. William C. Christenson, Director
Westboro	New England Power Service Company	Utilization of Nursing Personnel in a Mobile Health Unit	Mrs. Arleen Hayes, Assistant Director of Nursing
Michigan			
Dearborn	Henry Ford Community College, Nursing Division	New Media Approaches to Nursing Education	Miss Eleanor A. Tourtillott, Coordinator of Nursing
Missouri			
Kansas City	The Children's Mercy Hospital	Pediatric Motel Hospital Complex	Mrs. Dean Cowles, Director of Nursing
	Research Hospital and Medical Center, School of Nursing	Outstanding Example of a Good Diploma Program	Mr. Robert Adams, Executive Director; Mrs. Teresa L. Mitchell, Director, School of Nursing

TABLE H-1. SITE VISIT DATA

New Jersey

Newark	Rutgers University College of Nursing	Graduate Program in Advanced Psychiatric Nursing	Dr. Hildegard E. Peplau, Professor of Psychiatric Nursing
Perth Amboy	Perth Amboy General Hospital	Nursing Utilization Study	Mr. Robert Hoyt, Director Miss Mary Konyk, Director, Nursing Service Miss Suzanne Law, Director, Nursing Education

New York

Albany	Albany Medical Center Hospital	No Problems in Nursing Student Recruitment, and Seven Day Week Hospital Service	Dr. Ferdinand Haase, Jr., Medical Director Mrs. Helen F. Middleworth, Director of Nursing Service and School of Nursing
New York	National Federation Licensed Practical Nurses	Role of the LPN in the Delivery of Health Care	Mrs. Etta Schmidt, Executive Secretary
	National Association for Practical Nurse Education and Service	Role of the LPN in the Delivery of Health Care	Miss Rose G. Martin, Executive Director
	American Association of Industrial Nurses, Inc.	General Data Collection Regarding Nurses in the Industrial Setting	Miss Helen C. Rush, Executive Director

TABLE H-1. SITE VISIT DATA

New York (continued)		
Cornell University— New York Hospital School of Nursing	Role of Nurse in Health Maintenance Service Project and Use of Clinical Nurse Specialists	Dr. Ruth Kelly, Associate Dean Dr. Laura L. Simms, Head, Surgical Nursing Mrs. Mamie Wang, Outpatient Nursing Department
New York Medical College, Graduate School of Nursing	Nurse Generalist Program at the Graduate Level, Clinical Specialty Program in Neurological and Neurosurgical, and Master of Science in Maternity Nursing and Infant Health	Dr. Frances Reiter, Dean
Bronx Community College, Nursing Center	Use of Television in a Clinical Setting, and Success in Attracting and Retaining Minority Group Students	Dr. Beatrice Perlmutter, Chairman, Department of Nursing
Roosevelt Hospital	Hospital Involvement in Community Projects	Mr. Peter Terenzio, Executive Vice President
Montefiore Hospital and Medical Center Montefiore-Morrisania-Martin Luther King Community Center	Orientation Programs for New Staff Nurses Expanded Role of Public Health Nurse	Miss Catheryn Welch, Director Inservice Education Miss Chris Barth, Public Health Nurse
Albert Einstein College of Medicine, Lincoln Hospital	Health Careers Program	Dr. Tom Levin, Assistant Professor of Psychiatry and Community Health

TABLE H-1. SITE VISIT DATA

New York (continued)	Montefiore Hospital Loeb Center for Nursing and Rehabilitation	The R. N. Totally Responsible for all Patient Care	Miss Genrose Alfano, Director Loeb Center
	Visiting Nurse Service of New York	Proposed Expanded Services That Would Affect Nurse Role	Mrs. Eva M. Reese, Executive Director
	New York University, School of Nursing	Doctoral (Ph.D.) Program in Nursing	Dr. Martha E. Rogers, Head Division of Nurse Education
	Helene Fuld School of Nursing of the Hospital for Joint Diseases and Medical Center	An Experimental Program for LPN's To Become R.N.'s in 15 Months	Miss Justine Hannan, Director of Nursing and Nursing Education
	Western Electric Corp.	Delivery of Individual Comprehensive Health Care in the Occupational Setting	Miss Jeanne Healy, Nursing Service Director
	New York City Department of Health - Bureau of Public Health Nursing	Utilization of Nursing Personnel in School Health Programs	Miss Margaret J. O'Brien, Associate Director
	Beth Israel Medical Center, Gouverneur Health Services Program	Social Health Worker in a Comprehensive Community Health Setting	Dr. Anthony Kovner, Associate Director
	National League for Nursing	Aspects of Practical Nursing - Practice and Education	Mrs. Margery Low, Executive Secretary, Council of Practical Nurse Education

TABLE H-1. SITE VISIT DATA

New York (continued)	Beth Israel Medical Center - Beth Israel Hospital	Graduate Nurse Refresher Program	Mrs. Rose Muscatine Hauer, Director of Nursing Service and School of Nursing
Rochester	Eastman Kodak Company	Nursing's Role in Industrial Health Care	Dr. William L. Sutton, Corporate Medical Director
	Rochester General Hospital	Mental Health Center, Overview of Nursing Service Administration	Mrs. Marguerite Koderl, Director of Nursing Services
	Rochester State Hospital	Observation of Nursing Role in a Psychiatric Hospital	Miss Ruth Lewis, Chief, Nursing Services
	Strong Memorial Hospital and The University of Rochester Department of Nursing	Major Resource Institution for Study Staff	Mrs. Betty Deffenbaugh, Acting Director of Nursing Service Miss Eleanor Hall, Chairman, Department of Nursing
	Genesee Region Health Planning Council	Delivery of Health Care in an Eleven County Area	Mr. Walter Wenkert, Director
Troy	Russell Sage College Department of Nursing	Classical Nursing Education Program	Dr. Evelyn Elwood, Director of Masters Program Miss Marjory Keenan, Associate Professor, Medical-Surgical Nursing Miss Rosalind Wang, Associate Professor, Maternal and Child Health

TABLE H-1. SITE VISIT DATA

North Carolina

City	Institution	Description	Contact
Charlotte	Charlotte Memorial Hospital	Centralized Computer-Nursing Services, and Unique Concept in Outpatient Services	Mr. John W. Rankin, Director Mr. Eugene J. Smith, Director of Nursing
Durham	Duke University Medical Center	Physician's Assistant Program	Dr. D. Robert Howard, Director, Physician's Assistant Program
Raleigh	North Carolina State Board of Health	Community Health Aides for Rural Areas	Dr. W. Burns Jones, Jr., Assistant State Health Director

Ohio

City	Institution	Description	Contact
Cleveland	Case Western Reserve - Frances Payne Bolton School of Nursing	Joint Appointment in Nursing Education and Nursing Service and Extensive Ongoing Research in Nursing	Dr. Rozella M. Schlotfeldt, Dean Dr. Jannetta MacPhail, Director, Nursing Demonstration Project
Columbus	Ohio State University	Hospital Systems Research Group	Mr. Daniel Howland, Professor in Business Organization

Pennsylvania

City	Institution	Description	Contact
Hershey	The Milton S. Hershey Medical Center	Nursing Functions in Department of Family and Community Medicine	Mr. John Russell, Hospital Administrator
Philadelphia	Pennsylvania Hospital School of Nursing	Male Students in a School of Nursing	Dr. S. F. Mannino, Director

TABLE H-1. SITE VISIT DATA

Tennessee

Nashville
Vanderbilt University School of Nursing — A Patient Care Model Unit, Major Revision in Baccalaureate Curriculum and New Graduate Program in Medical and Surgical Nursing — Dr. Luther Christman, Dean; Mrs. Sara Archer, Director of Graduate Program in Medical and Surgical Nursing

Veterans Administration Hospital — Center for Excellence in Nursing — Dr. William S. Coppage, Jr., Chief of Staff; Miss Margaret Buchanan, Associate Chief, Nursing Service

Virginia

Alexandria
American Association of Medical Clinics — General Data Collection, Nursing in the Medical Clinic Setting — Dr. Edward M. Wurzel, Director

Washington

Seattle
University of Washington School of Nursing — Evaluation of Video Tapes in Nursing Education — Dr. Madeleine Leininger, Dean; Mrs. Stella Hay, Associate Professor and Project Director of Videotapes in Nursing

University of Washington Hospital — Extensive Use of Clinical Specialists and Team Leader Nursing Project — Mrs. Ruth Fine, Director, Nursing Service

The Children's Orthopedic Hospital and Medical Center — A Program for Training Inactive Nurses as Pediatric Assistants — Dr. Abraham B. Bergman, Director of Outpatient Services

APPENDIX I

THE MEASUREMENT AND EVALUATION OF STUDENT AND FACULTY PERCEPTIONS OF NURSING EDUCATION ENVIRONMENTS: A SUMMARY REPORT*

Recent statements by authorities in the field of health care and by representatives of the nursing profession (U. S. P. H. S. No. 992, 1963; ANA Committee on Education, 1965) have stressed a clear distinction between the levels of competency expected of the graduates of the three types of nursing education programs. These statements have found widespread acceptance and have resulted in policy changes in the recruitment and advancement of practicing nurses by employing agencies (Report of The Committee on Nursing, 1969, p. 4) and in a decline in the number of nursing education programs which grant a diploma (ANA 1968). The statements assert that the graduates of four-year baccalaureate nursing programs are professionally qualified for leadership roles in the practice of nursing, and that graduates of two-year associate degree programs, or three-year diploma programs are technically qualified for staff nursing duties. These differences in nursing competency are founded upon the assumption of differences in the quality, structure, and environment of the different nursing programs.

The fundamental purpose of this study was to investigate and compare six selected dimensions of the environments of nursing schools as perceived by nursing students and faculty to determine whether such differences can be empirically demonstrated. The environmental dimensions examined were defined by the six factors in the Medical School Environment Inventory (MSEI) (Hutchins 1962; Hutchins and Nonneman 1966). The data of the study consisted of the responses

*This appendix and related research are the work of William R. Johnson in partial completion of requirements for a doctoral degree in education at the University of Rochester, 1970.

287

of senior students and faculty members of a national sample of 212 nursing schools under study by the National Commission for the Study of Nursing and Nursing Education. These responses were examined to determine the differences between the perceived environments of the three types of nursing schools.

Questions and Hypotheses

In this study, a single basic question was asked. Do the environments of associate degree schools (AD), diploma schools (DI), and baccalaureate degree schools (DE) differ sufficiently to be distinguishable through the perceptions of graduating students and faculty members? The question was answered by testing several null hypotheses which distinguish between the perceptions of individuals, disregarding their association with specific schools, and the perceptions of school environments, independently of the perception of individuals.

Limitations and Significance

It was recognized that the findings of this study are limited to the data produced by the instrument used to measure perceptions of the nursing school environment. It was assumed that this instrument was a valid tool for the measurement of meaningful differences between nursing school environments. Interpretation of the results of this study was limited to the portion of all possible perceptions of school environments represented by the data. Other, possibly more meaningful dimensions of comparison undoubtedly exist.

Although care was taken to insure representativeness in the sample of schools used in this study, it was recognized that the sample was not perfect in this respect. The sample was somewhat less representative of smaller schools than was desired. The sample of responding students and faculty was also subject to the loss of data due to non-response. These factors limited but did not necessarily invalidate generalizations which were made from the data.

The significance of this study is found in the unsubstantiated differences between the three basic nursing programs presently assumed by those charting the future growth of the nursing profession. These assumptions have led to proposals of fundamental change in the structure of the nursing profession, and the relationships of the basic nursing education programs. Substantiation of the existence of these differences is of vital importance to the charting of realistic policies and practices within the nursing community. An accurate description of the present parameters of similarities and differences between the three programs of nursing education is the only basis for appropriate planning.

Studies which measure the differences between types of nursing education programs by means of the perception of the nursing school environment are rare. While most of the studies which have been completed have also been limited, either in scope or content, in respect to the objectives of this study, the predominant impression is that of little differentiation between the types of nursing education investigated. When differences have been noted, they have been contradictory, or contrary to the differences anticipated by the authors. Taken together, these studies illustrate a need for a comprehensive, in-depth study of the differences and similarities of the three types of nursing education, with particular emphasis on the consequences for the students.

BACKGROUND OF THE INSTRUMENT

The Medical School Environment Inventory (MSEI) was constructed by Dr. Edwin B. Hutchins* while he was associated with the Association of American Medical Colleges. The MSEI was chosen as the basic instrument for this study after determining that it was the only instrument designed to measure a medically oriented educational environment (Lysaught, 1969). The items of the MSEI were of sufficient generality to require only minor changes for use with schools of nursing. The revised MSEI was called the Nursing School Environment Inventory (NSEI).

Dr. Hutchins adapted the items of original version of the MSEI from the Stern and Pace College Characteristics Index (CCI), (Pace and Stern, 1957). Interest in the interaction process approach to the measurement of student environment is reflected in the work of several researchers: Pace and Stern, 1958; Nunnally and Thistlewaite, 1963; Thistlewaite, 1963; Astin, 1963; and Halpin and Croft, 1963.

The original version of the MSEI (Hutchins, 1961) consisted of 180 items divided arbitrarily into 18 ten-item scales. This prototype was administered to 1901 entering freshmen from 25 medical school participants in the American Association of Medical Colleges Longitudinal Study. The instrument was found to measure differences between schools effectively. Subsequent factor analysis (Hutchins and Wolins, 1963) reduced the NSEI to 69 items arranged in six empirical factors.

The first factor was called General Esteem (GE). It appeared to be a general factor, and was composed of statements of a clear-cut good or bad nature.

The second factor was labeled Academic Interest and Enthusiasm (AE). Its high end described an environment where students seek academic excellence, and the faculty is enthusiastic about subject matter.

Factor three was called Extrinsic Motivation (EM). The high end of this factor described an environment where discipline is strict. There is faculty pressure to achieve, students are closely supervised by faculty, and encouraged to work together to avoid clinical mistakes. Formal group structure among students operates to inhibit hostilities. A climate of external motivational pressure is suggested.

Factor four was called Breadth of Interest (BI). The high end of this scale described an environment in which students and faculty share interests beyond the boundaries of medicine, in the philosophy of science, behavioral sciences and social activities.

* Dr. Hutchins, who is presently associated with the University of Iowa, has given his permission to use his instrument in this study.

Factor five was called Intrinsic Motivation (IM). The high end of this scale described an environment in which students are not pressured into achieving or conforming. They behave and are treated like adults. They do not study together, or engage in hazing or teasing. Individual pursuit of knowledge is encouraged.

The sixth and final factor was called Encapsulated Training (ET). The high end of this scale described an environment where instruction is well organized, with little divergence from a prescribed curriculum, and generally deals with facts rather than generalizations or abstractions.

The construct validity of the MSEI has been reported in a study by Hutchins and Nonneman (1966) in which a five year longitudinal sample was used to calculate test-retest reliabilities for all six scales. The between schools reliabilities, based on school means, ranged from 0.98 for IM to 0.76 for EM. The reliabilities reported were quite adequate, indicating a stable ordering of schools on all six factors.

The Sample of Schools

The objective of the NCSNNE in the selection of schools sample was to construct the sample so as to maintain representativeness by school type and geographic region. The nine regional divisions of the ANA, provided the geographic sampling units for the selection of schools. It was arbitrarily decided that 25 percent of the AD and DE schools from each region would be chosen. Because they were more numerous, a sample of 20 percent of the DI schools of each region was deemed sufficient.

Original Sample of Schools

The NCSNNE obtained a list of 253 nursing schools compiled in 1961 for use of a sample in the NLN Nurse Career Pattern Study (NLN, Unpublished). This list had been constructed by random assignment from a list of all nursing schools known to exist in 1961. The NLN sample was found to be satisfactory when tested for representativeness (Tate, 1969).

Revised Sample

The NCSNNE modified the NLN sample, adding and deleting schools to compensate for those which has ceased to exist, or were known to be unwilling to participate in the NCSNNE study, and to achieve the proportionate regional representation considered desirable for this study. An attempt was made to balance additions and deletions in respect to the school characteristics of the original NLN sample as much as possible.

The revised version of the NLN sample consisted of 283 schools of nursing, of which 194, or 75.6 percent, had been retained from the original sample. The revised sample could not be considered a wholly random sample, although the revisions had increased regional representativeness.

The revised version of the NLN sample constituted the sample of schools contacted by the NCSNNE for participation in this study of nursing school environments.

Final Sample

The final sample of schools consisted of those schools from the revised sample which actually contributed data to the study. Of the 283 schools of nursing contacted by the NCSNNE, 212, or 74.9 percent ultimately returned usable data. Further analysis revealed that the final sample did not represent each ANA region equally, although the national sample was found to be adequate. As a result, inter-regional comparisons were not made.

It was also found that individual senior and faculty response was subject to the attrition due to non-response typical of surveys employing the mailed questionnaire technique (Kerlinger, 1965, p. 397). As a whole, the sample suffered a loss of approximately 50 percent due to the non-response of individuals.

In all, 1789 faculty members, and 5267 senior nursing students returned usable data.

Statistical Procedures

Since the objective of this study was to demonstrate the presence or absence of meaningful differences between the environments of the three types of nursing schools, and to demonstrate something of the quality of the differences between them, it was decided that meaningful differences would be evident on a nationwide basis, and that these differences should be large enough to have obvious consequences in the determination of the characteristics of the school's graduates. To this end, both descriptive statistics, and inferential techniques were chosen for analysis of the data.

The descriptive techniques used consisted of a direct comparison of the ranges, means, medians, and standard deviations of each of the score distributions for each factor of the NSEI, analyzed by school type, and respondent category — i.e. senior students and faculty.

Inferential technique consisted of analysis of variance of each group of factor scores, and the direct application of T tests between appropriate pairs of contrasting groups. Significant differences determined by appropriate F ratios, in which Ho was rejected at the 0.05 level of probability, were examined for their meaning.

Each NSEI factor was treated as a separate variable, with comparisons made between each sample group on each factor separately. No comparisons between different factor scores were attempted.

The data was divided into two sets, one consisting of the scores of individuals, disregarding the specific school, the others consisting of mean scores for each participating school. In the first set the individual was thus the measured unit, in the second set, the school became the measured unit. This study was primarily concerned with the school means, although the factor scores of individuals were also examined.

Analysis of the Data

In this section, the results of six analyses of variance and 54 T tests are reported.

Each analysis of variance tested the general null hypothesis of no differences on each of the six NSEI factor scores for faculty members and senior students compared within and between each of the three basic types of nursing schools. Each of the T statistics tests a specific null hypothesis of no difference between each of the pairs of faculty and senior student groups between and within the three basic types of nursing schools for each of the six factors of the NSEI.

Both individual and school mean scores were used as the measured unit. The differences between the distributions of individual scores and school means were expressed largely as increased variance and range for the individual scores. The means of these two sets of distributions are not meaningfully different. For this reason, as well as the fact that the school was the principal focus of this investigation, the school means are examined here. The specific null hypotheses to be examined were:

1. There are no differences among the school environments of each of the three basic nursing programs as measured by the perceptions of the faculty members of each school.

2. There are no differences among the school environments of each of the three basic nursing programs as measured by the perceptions of the senior students of each school.

3. There are no differences within each of the three basic nursing programs between the school environment as measured by the perceptions of faculty members of each school and as measured by the perceptions of the senior students of each school.

Analyses of Variance

Tables I-1 through I-6 present the data and results of six analyses of variance performed for each NSEI factor.

Each of the reported F ratios tests a hypothesis which must be explicitly expressed, each hypothesis being related to the general hypotheses of this study. The row, or Faculty-Student F ratios compare the differences between senior students and faculty members, disregarding the distinction between school types. The column, or Schools F ratios compare the differences between the three types of nursing schools, disregarding the distinctions between faculty and students. The Interaction F ratio tests the existence of systematic differences among each of the cells of the analysis of variance table which are not accounted for in the row and column comparisons.

Results Based On School Mean Factor Scores

Tables I-1 through I-6 present data and analyses based on the mean factor scores for senior students and for faculty members for each school in the sample. Two mean scores for each school on each NSEI factor are reported. This data reduction removed the variance caused by individual differences. The remaining variance in school means can more definitely be assigned to actual differences between school environments rather than differences between individual perceptions of these environments.

The explicit null hypotheses tested by the analyses of variance of the school mean factor scores were as follows:

1. There are no differences between the environments of all types of nursing schools for faculty and senior students as measured by the perceptions of each group. (Ho Faculty-Student)

2. There are no differences among the environments of each of the three basic types of nursing schools, as measured by the combined perceptions of both faculty members and senior students of each school. (Ho Schools)

3. There are no differences between and among the environments of the three basic types of nursing schools as measured separately by the perceptions of the faculty members of each school and the senior students of each school. (Ho Interaction)

The results of the analysis of variance of the school mean factor scores for the NSEI factor *General Esteem* are presented in Table I-1.

The factor *General Esteem* measures the clearly good and bad things about the nursing school environment, exemplified by cordial faculty student relationships, a regard for intellectual pursuits, a valued curriculum, and an institutional concern for the student and her problems.

The environment is appreciably better for faculty members, with a row mean factor score of 57.67, than for senior students, with a row mean factor score of 54.81. Column means suggest that AD schools possess environments characterized by greater esteem than those of DE and DI schools, with means of 58.10, 57.01, and 55.10 respectively. The small, but significant F for interaction effects suggests that further differences exist between the subgroups.

The results of the analysis of variance for the school mean factor scores for the NSEI factor *Academic Enthusiasm* are presented in Table I-2.

TABLE I-1. ANALYSIS OF VARIANCE OF SCHOOL MEAN NSEI FACTOR SCORES FOR THE FACTOR *GENERAL ESTEEM*

Mean Factor Scores of Students and Faculty, Classified by School Types

	AD		DI		DE		Row Summary	
	Mean	N	Mean	N	Mean	N	Mean	N
Faculty	55.556	50	56.955	107	58.410	44	57.672	201
Student	57.651	51	53.153	111	55.666	46	54.812	208
Column Summary	58.099	101	55.091	218	57.008	90		

Analysis of Variance Table for NSEI Factor Scores For Students, Faculty, and School Types

Source of Variation	Sums of Squares	Degrees of Freedom	Mean Square	F
Faculty-Student	541.9783	1	541.9783	28.7995[a]
School Types	561.0733	2	280.5367	14.9071[a]
Interaction	125.9336	2	62.9668	3.3459[c]
Within	7584.0547	403	18.8190	

a = Significant at or beyond the 0.001 level.
b = Significant at or beyond the 0.01 level.
c = Significant at or beyond the 0.05 level.

TABLE I-2. ANALYSIS OF VARIANCE OF SCHOOL MEAN NSEI FACTOR SCORES FOR THE FACTOR *ACADEMIC ENTHUSIASM*

Mean Factor Scores of Students and Faculty, Classified by School Types

	AD		DI		DE		Row Summary	
	Mean	*N*	*Mean*	*N*	*Mean*	*N*	*Mean*	*N*
Faculty	30.432	50	30.122	107	31.356	44	30.469	201
Student	30.678	51	29.160	111	29.796	46	29.673	208
Column Summary	50.556	101	29.632	218	30.559	90		

Analysis of Variance Table for NSEI Factor Scores For Students, Faculty, and School Types

Source of Variation	*Sums of Squares*	*Degrees of Freedom*	*Mean Square*	*F*
Faculty - Student	50.5612	1	50.5612	10.4233[a]
School Type	66.7708	2	33.3834	6.8825[b]
Interaction	49.5417	2	24.7709	5.1066[b]
Within	1954.8617	403	4.8508	

a = Significant at or beyond the 0.001 level.
b = Significant at or beyond the 0.01 level.
c = Significant at or beyond the 0.05 level.

The factor *Academic Enthusiasm* measures perceptions of a nursing school environment characterized by active student competition, interested and enthusiastic instructors, and an emphasis on fundamental theory in course work.

The results of the analysis of variance suggest the nursing school environment differs for faculty members and senior students. The environment is appreciably more oriented toward enthusiasm for academic matters for faculty, with a row mean factor score of 30.47, than for senior students, with a row mean of 29.67. Column means suggest that AD and DE school environments are equally characterized by this quality, both having means of 30.56. DI school environments are characterized less by this quality, with a mean of 29.63. The significant F for interaction suggests that small systematic differences exist between the subgroups.

The results of the analysis of variance for the school mean factor scores for the NSEI factor *Extrinsic Motivation* are presented in Table I-3.

The factor *Extrinsic Motivation* measures aspects of the nursing school environment related to pressures for group conformance to prescribed norms of behavior. Such perceived phenomena as strict enforcement of rules, faculty intolerance of mediocrity, strong student leadership, and a reliance of students on group consensus for standards of behavior, contribute to high scores on this factor.

The results of the analysis of variance suggest that the nursing school environment is the same for both faculty members and for senior nursing students, with row mean factor scores of 29.21 and 29.18 respectively. The environments of DI schools are more oriented to the characteristics of *Extrinsic Motivation* than the environments of AD and DE schools, with column mean factor scores of 29.48, 28.93, and 28.80 respectively. The non-significant F for interaction suggests that the differences between the subgroups can be attributed to environmental differences within the schools common to both students and faculty.

The results of the analysis of variance of the school mean factor scores for the NSEI factor *Breadth of Interest* are presented in Table I-4.

The factor *Breadth of Interest* measures the tendency for a school environment to reflect interests beyond the boundaries of nursing. Since more than half of the items of this scale were negatively weighted, a high score required the respondent to disagree with the items. The environment is perceived as *not* being characterized by students who are concerned only with the work at hand, or by little faculty concern for the humanities and the broader social implications of nursing.

The results of the analysis of variance suggest that the nursing school environment for faculty members differs from the environment for senior students, reflecting a greater interest in non-nursing activities for faculty members, with row mean factor scores of 16.80 and 15.55 respectively. The environment of DE schools reflect wider interests than the environments of AD and DI schools, with column mean factor scores of 17.23, 16.47, and 15.57, respectively. The non-significant F for interaction suggests that the differences between student and faculty environments is consistent among school types.

TABLE I-3. ANALYSIS OF VARIANCE OF SCHOOL MEAN NSEI FACTOR SCORES FOR THE FACTOR *EXTRINSIC MOTIVATION*

Mean Factor Scores of Students and Faculty, Classified by School Types

	AD Mean	N	DI Mean	N	DE Mean	N	Row Summary Mean	N
Faculty	28.955	50	29.559	107	28.664	44	29.213	201
Student	28.905	51	29.411	111	28.934	46	29.181	208
Column Summary	28.930	101	29.484	218	28.802	90		

Analysis of Variance Table for NSEI Factor Scores For Students, Faculty, and School Types

Source of Variation	Sums of Squares	Degrees of Freedom	Mean Square	F
Faculty - Student	0.0516	1	0.0516	0.0179^{ns}
School Type	31.0798	2	15.5399	5.3891^{b}
Interaction	2.7899	2	1.3950	0.4838^{ns}
Within	1162.0859	403	2.8836	

a = Significant at or beyond the 0.001 level.
b = Significant at or beyond the 0.01 level.
c = Significant at or beyond the 0.05 level.

TABLE I-4. ANALYSIS OF VARIANCE OF SCHOOL MEAN NSEI FACTOR SCORES FOR THE FACTOR *BREADTH OF INTEREST*

Mean Factor Scores of Students and Faculty, Classified by School Types

	AD		DI		DE		Row Summary	
	Mean	*N*	*Mean*	*N*	*Mean*	*N*	*Mean*	*N*
Faculty	16.805	50	16.376	107	17.816	44	16.798	201
Student	16.150	51	14.801	111	16.675	46	15.546	208
Column Summary	16.474	101	15.574	218	17.233	90		

Analysis of Variance Table for NSEI Factor Scores For Students, Faculty, and School Types

Source of Variation	*Sums of Squares*	*Degrees of Freedom*	*Mean Square*	*F*
Faculty - Student	111.0011	1	111.0011	24.0979^a
School Type	161.1143	2	80.5572	17.4886^a
Interaction	12.3888	2	6.1929	1.3445^{ns}
Within	1856.3248	403	4.6063	

a = Significant at or beyond the 0.001 level.
b = Significant at or beyond the 0.01 level.
c = Significant at or beyond the 0.05 level.

The results of the analysis of variance of the school mean factor scores for the NSEI factor *Intrinsic Motivation* are presented in Table I-5.

The factor *Intrinsic Motivation* is defined by items which describe an environment in which students are not pressured into achieving or conforming. Seven of the nine items of the scale were weighted negatively, requiring high-scoring respondents to disagree with the items. The environment is perceived as *not* being characterized by frequent, unannounced examinations, hazing, teasing or practical joking, and the assignment of seats in lecture rooms.

The results of the analysis of variance suggest that the nursing school environment for faculty members differs from the environment experienced by senior students. Faculty members appear to experience less pressure to achieve or conform than senior students, with row mean factor scores of 16.27 and 15.68 respectively. The column means suggest that DE school environments are characterized by the least pressure for achievement or conformity, followed by AD and DI schools with mean factor scores of 17.61, 16.18, and 15.19, respectively. The non-significant F for interaction suggests that the differences for faculty members and senior students are consistent between school types.

The results of the analysis of variance of the school mean factor scores for the NSEI factor *Encapsulated Training* are presented in Table I-6.

The results of the analysis of variance suggest that the nursing school environment of faculty members is more characterized by prescribed instructional procedures than the school environments of senior students. The respective row means are 19.85 and 17.97. The column means suggest that AD school environments are more characterized by prescribed instructional procedures than DI and DE schools, with factor means of 19.53, 19.14, and 17.56 respectively. The non-significant F for interaction suggests that the student-faculty environmental differences are stable between the three types of nursing schools.

T Tests

The data and analyses presented in Tables I-7 through I-12 relate to the general hypotheses posed at the beginning of this section. These hypotheses are tested by a series of T statistics which compare pairs of means of the six groups of the sample population for each of the NSEI factors.

While the analyses of variance reported allowed gross comparisons between students and faculty, as well as between the school types, the T statistic tests the significance of differences between specific subgroups. The results of these comparisons also allow a meaningful ordering of the mean factor scores in terms of their real or significant differences.

Each mean comparison is related to a separate null hypothesis, just as every F ratio was related to a specific null hypothesis. There is a close relationship between the null hypotheses of the analyses of variance and those associated with each T

TABLE I-5. ANALYSIS OF VARIANCE OF SCHOOL MEAN NSEI FACTOR SCORES FOR THE FACTOR *INTRINSIC MOTIVATION*

Mean Factor Scores of Student and Faculty, Classified by School Types

	AD		DI		DE		Row Summary	
	Mean	N	Mean	N	Mean	N	Mean	N
Faculty	16.395	50	15.648	107	17.625	44	16.267	201
Student	15.978	51	14.755	111	17.590	46	15.684	208
Column Summary	16.184	101	15.193	218	17.607	90		

Analysis of Variance Table for NSEI Factor Scores For Students, Faculty, and School Types

Source of Variation	Sums of Squares	Degrees of Freedom	Mean Square	F
Faculty - Student	17.6709	1	17.6709	6.0079^{c}
School Type	342.6882	2	171.3440	58.2546^{a}
Interaction	10.8279	2	5.4140	1.8407^{ns}
Within	1185.3427	403	2.9413	

a = Significant at or beyond the 0.001 level.
b = Significant at or beyond the 0.01 level.
c = Significant at or beyond the 0.05 level.

TABLE I-6. ANALYSIS OF VARIANCE OF SCHOOL MEAN NSEI FACTOR SCORES FOR THE FACTOR *ENCAPSULATED TRAINING*

Mean Factor Scores of Students and Faculty,
Classified by School Types

	AD		DI		DE		Row Summary	
	Mean	N	Mean	N	Mean	N	Mean	N
Faculty	20.114	50	20.237	107	18.587	44	19.853	201
Student	18.963	51	18.081	111	16.582	46	17.966	208
Column Summary	19.533	101	19.139	118	17.562	90		

Analysis of Variance Table for NSEI Factor Scores
For Students, Faculty, and School Types

Source of Variation	Sums of Squares	Degrees of Freedom	Mean Squares	F
Faculty - Student	275.5541	1	275.5541	94.3164[a]
School Type	251.5775	2	125.7888	43.0548[a]
Interaction	17.2116	2	8.6058	2.9456[ns]
Within	1178.4023	403	2.9216	

a = Significant at or beyond the 0.001 level.
b = Significant at or beyond the 0.01 level.
c = Significant at or beyond the 0.05 level.

test. Ho Faculty-Student under the conditions of the T tests, is resolved into three separate null hypotheses: Ho AD Faculty-Student; Ho DI Faculty-Student; and Ho DE Faculty-Student. Similarly, Ho Schools is resolved into six null hypotheses: Ho Student AD-DI; Ho Student AD-DE; Ho Student DI-DE; Ho Faculty AD-DI; Ho Faculty AD-DE; and Ho Faculty DI-DE. Ho Interaction is not related to the T tests reported here, since comparisons of senior student-faculty differences between different school types does not correspond to the actual organization of nursing schools.

The F ratios also have statistical relationships to the T statistics reported here. Significant T statistics associated with non-significant F ratios are suspect as chance events, because of the large number of T statistics and F ratios being calculated.

Results Based On School Mean Factor Scores

Tables 1-7 through 1-12 present data and results based on the mean factor scores for each school in the sample for faculty members and senior students. The school mean scores are considered as measurements of the environments of the schools rather than the perceptions of the individual inhabitants of the schools.

The explicit null hypotheses under examination when using the school as the measured unit are as follows:

1. There is no difference between the nursing school environments of AD faculty members and AD senior students.

2. There is no difference between the nursing school environments of DI faculty members and DI senior students.

3. There is no difference between the nursing school environments of DE faculty members and DE senior students.

4. There is no difference between the nursing school environments of AD faculty members and DI faculty members.

5. There is no difference between the nursing school environments of AD faculty members and DE faculty members.

6. There is no difference between the nursing school environments of DI faculty members and DE faculty members.

7. There is no difference between the nursing school environments of AD senior students and DI senior students.

8. There is no difference between the nursing school environments of AD senior students and DE senior students.

9. There is no difference between the nursing school environments of DI senior students and DE senior students.

The data and results of the T tests for the significance of the differences between the mean school scores for the NSEI factor *General Esteem* are presented in Table I-7.

The NSEI factor *General Esteem* measures the clearly good and bad things about the nursing school environment.

TABLE I-7. T-TEST COMPARISONS OF MEANS OF NURSING SCHOOL MEAN NSEI FAC-
TOR SCORES AMONG AND BETWEEN STUDENT AND FACULTY GROUPS FROM AD,DI,
DE SCHOOLS FOR THE FACTOR *GENERAL ESTEEM*

	Means, Standard Deviations, and Standard Error of Mean			
		AD	*DI*	*DE*
Faculty	N	50	107	44
	Mean	58.5557	56.9555	58.4103
	Std. Dev.	4.7432	4.3909	3.9710
	Std. Error	0.6776	0.4265	0.5986
Students	N	51	111	46
	Mean	57.6511	53.1532	55.6664
	Std. Dev.	3.6501	4.4673	4.1904
	Std. Error	0.5162	0.4259	0.6247

T-Tests

Comparison Groups		*Standard Error of Difference*	*T-Statistic*	*Degrees of Freedom*	*Probability*
AD	Faculty-Student	0.8946	1.0647	99	0.2896^{ns}
DI	Faculty-Student	0.6029	6.3062	216	0.0000
DE	Faculty-Student	0.8710	3.1501	88	0.0022
Faculty	AD-DI	0.7769	2.0598	155	0.0419
	AD-DE	0.9191	0.1583	92	0.8746^{ns}
	DE-DI	0.7703	−1.8885	149	0.0609^{ns}
Student	AD-DI	0.7195	6.2511	160	0.0000
	AD-DE	0.8045	2.4669	95	0.0154
	DE-DI	0.7744	−3.2455	155	0.0014

The environments of AD schools, as measured by the factor *General Esteem* are the same for senior students and faculty members. Senior students of DI schools experience an environment significantly less characterized by the qualities of *General Esteem* than that experienced by faculty members. Similar differences in environment, as measured by *General Esteem*, exist for senior students and faculty members of DE schools.

TABLE I-8. T-TEST COMPARISONS OF MEANS OF NURSING SCHOOL MEAN NSEI
FACTOR SCORES AMONG AND BETWEEN STUDENT AND FACULTY GROUPS FROM
AD, DI, DE SCHOOLS, FOR THE FACTOR *ACADEMIC ENTHUSIASM*

Means, Standard Deviations, and Standard Error of Mean				
		AD	*DI*	*DE*
Faculty	N	50	107	44
	Mean	30.4325	30.1219	31.3558
	Std. Dev.	2.5429	2.4402	2.2693
	Std. Error	0.3633	0.2370	0.3421
Students	N	51	111	46
	Mean	30.6781	29.1604	29.7960
	Std. Dev.	1.7134	2.0933	1.6918
	Std. Error	0.2423	0.1996	0.2522

T-Tests

Comparison Groups		*Standard Error of Difference*	*T-Statistic*	*Degrees of Freedom*	*Probabilty*
AD	Faculty-Student	0.4350	−0.5646	99	0.5737^{ns}
DI	Faculty-Student	0.3090	3.1119	216	0.0021
DE	Faculty-Student	0.4255	3.6660	88	0.0004
Faculty					
	AD-DI	0.4264	0.7283	155	0.4676^{ns}
	AD-DE	0.5054	−1.8271	92	0.0709^{ns}
	DE-DI	0.4312	−2.8616	149	0.0048
Student					
	AD-DI	0.3373	4.4994	160	0.0000
	AD-DE	0.3500	2.5205	95	0.0134
	DE-DI	0.3502	−1.8153	155	0.0714^{ns}

Faculty members of DI schools experience an environment less characterized by *General Esteem* than that of AD faculty members. The environments of AD faculty members and DE faculty members are similar in respect to these characteristics, while DI faculty environment is least characterized by these qualities.

TABLE I-9. T-TEST COMPARISONS OF MEANS OF NURSING SCHOOL MEAN NSEI FAC-
TOR SCORES AMONG AND BETWEEN STUDENT AND FACULTY GROUPS FROM AD,
DI, DE SCHOOLS, FOR THE FACTOR *EXTRINSIC MOTIVATION*

		Means, Standard Deviations, and Standard Error of Mean		
		AD	DI	DE
Faculty	N	50	107	44
	Mean	28.9548	29.5589	28.6642
	Std. Dev.	2.0920	1.6958	1.4068
	Std. Error	0.2988	0.1647	0.2121
Students	N	51	111	46
	Mean	29.9049	29.4112	28.9341
	Std. Dev.	1.6566	1.6432	1.5382
	Std. Error	0.2343	0.1567	0.2293

T-Tests

Comparison Groups		*Standard Error of Difference*	*T-Statistic*	*Degrees of Freedom*	*Probability*
AD	Faculty-Student	0.3789	0.1316	99	0.8955[ns]
DI	Faculty-Student	0.2272	0.6485	216	0.5174[ns]
DE	Faculty-Student	0.3146	−0.8577	88	0.3934[ns]
Faculty	AD-DI	0.3157	−1.9129	155	0.0576[ns]
	AD-DE	0.3769	0.7709	92	0.4427[ns]
	DI-DE	0.2915	3.0687	149	0.0026
Student	AD-DI	0.2804	−1.8062	160	0.0728[ns]
	AD-DE	0.3291	0.0886	95	0.9296[ns]
	DI-DE	0.2848	1.6768	155	0.0956[ns]

The environment experienced by AD students is more highly characteristic of *General Esteem* than the environments of DE or DI schools. DI school environments for senior students are least characterized by these qualities.

TABLE I-10. T-TEST COMPARISONS OF MEANS OF NURSING SCHOOL MEAN NSEI
FACTOR SCORES AMONG AND BETWEEN STUDENT AND FACULTY GROUPS FROM
AD, DI, DE SCHOOLS, FOR THE FACTOR *BREADTH OF INTEREST*

			Means, Standard Deviations, and Standard Error of Mean		
			AD	*DI*	*DE*
Faculty		N	50	107	44
		Mean	16.8054	16.3761	17.8162
		Std. Dev.	2.3408	2.2048	2.0358
		Std. Error	0.3344	0.2141	0.3069
Students		N	51	111	46
		Mean	16.1496	14.8011	16.6750
		Std. Dev.	2.0311	2.1274	1.9059
		Std. Error	0.2872	0.2028	0.2841

T-Tests

Comparison Groups		*Standard Error of Difference*	*T-Statistic*	*Degrees of Freedom*	*Probability*
AD	Faculty-Student	0.4402	1.4897	99	0.1395^{ns}
DI	Faculty-Student	0.2948	5.3431	216	0.0000
DE	Faculty-Student	0.4202	2.7146	88	0.0080
Faculty	AD-DI	0.3877	1.1072	155	0.2699^{ns}
	AD-DE	0.4604	−2.1955	92	0.0306
	DE-DI	0.3889	−3.7033	149	0.0003
Student	AD-DI	0.3571	3.7768	160	0.0002
	AD-DE	0.4053	−1.2963	95	0.1980^{ns}
	DE-DI	0.3644	−5.1421	155	0.0000

The data and results of the T tests for the significance of the differences between the mean school scores for the NSEI factor *Academic Enthusiasm* are presented in Table I-8.

TABLE I-11. T-TEST COMPARISONS OF MEANS OF NURSING SCHOOL MEAN NSEI FACTOR SCORES AMONG AND BETWEEN STUDENT AND FACULTY GROUPS AND AD, DI, DE SCHOOLS, FOR THE FACTOR *INTRINSIC MOTIVATION*

		Means, Standard Deviations, and Standard Error of Mean		
		AD	*DI*	*DE*
Faculty	N	50	107	44
	Mean	16.3948	15.6481	17.6246
	Std. Dev.	1.7496	1.5638	1.3959
	Std. Error	0.2499	0.1519	0.2104
Students	N	51	111	46
	Mean	15.9776	14.7550	17.5896
	Std. Dev.	1.9457	1.5940	2.1361
	Std. Error	0.2752	0.1520	0.3178

T-Tests

Comparison Groups		Standard Error of Difference	T-Statistic	Degrees of Freedom	Probability
AD	Faculty-Student	0.3721	1.1210	99	0.2650[ns]
DI	Faculty-Student	0.2149	4.1559	216	0.0001
DE	Faculty-Student	0.3865	0.0906	88	0.9280[ns]
Faculty	AD-DI	0.2802	2.6650	155	0.0085
	AD-DE	0.3330	−3.6930	92	0.0004
	DE-DI	0.2734	−7.2289	149	0.0000
Student	AD-DI	0.2915	4.1943	160	0.0001
	AD-DE	0.4188	−3.8491	95	0.0002
	DE-DI	0.3124	−9.0743	155	0.0000

The NSEI factor *Academic Enthusiasm* measures a nursing school environment characterized by a high regard and enthusiasm for academic achievement.

The faculty environment of AD schools is substantially the same as that of AD senior students in respect to the qualities measured by *Academic Enthusiasm*. The environments of both DI and DE schools are significantly more characterized

TABLE I-12. T-TEST COMPARISONS OF MEANS OF NURSING SCHOOL MEAN NSEI
FACTOR SCORES AMONG AND BETWEEN STUDENT AND FACULTY GROUPS FROM
AD, DI, DE SCHOOLS, FOR THE FACTOR *ENCAPSULATED TRAINING*

	Means, Standard Deviations, and Standard Error of Mean			
		AD	*DI*	*DE*
	N	50	107	44
	Mean	20.1148	20.2367	18.5874
Faculty	Std. Dev.	1.7151	1.3154	1.1145
	Std. Error	0.2450	0.1278	0.1680
	N	51	111	46
	Mean	18.9634	18.0808	16.5816
Students	Std. Dev.	1.9189	2.0552	1.7056
	Std. Error	0.2714	0.1960	0.2542

T-Tests

Comparison Groups		*Standard Error of Difference*	*T-Statistic*	*Degrees of Freedom*	*Probability*
AD	Faculty-Student	0.3660	3.1447	99	0.0022
DI	Faculty-Student	0.2358	9.1447	216	0.0000
DE	Faculty-Student	0.3086	6.4997	88	0.0000
Faculty	AD-DI	0.2508	−0.4878	155	0.6264[ns]
	AD-DE	0.3061	4.9886	92	0.0000
	DE-DI	0.2272	7.2581	149	0.0000
Student	AD-DI	0.3427	2.5753	160	0.0109
	AD-DE	0.3741	3.3662	95	0.0000
	DE-DI	0.3458	4.3359	155	0.0003

by these qualities for faculty members than for senior students. The greatest
discrepancy exists in the DI schools.

The environmental qualities of *Academic Enthusiasm* are substantially the same for faculty members in all three types of schools. DE faculty environment is most characterized by these qualities, while DI faculty environments are least so characterized.

Senior students of DE and DI schools experience similar environments with respect to *Academic Enthusiasm*, while AD senior student environments seem to be best described by these characteristics.

The data and results of the T tests for the significance of the differences between the mean school scores for the NSEI factor *Extrinsic Motivation* are presented in Table I-9.

The NSEI factor *Extrinsic Motivation* measures aspects of the nursing school environment related to pressure for group conformance to prescribed norms of behavior.

Of the nine T tests performed, only one, testing Ho Faculty DI-DE, was significant, indicating substantial similarity between the three types of nursing school environments for both faculty members and senior students. Several probabilities approached significance, suggesting that AD and DE school environments are similar in respect to *Extrinsic Motivation*, while DI school environments are somewhat more characterized by these qualities.

The data and results of the T tests for the significance of the differences between the mean school scores for the NSEI factor *Breadth of Interest* are presented in Table I-10.

The NSEI factor *Breadth of Interest* measures the tendency for a nursing school environment to reflect interests beyond the boundaries of nursing.

The results indicate that the environments of AD schools are relatively homogeneous for faculty members and senior students in respect to the qualities measured by *Breadth of Interest*. The environments for faculty members of both DE and DI schools are more characterized by these qualities than for senior students.

The environments of AD and DI schools are similar for faculty members with respect to *Breadth of Interest*, while the faculty environment of DE schools seem to be characterized by more of these qualities.

In contrast, the senior student environments of AD and DE schools are similar, while the senior student environments of DI schools are deficient in these qualities.

The data and results of the T tests for the significance of the differences between the school mean scores for the NSEI factor *Intrinsic Motivation* are presented in Table I-11.

The NSEI factor *Intrinsic Motivation* measures aspects of the nursing school environment which do not pressure students into achieving or conforming.

Faculty members and senior students of DE schools share environments which are very similar with respect to the characteristics of *Intrinsic Motivation*. The same similarity of environment is found in AD schools to a lesser degree. The faculty environment of DI schools is more strongly characterized by the qualities of *Intrinsic Motivation* than the environments of the senior students of DI schools.

The nursing school environments for faculty members differ among all three types of schools with respect to the characteristics measured by *Intrinsic Motivation*. DE faculty members experience these environmental characteristics to the greatest degree, while DI faculty members experience them the least.

The nursing school environments of senior students differ in a pattern similar to that for faculty members with respect to *Intrinsic Motivation*.

The data and results of the T tests for the significance of the differences between the school mean scores for the NSEI factor *Encapsulated Training* are presented in Table I-12.

The NSEI factor *Encapsulated Training* measures aspects of a nursing school environment in which instruction is well organized, with little divergence from a prescribed curriculum.

The nursing school environments of faculty members are more characterized by the qualities measured by *Encapsulated Training* than the environments of senior students in all three types of nursing schools. AD schools provide environments for faculty and students which are most similar with respect to *Encapsulated Training*. Faculty and senior student environments of DI schools are most divergent.

Faculty members of AD schools experience an environment similar to that experienced by DI faculty with respect to *Encapsulated Training*. DE school faculty experience significantly less of these qualities.

Senior students of all three types of nursing schools experience significantly different environments with respect to *Encapsulated Training*. DE senior student environments are least characterized by these qualities, while DI student environments are measured as characterized most by the qualities of *Encapsulated Training*.

CHARACTERISTICS OF THE SCHOOL MEANS DATA

Figures I-1 through I-6 present the distribution of school means for each subgroup of the sample for each scale of the NSEI. This data was presented graphically to provide a direct comparison of the many distributions generated by this study. The figures also provide a means of verifying the assumptions of homogeneous variance and normal distributions of data which have been made in the preceding calculations. The statistical robustness of the analysis of variance and T test techniques allow relatively large departures from these assumptions. Such departures should be detected by visual inspection of the data presented in Figures I-1 through I-6.

Figures I-1 through I-6 were constructed by representing the range of each distribution of NSEI factor scores with a horizontal line drawn in reference to a common scale which appears at the bottom of each figure. The units of each of these scales are equal. The small vertical lines above each line representing the range correspond to the values of the quartiles of each distribution, with the center and longest of these vertical lines representing the median. Similarly, the longest vertical line below each range line represents the mean of the distribution, with the shorter vertical lines to the right and left of this mark representing the range of one standard deviation above and below the mean.

The figures are read vertically, comparing means with medians and inter-quartile ranges with standard deviations within and between each distribution. When the mean and median are in close agreement and the inter-quartile range is exceeded by the range of two standard deviations, the distribution can be assumed to approximate the normal distribution. Gross differences in the standard deviations of the distributions can also be detected by inspection.

Inspection of the thirty-six distributions presented in Figures I-1 through I-6 reveals that only one distribution departs seriously from normality. The AD Faculty mean score distribution for the NSEI factor *General Esteem*, found in Figure I-1, appears to be positively skewed. None of the remaining distributions appear to depart from normality to such a degree as to invalidate the conclusions drawn from the T tests performed. In addition, the variances of the distribution of mean scores for each of the NSEI factors appear to be sufficiently similar to justify the conclusions based on the results of the analyses of variance.

An additional feature of the data presented in Figures I-1 through I-6 is the similarity of the distributions for each of the NSEI factors. Although the differences between these distributions are generally significant statistically, the means actually occur within a relatively restricted range of the total possible score for each factor. In addition, the distributions overlap to a significant extent, with many schools of different types sharing the same factor scores. In fact, using the lowest first quartile score for each factor as a comparison point reveals that it is reasonable to state that at least one-half of the schools of each type possess environments which are similar as measured in this study.

The similarity between school types revealed by this data is of fundamental interpretive importance.

A presentation of the factor score distribution based on individual scores was not made because of the redundancy of such data.

Summary of the Analysis

The analyses of variance results indicated that the NSEI was more efficient in discriminating between the environments of faculty members and of senior students than between the environments of different school types. With the exception of the factors *Extrinsic Motivation* and *Intrinsic Motivation*, the F ratios for faculty-student comparisons were larger than those for school type comparisons. The single exception, *Extrinsic Motivation*, did not produce significant differences between students and faculty, nor did it provide strong evidence for differences between school types. Of the six NSEI factors, *Encapsulated Training* produced the largest faculty-student differences. *Intrinsic Motivation* produced the largest differences between school types.

The evidence for environments within the same school which differ for faculty members and senior students should not be surprising.

The results of the T tests confirmed that faculty members and senior students of DE and DI schools did not share similar environments as measured by the NSEI, with the exception of the characteristics measured by *Intrinsic Motivation*. However, the senior students and faculty members of AD schools appeared to share similar environments, as measured by the NSEI, with the exception of the characteristics measured by the factor *Extrinsic Motivation*. In general, faculty members tended to endorse more of the items of the NSEI than senior students, even when these differences failed to reach sufficient magnitude for statistical significance.

Comparisons between school types for faculty members and senior students followed complex patterns, in which generalizations cannot be made without qualification.

AD senior students appeared to share the most desirable nursing school environments as measured by the NSEI, with the highest mean scores for the factors *General Esteem, Academic Enthusiasm* and *Encapsulated Training*. The AD senior student environments were also quite similar to the environments of DE senior students, sharing similar mean scores for the factors *General Esteem, Breadth of Interest* and *Extrinsic Motivation*. In contrast, AD faculty members, the only faculty group which shared a substantially common environment with their senior students, also found their school environments similar to those of DI faculty members, with similar scores for the factors *Academic Enthusiasm, Encapsulated Training* and *Breadth of Interest*.

Senior students of DE schools also found their environments favorable, with high factor scores for *Breadth of Interest* and *Intrinsic Motivation*. Surprisingly, the characteristics of *Academic Enthusiasm* were relatively absent from the environments of DE senior students, which resembled those of DI students for this factor. DE schools possessed the most favorable environments for faculty members, particularly if low scores for the factors *Extrinsic Motivation* and *Encapsulated Training* are considered as reflecting desirable environmental qualities.

Senior students of DI schools experienced the least favorable environments of any group. DI faculty members were significantly more aware of the positive qualities of their schools than senior students, but also experienced the least desirable environments among faculty groups.

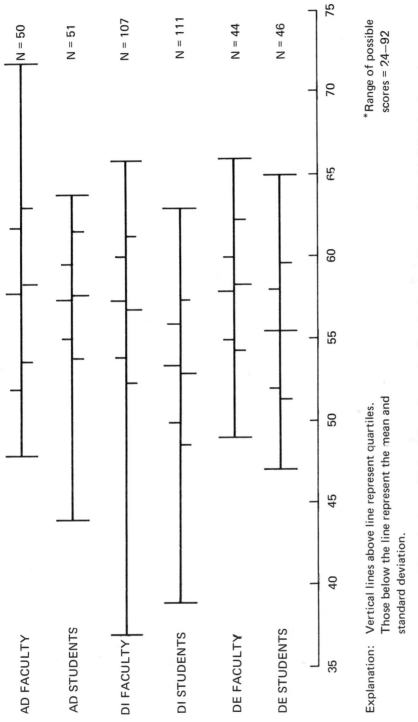

AD FACULTY   N = 50

AD STUDENTS   N = 51

DI FACULTY   N = 107

DI STUDENTS   N = 111

DE FACULTY   N = 44

DE STUDENTS   N = 46

35   40   45   50   55   60   65   70   75

Explanation: Vertical lines above line represent quartiles.
               Those below the line represent the mean and
               standard deviation.

*Range of possible
 scores = 24–92

Figure I-1. Comparison of Distributions of School Mean Scores for Faculty-Student Groups of AD, DI, DE Schools on the NSEI Factor General Esteem*

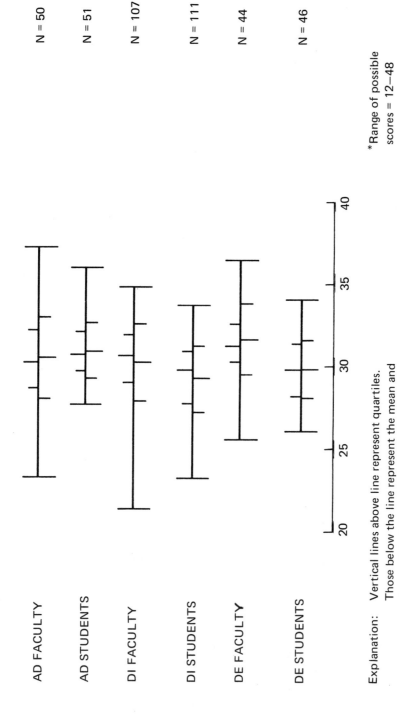

Figure I-2. Comparison of Distributions of School Mean Scores for Faculty-Student Groups of AD, DI, DE Schools on the NSEI Factor Academic Enthusiasm*

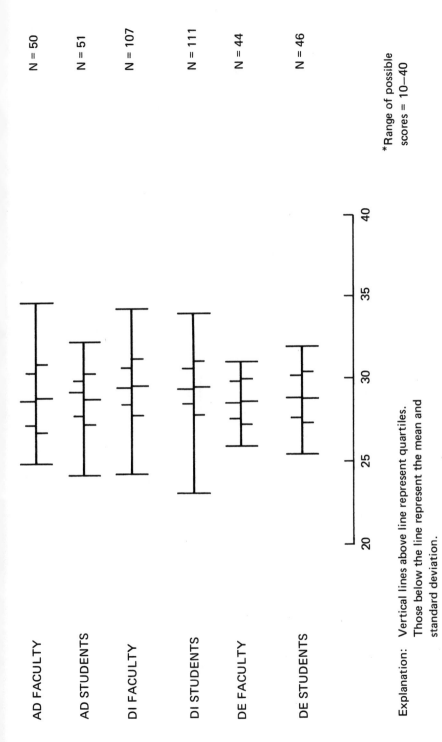

Explanation: Vertical lines above line represent quartiles. Those below the line represent the mean and standard deviation.

Figure I-3. Comparison of Distributions of School Mean Scores for Faculty-Student Groups of AD, DI, DE Schools on the NSEI Factor Extrinsic Motivation*

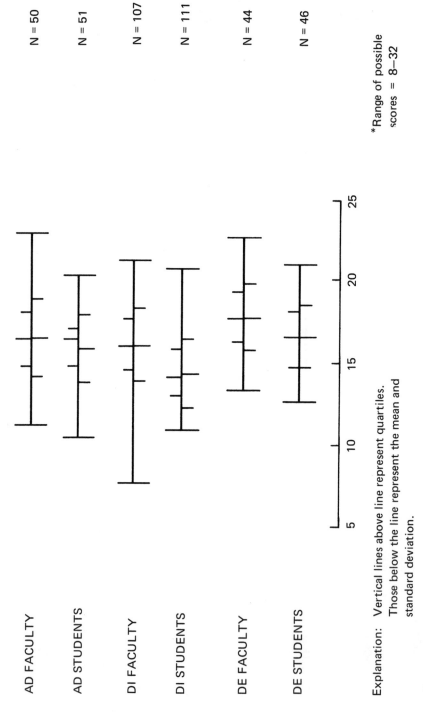

N = 50

N = 51

N = 107

N = 111

N = 44

N = 46

AD FACULTY

AD STUDENTS

DI FACULTY

DI STUDENTS

DE FACULTY

DE STUDENTS

*Range of possible scores = 8–32

Explanation: Vertical lines above line represent quartiles.
                      Those below the line represent the mean and
                      standard deviation.

Figure I-4. Comparison of Distributions of School Mean Scores for Faculty-Student Groups of AD, DI, DE Schools on the NSEI Factor Breadth of Interest

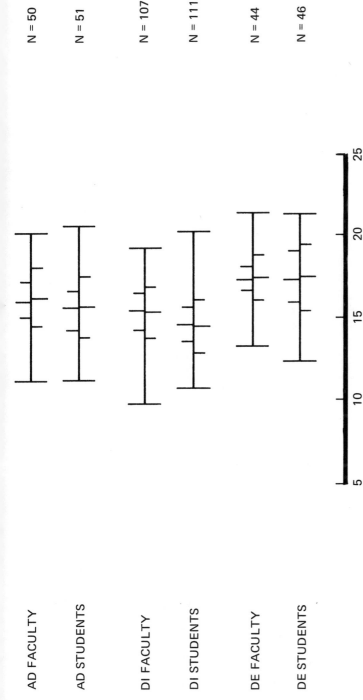

AD FACULTY   N = 50

AD STUDENTS   N = 51

DI FACULTY   N = 107

DI STUDENTS   N = 111

DE FACULTY   N = 44

DE STUDENTS   N = 46

*Range of possible scores = 9–36

Explanation: Vertical lines above line represent quartiles. Those below the line represent the mean and standard deviation.

*Figure I-5. Comparison of Distributions of School Mean Scores for Faculty-Student Groups of AD, DI, DE Schools on the NSEI Factor Intrinsic Motivation**

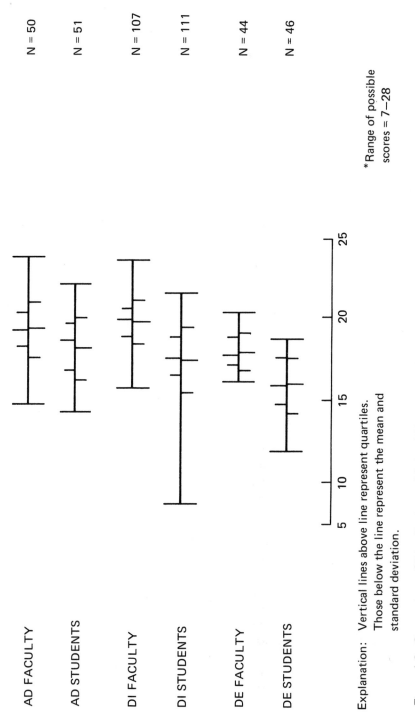

Figure I-6. Comparison of Distributions of School Mean Scores for Faculty-Student Groups of AD, DI, DE Schools on the NSEI Factor Encapsulated Training*

While the differences in the environments of the three types of schools, as measured by the NSEI were striking, it should be borne in mind that the variations of individual school environments within each school type caused considerable overlap between school types. In general, more similarity than differences existed between school types. Thus a majority of the schools in this study could be seen to possess similar environments, rendering all-or-nothing generalizations about the differences between these school environments invalid. Care must be exercised in the application of these findings to specific schools.

Summary of the Study

The basic purpose of this study was to investigate and compare the environments of the three basic types of nursing schools as perceived by their senior students and faculty members, in order to determine the degree and quality of the differences between and among them. It is commonly held by the nursing profession that the graduates of baccalaureate degree programs are qualified as professional nurses and able to assume leadership roles in nursing practice, while graduates of associate degree programs and diploma programs are qualified as technical nurses, but not qualified for leadership roles on the nursing team, or for roles in nursing education. At least in part, these differences in proficiency levels are attributed to differences in the educational environments which mold the characteristics of their graduates. This study was designed to determine whether such differences could be demonstrated by empirical methods, as well as to investigate the nature of such differences.

The instrument chosen for use in this study was based on the Medical School Environment Inventory (MSEI), a 69-item questionnaire devised to evaluate six dimensions of medical school environments as perceived by medical students. The MSEI was validated by demonstrating significant correlations between its factor scores and criterion variables associated with medical schools and students which closely resemble the characteristics believed to distinguish professional nurses and their educational environments from technical nurses. The MSEI, with very minor modifications, was renamed the Nursing School Environment Inventory (NSEI). In this study the NSEI was assumed to have face validity based on the appropriateness of the items for the measurement of nursing school environments.

The subjects of this study consisted of 5,267 senior students and 1,789 faculty members from a representative national sample of 212 nursing schools.

The data was analyzed for differences and similarities between and among senior students and faculty members of each of the three types of nursing programs. Separate analyses were carried out for individual responses and for school mean scores on each of the six NSEI factors. The statistical procedures employed consisted of analyses of variance and the T statistic.

The relatively high levels of significance at which most of the various null hypotheses tested with these techniques could be rejected reflect the magnitude of the environmental differences measured by the NSEI, and can be interpreted as an indication of the success of the instrument in distinguishing between the environments of nursing schools as well as evidence of actual differences between the environments being measured.

The pattern of measured differences between the three types of nursing programs, while somewhat complex, tended to support the expectation that DE schools possessed environments more nearly ideal for the development of professional graduates than those of DI schools. AD schools tended to resemble DE schools with the exceptions of the factors *General Esteem, Academic Enthusiasm* and *Encapsulated Training*. Both senior students and faculty members of AD schools were more aware of the positive qualities of their schools and academic work than DE students and faculty. AD schools also ranked highest on the factor *Encapsulated Training*, which described a circumscribed and defined curriculum unlike that considered desirable for the development of professional nurses. DE schools ranked lowest on this factor, as might be expected.

The NSEI proved to be efficient in distinguishing between the environments of faculty members and students. In general, faculty environments followed the same school type pattern as did senior student environments. Faculty members tended to perceive more of the characteristics of each NSEI factor in their environments than did their senior students. The environments for faculty members and senior students of AD schools were very similar, in contrast to the other school types. While AD senior student environments tended to resemble DE senior student environments, AD faculty environments resembled DI faculty environments.

While the data of this study demonstrated significant trends toward meaningfully discernible differences between the environments of the three types of nursing schools, they also yielded evidence for substantial similarity between the environments of many of the same schools. These similarities must be taken into account when generalizations are made concerning differences between types of nursing education.

Interpretation of the Results

The differences between the professional graduate nurse and the technical graduate nurse are often described as personality characteristics attributed to differences in their educational programs. Professional graduate nurses are products of DE programs and are said to possess such traits as self-confidence, self-respect, independence of judgment, leadership potential, scholarly interests, and a firm intellectual understanding of the theoretical bases of nursing practice (Brown, 1948, 1965; Rogers, 1964). While this study made no attempt to assess the relationships of the environmental qualities measured by the NSEI to these qualities, tentative inferences can be drawn from the validation studies conducted in medical schools for the MSEI.

Table I-13 compares the patterns of high and low mean school scores for each of the NSEI factors for the three types of nursing schools.

TABLE I-13. PATTERN OF HIGH AND LOW SCORES FOR AD, DI, AND DE SCHOOLS ON THE SIX FACTORS OF THE NSEI

School Type	GE	AE	EM	BI	IM	ET
AD	+	+	+	−*		+
DI	−	−		−	−	
DE			−	+	+	−

+ = highest school mean factor score
− = lowest school mean factor score
* = non-significant difference between the highest (+*) or the lowest (−*) factor score

Table I-14 presents a summary of significant correlations of each of the six factors of the MSEI with measurements of a variety of aspects of medical school environments, as reported by Hutchins. The last column of Table I-14 shows which of the patterns of NSEI factor scores found in Table I-14 matches the pattern of NSEI factor scores found by Hutchins for each variable. Inspection of these patterns reveals that the NSEI factor scores of DE schools most closely match the patterns of MSEI factor scores correlated with desirable criterion characteristics of medical schools. While the comparisons of Table I-14 are speculative at best, it is not unreasonable to assume that excellence in the profession of nursing shares commonalities with the profession of medicine.

Table I-14 was constructed to illustrate the major interpretation of the results of this study. When the environments of the three basic types of nursing schools are examined through the perceptions of faculty members and senior students, the environments of DE schools tend to be those most likely to produce graduates which conform to the commonly held expectations for professional nurses.

An apparent contradiction to this interpretation exists in the higher rank of AD schools on the factors *General Esteem* and *Academic Enthusiasm*. The most likely interpretation of this discrepancy is based on the Hutchin's data, which indicated that these factors were unlikely to be associated with known criteria of excellence in medical education. It is therefore possible that the discrepancy is irrelevant. It is also possible, as suggested by the Fox and Diamond (1964) study, that the impact of clinical experience is such as to reduce the enthusiasm of student nurses for their academic environments. AD programs probably devote the least time to clinical experience, while DI programs include the greatest amount of practical experience.

TABLE I-14. SIGNIFICANT CORRELATIONS BETWEEN MEAN SCORES OF 6 MSEI SCALES AND 42 SELECTED CRITERION VARIABLES ARRANGED BY MSEI FACTOR PATTERNS COMPARED TO FACTOR SCORE PATTERNS OF AD, DI, AND DE SCHOOLS

	GE	AE	EM	BI	IM	ET	School Type
Size of Student Body (1)	—*						DI
Theoretical (3)					+		DE
Aestheticism Factor (2)					+*		DE
Deference (4)					—*		DI
Percent Research Fellows (1)	+				+*		DE-AD
Abasement (4)						+*	AD
Nurturance (4)						+*	AD
Aggression (4)						—*	DE
Endurance (4)				+*			DE
Succorance (4)			+				AD
Achievement (4)					+	—	DE
Total School Expenditure (1)					+*	—*	DE
Order (4)					—*	+*	
Religion (3)					—	+	
Change (4)	—		—	—			DI
Artistic Orientation (2)				+	+		DE
Total Attrition (1)				—*	—*		DI
Academic Attrition (1)	—			—*	—*		DI
Pragmatism Factor (2)	—*			—*	—		DI
Conventional Orientation (2)				—	—*	+	DI-AD
Economic (3)			+		—*		DI
Social Orientation (2)			+		—		
Dominance (4)			—		+		DE
Enterprising Orientation (2)			—		+		DE
Research $/Faculty (1)			—		+*		DE
Private(1) vs. Tax(0) (1)			—		+		DE
MCAT —Verbal			—		+*	—*	DE
Quantitative			—		+*	—*	DE
Modern Society			—		+*	—*	DE
Science			—		+*	—*	DE
Faculty Size (1)			—		+*	—*	DE
Autonomy (4)	—		—		+	—*	DE
Aesthetic (3)			—	*	+*	—*	DE
Scientific Orientation (2)	+			+	+*	—	DE
Historical Percent Grads in Med. Ed. (1)	+			+*	+*	—*	DE
Status Factor (2)	+		—	+	+*	—	DE
Faculty/Student Ratio (1)	+*		—	+	+*	—	DE

TABLE I-14. SIGNIFICANT CORRELATIONS BETWEEN MEAN SCORES OF 6 MSEI
SCALES AND 42 SELECTED CRITERION VARIABLES ARRANGED BY MSEI FACTOR
PATTERNS COMPARED TO FACTOR SCORE PATTERNS OF AD, DI, AND DE SCHOOLS

	GE	AE	EM	BI	IM	ET	*School Type*
Percent Students Out of State (1)	+		−	+*	+		DE
SP/RT (1)	+		−	+	+*		DE
G/SP (1)	−		+	−	−*		DI
Intellectual Factor (2)	+		−		+		DE
Affiliation (4)	+	+		+			AD
Total Number of Correlations:	15	1	20	16	34	19	105#

Variable Codes: 1 = Objective Medical School Data
  2 = Astin Variables
  3 = Allport-Vernon-Lindzey Study of Values
  4 = Edward's Personal Preference Schedule

*Correlations significant beyond the 0.01 level.
 All others between 0.05 and 0.01.
#Grand total of all correlations.

Data taken from Hutchins, 1962, 1963, 1965.

It was not surprising to find that faculty members generally rate their environments more favorably than senior students. However, there were two exceptions to this trend which are worthy of interpretation. The characteristics measured by the NSEI factors *Extrinsic Motivation* and *Encapsulated Training* would generally be considered as undesirable in a school environment. Yet faculty members were more aware of these negative characteristics than their students.

The items of *Extrinsic Motivation* stressed the responsibility of faculty members for the activities of their students in such matters as patient safety in clinical experience, ethical behavior, and idealistic student deportment. Faculty members may well endorse these items as legitimate expectations for themselves and their students. Similarly, the items of *Encapsulated Training* tended to stress organization, planning and detail in the presentation of instruction. Faculty members probably view such activities as good instruction and careful curriculum planning rather than as "spoon feeding". The environmental press measured by *Extrinsic Motivation* and *Encapsulated Training* was not the same for faculty members as for senior students.

It is possible that the sensitivity of the NSEI to differences in faculty and student environments may be explained by similar qualitative differences, rather than quantitative environmental differences. The possibility that students and faculty view similar phenomena in their school environments from differing value premises has already been suggested in the literature: Davis and Olesen, 1964, 1965;

Olesen and Davis, 1966; Siegel, 1968. Such differences may have unpredictable and possibly adverse effects upon students and faculty alike, particularly if they are not identified. The methodology embodied by the NSEI may hold promise for the accurate identification of such differences.

The distribution of scores for each of the NSEI factors revealed that many schools were similar regardless of type. These schools may have equal capacity for producing graduates who possess potential for successful performance as professional nurses, at least to the extent that school environment alone can contribute to this potential. It would be unwise to arbitrarily divest these AD and DI schools of responsibility for the development of professional potential in their graduates, just as it would be unwise to bar their graduates from full professional development after graduation, on the basis of the source of their training.

Recommendations

The NSEI was an adaptation of an instrument originally designed for use with medical schools and students. In spite of the fact that it possessed only face validity for use in this study, it proved an effective instrument. It is therefore recommended that this methodology be further refined for more precise use with nursing school environments. Research designed to investigate the significance and nature of the differences between student and faculty press factors should be undertaken. The dimensions of nursing school environments relevant to the optimum development of desirable characteristics of nursing graduates should be precisely identified. Efforts should also be made to provide an empirical basis for distinguishing between professional and technical nurses.

Presently, the criteria of educational background may be the most precise means of differentiating between levels of proficiency within the nursing profession. However, this study has shown that at least as much variation exists within each type of nursing education as between them. It is therefore recommended that research be undertaken to provide a more precise definition of the professional and technical levels of proficiency in the nursing profession in order to allow the conservation and strengthening of the present educational resources of the nursing profession, and to provide continuity in the development of professional talent in nursing. Well-defined guide lines for distinguishing between technical and professional levels of nursing education and activities would also aid young people in choosing appropriate goals and educational programs for entry into the nursing profession. Such clarification would additionally provide a more precise and meaningful frame of reference for the evaluation of nursing school environments.

This study initially entertained the possibility of making further comparisons between school types on a regional basis. Examination of the regional characteristics of the sample precluded such comparisons. However, regional variations in the quality and character of nursing education are of interest to the nursing profession, since it is desirable to maintain uniform standards of quality in all nursing education programs. Furthermore, regional health requirements vary from industrial to rural environments, among socio-economic levels, and according to the age distribution of local populations. These regional differences create unique demands upon local nursing schools which should be reflected in regional differences between nursing programs. The success of the present study suggests that further investigation of nursing environments on a regional basis could be undertaken. Such a study should employ a more precise methodology, and more refined goals than were utilized in the present study.

BIBLIOGRAPHY

Allport, G. W., Vernon, P. E., and Lindzey, G. *Study of Values.* Boston: Houghton, Mifflin Co. 1951.

American Nurses' Association, Committee on Education. "First Position on Education for Nursing." *Americal Journal of Nursing.* 65:106-111. (December, 1965).

American Nurses' Association. *Facts About Nursing: A Statistical Summary,* 1968 Edition, New York. 1968.

Astin, A. *Who Goes Where to College?* Chicago: Science Research Associates, Inc. 1965.

———: "Further Validation of the Environmental Assessment Technique." *Journal of Educational Psychology.* 54:217-226. 1963.

Brown, E. L. *Nursing for the Future.* New York: The Russell Sage Foundation. 1948.

———: *Prospectus: Better Nursing Education for Improved Patient Care and Health Guidance.* Mimeographed. Submitted to the ANA and NLN, October, 1965.

Brown, N. W. "A Study of the Interests of Baccalaureate Registered Nurses in Relation to Aptitudes, Achievement and Attitudes and the Development of an Occupational Scale for the Strong Vocational Interest Blank." *Dissertation Abstracts.* 27:1-B, 209. 1966.

Corwin, R. G. and Taves, M. J. "Nursing and Other Health Professions." In Freeman, Levine, and Reever (Eds.). *Handbook of Medical Sociology.* Englewood Cliffs: Prentice Hall. 1963.

Cunningham, E. B. *Today's Diploma Schools of Nursing.* New York: National League for Nursing, Department of Diploma and Associate Degree Programs. 1963.

Davis, A. J. "Self Concept, Role Expectations and Occupational Choice in Nursing and Social Work." *Nursing Research.* 18:1,55-89. 1969.

Davis, F. and Olesen, V. L. "Baccalaureate Students' Image of Nursing: A Study of Change, Consensus and Consonance in the First Year." *Nursing Research.* 13:8-15. (Winter 1964).

——— and ———: "The Career Outlook of Professionally Educated Women: The Case of the Collegiate Student Nurse." *Psychiatry.* 26:4,334-345. 1965.

Dustan, L. C. "Characteristics of Students in Three Types of Nursing Education Programs." *Nursing Research.* 13:159-166. (Spring 1964).

Edwards, A. L. *Edwards Personal Preference Schedule.* New York: The Psychological Corp. 1953.

Flexner, A. *Medical Education in the United States and Canada: A Report to the Carnegie Foundation for the Advancement of Teaching.* 1910.

Fox, D. J., Diamond, K., and Associates. *Satisfying and Stressful Situations in Nursing Education.* New York: Bureau of Publications, Columbia University. 1964.

Gartner, S. R. "Nursing Majors in 12 Western Universities: A Comparison of Registered Nurse Students and Basic Senior Students." *Nursing Research.* 17:121-128. (March-April 1968).

Goldmark, J. A. *Nursing in the United States.* Report of the committee for the study of nursing education and a report of the survey of Josephine Goldmark. New York: The Macmillan Co. 1923.

Guilford, J. P. *Fundamental Statistics in Psychology and Education.* New York: McGraw-Hill Book Company. 1965.

Halpin, A. W. and Croft, D. B. *The Organizational Climate of Schools.* Chicago; Midwest Administration Center, The University of Chicago. 1963.

Hutchins, E. B."The 1960 Medical School Graduate: His Perceptions of His Faculty, Peers and Environment." *Journal of Medical Education.* 36:4, 322-329. (April 1961).

———: *The Medical School Environment Inventory.* 1962.

———: *The Measurement of Student Environment and Its Relation to Career Choice in Medicine.* Mimeographed. The Association of American Medical Colleges. 1962.

——— and Wollins, L. "Factor Analysis of Statements Describing Student Environment in American Medical Colleges." Paper read at the thirty-first annual meeting of the Midwestern Psychological Association. Chicago. May 3, 1963.

———: "The AAMC Longitudinal Study: Implications for Medical Education." *Journal of Medical Education.* 29:265-277.1964.

———: "The AAMC Study of Medical Student Attrition: Overview and Major Findings." *Journal of Medical Education. 40:913-920. 1965*

——— and Nonneman, A. J. *Construct Validity of an Environmental Assessment Technique for Medical Schools. Technical Report No. 1661.* Evanston: Office of Basic Research, Division of Education, The Association of American Medical Colleges.1966.

Kerlinger, F. *Foundations of Behavioral Research, Educational and Psychological Enquiry.* New York: Holt, Rinehart and Winston. 1965

Kish, L. *Survey Sampling.* New York: John Wiley and Sons, Inc. 1965.

Klahn, J. E. "An Analysis of Selected Factors and Success of First Year Student Nurses." *Dissertation Abstracts.* 27:9-A, 2888. 1967.

Knudsin, E. G. "Public Health Nurses: Interest in Occupational Advancement." *Nursing Research.* 17:4, 327-335. (July-August 1968).

Levitt, E. E., Lubin, B., and Zuckerman, M. "The Student Nurse, the College Woman and the Graduate Nurse: A Comparative Study." *Nursing Research.* 11:2, 80-82. 1962.

Lysaught, J. P. Director, National Commission for the Study of Nursing and Nursing Education. Personal communication. 1969.

McNemar, Q. *Psychological Statistics.* New York: John Wiley and Sons, Inc. 1949.

Murray, H. A. *Explorations in Personality.* New York: Oxford University Press. 1938.

Nunnally, J. C., Thistlewaite, D. L., and Wolfe, S. "Factored Scales for Measuring Characteristics of College Environments." *Educational and Psychological Measurement.* 23:239-248. 1963.

Olesen, V. L. and Davis, F. "Baccalaureate Students' Images of Nursing: A Follow-up Report." *Nursing Research.* 15:239-248. 1963

Pace, C. R. and Stern, G. C. *College Characteristics Index.* Syracuse. 1957.

———: "An Approach to the Measurement of Psychological Characteristics of College Environments." *Journal of Educational Psychology.* 49:269-277. 1958.

Popham, J. W. *Educational Statistics: Use and Interpretation.* New York: Harper and Row. 1967.

Psathos, G. and Plapp, J. "Assessing Effects of a Nursing Program: A Problem in Design." *Nursing Research.* 17:4, 337-342. (July-August 1968).

Report of the Committee on Nursing. Rochester: University of Rochester Medical Center. 1969. Unpublished.

Roberts, M. M. *American Nursing: History and Interpretation.* New York: The Macmillan Co. 1954.

Roeme, M. E. "An Analysis of Role Behavior, Role Expectations, Role Conflict, Job Satisfactions and Coping Patterns of Associate Degree, Diploma and Baccalaureate Degree Graduates in Beginning Nursing Positions." *Dissertation Abstracts.* 27:6-B, 2001. 1966.

Rogers, M. E. *Reveille in Nursing.* Philadelphia: F. A. Davis Company. 1964.

Sanazarro, P. J. "Class Size in Medical School." *Journal of Medical Education.* 41:11, 1017-1029. 1966.

——— and Hutchins, E. B. "The Origin and Rationale of the Medical College Admissions Test." *Journal of Medical Education.* 34:1044-1050. 1963.

Siegel, H. "Professional Socialization in Two Baccalaureate Programs." *Nursing Research.* 17:5, 403-407. (September-October 1968).

Stephan, F., and McCarthy, P. *Sampling Opinions, An Analysis of Survey Procedure.* New York: John Wiley and Sons Inc. 1958.

Stern, G. G. "Student Ecology and the College Environment." *Journal of Medical Education.* 40:2, 132-153. 1965.

———: "B = f(P, E)." *Journal of Projective Techniques and Personality Assessment.* 28:161-168. 1964.

Tate, B. Research Associate, National League for Nursing. Personal communication to the NCSNNE. 1969.

Thistlewaite, D. L. "College Environments and the Development of Talent." *Science.* 130:71-76. 1963.

United States Public Health Service. Report of the Surgeon General's Consultant Group on Nursing. *Toward Quality in Nursing: Needs and Goals.* Publication Number 922. (February 1963).

Winer, B. J. *Statistical Principles in Experimental Design.* New York: McGraw-Hill Book Company. 1962.

Yates, F. *Sampling Methods for Censuses and Surveys.* New York: Hafner Publishing Company. 1960.

APPENDIX J
FACULTY QUESTIONNAIRES: SUMMARY AND FINDINGS

Over the course of the study, the Commission and staff have been bombarded with a great deal of anecdotal evidence regarding nursing faculty in basic preparatory nursing programs in the United States. Much of this "evidence" has appeared in the form of generalizations, two of the more common being: there exists a shortage of qualified faculty in all types of basic nursing programs; important differences exist in the background, education and career activities of faculty members in the three basic programs preparing students for nursing in the United States.

There have been few objective data to support such generalizations although they are commonly accepted as truisms by the nursing profession. The Commission felt it to be most important that nursing faculty, by means of a stratified, random sample, be allowed to confirm or deny these generally held assumptions. Thus, by the end of the year 1968, as a portion of Phase III of the study, a questionnaire was developed by the staff, designed to indicate the background, education and career activities of faculty members in institutions preparing basic students for nursing. (For a copy of the questionnaire, see Appendix R.)

SAMPLING

The objective of the NCSNNE in selecting schools to participate was to construct a sample that would maintain representativeness by both program type and geographic region. The nine area divisions of the ANA provided natural geographic sampling units for the selection of schools. After study the decision was that 25 percent of the associate degree and baccalaureate programs for each region would be included, together with 20 percent of the diploma programs since these last were far more numerous.

The staff was provided a list of 253 nursing schools compiled in 1961 for use as a random sample in the NLN Nurse Career Pattern Study (NLN, Unpublished). This list had been constructed by random drawing from a list of all known nursing schools in 1961 and was found to be a valid and satisfactory representation when tested.[1]

To maintain the proportionate regional representation considered desirable, the NCSNNE modified the NLN sample by adding and deleting schools to compensate for those which had ceased to exist and also for the growth in numbers of collegiate programs. The revised version of the NLN sample consisted of 278 schools and appeared under scrutiny to be a valid, national sample.

The final sample, of course, consisted of those schools which actually contributed data to the study. Of the 278 schools of nursing contacted by the Commission, 228 or 82 percent returned useable data. Of the 228 nursing programs, 123 were diploma, 57 associate degree, and 48 baccalaureate. Thus, there was an approximate 80 percent return by the hospital schools of nursing and the associate degree programs, and an approximate 88 percent return by the baccalaureate institutions.

The questionnaire used in this survey was an adaptation of an instrument employed in a study of home economics conducted in 1967 by Earl McGrath of the Institute of Higher Education at Columbia University. A similar questionnaire was used with his approval, and the adaptation was made by Herman Kauz, staff administrator of the NCSNNE group, who had served with the Institute and had taken part in the home economics study. The survey in that field was conducted without difficulty and produced a high rate of response.

Over 5,000 questionnaires were sent to full- and part-time faculty members with primary appointments in the departments of nursing in 278 basic nursing programs throughout the country. The staff estimated the number of nursing faculty at each institution by consulting the most recent school catalogs, after which the appropriate number of questionnaires was sent. Where the number was at variance with actual faculty membership, departments of nursing were asked to either request more questionnaires or return the surplus.

Although 82 percent of the schools contacted did respond, not all of the faculty members in each school completed individual questionnaires. We found that some faculty members were quite suspicious of forwarding questionnaires to the staff through their dean's office, and, also, that many of the faculty were highly sensitive to questions that involved areas of a "confidential" nature such as salary or institutional problems. In addition, a number of schools included in our sample did not fill out the questionnaires. One director of nursing education in a diploma program felt that the questionnaire was more "appropriate for collegiate faculty," while the chairman of a baccalaureate department felt the forms were "intended for hospital schools". The dean of a collegiate program "destroyed" the questionnaires because "of their ambiguity". Many of the remaining schools which did not fill out and return questionnaires chose not to participate either because their programs had recently closed or were about to do so. A small number of diploma programs reported that their academic year had ended. These examples, however, were the exception and no less than 228 schools and 2,949 faculty members (approximately 59 per cent) took the time and energy to complete the questionnaire. Because of their help, we were able to obtain some accurate data regarding commonly held assumptions about the nursing faculties.

OBJECTIVES AND FINDINGS

One of our primary objectives was to determine the levels of faculty preparation in the three different types of preparatory programs. The findings are presented in Table J-1:

TABLE J-1. ACADEMIC PREPARATION OF NURSE FACULTY

Highest Degree Attained	Percent of Diploma faculty	Percent of AD faculty	Percent of Baccalaureate faculty
RN	21.0	1.2	0.4
Associate Degree	0.6	0.7	-
Baccalaureate	57.1	35.4	14.2
Masters	20.7	62.4	78.2
Doctorate	0.1	0.2	7.3
Did not Answer	0.5	-	-

In most professions, a master's degree is considered to be the minimum requirement for a qualified faculty member. If this rule is applied to nursing, then we find approximately a 79 percent deficit in diploma faculty preparation, and a 14 percent deficit among baccalaureate faculty. A shortage of qualified and adequately prepared faculty in the three types of basic nursing programs is definitely supported in our findings; however, the shortage within the baccalaureate programs appears to be the least critical while the shortage within diploma programs appears certainly to be the most critical.

We next felt it necessary (in view of the educational deficit) to determine the amount of continuing education, both full- and part-time, being engaged in by faculty from the three types of programs in order to ascertain the percentages pursuing their academic/professional development. Table J-2 provides the results:

TABLE J-2. CONTINUING EDUCATION OF NURSE FACULTY

September 1966 — June 1968	Diploma	AD	Baccalaureate
Percent of faculty taking courses, part-time	30.0	34.0	19.0
Average number of part-time courses taken by each	3.5	.4	2.5
Percent of faculty as full-time students	14.0	15.0	23.0
Total percent of faculty taking courses, both full- and part-time	44.0	49.0	42.0
Percent of faculty not engaged in either full- or part-time study	56.0	51.0	58.0

In all three types of programs, less than half of the faculty queried was engaged in some sort of formal academic preparation during the preceding two years. Considering the deficit in faculty preparation that was found in our sample, this seemed like a rather small percentage continuing their education.

The faculty engaged in taking full- or part-time courses, however, appear to be pursuing their professional development seriously since, on the average, about 17 percent have been full-time students while another 28 percent were taking, on the average, 3½ courses each. It is the nearly 55 percent of the faculty who have not been enrolled in any academic courses that is startling, when such a pronounced deficit in faculty preparation exists, according to the results of our sample.

When asked, "In your opinion, what is the most serious problem facing nursing education today?", 22 percent of the faculty indicated the lack of qualified faculty, while the next highest percent (17 percent), discounting "miscellaneous", indicated that confusion among the different types of programs preparing nurses was the greatest problem. When questioned further as to what one change would most improve nursing education at their institution, 13 percent of the faculty listed "more and better qualified faculty", while the next highest percentage (6 percent) of any homogeneity mentioned "more facilities" (the percents for "miscellaneous" and "did not answer" were both higher than any one problem; see Table J-6).

In order to discover more about the career patterns and distribution of activities of faculties of diploma, associate degree and baccalaureate programs, we asked the subjects to account for all the years of their career, since receiving their RN, including periods of non-paid employment such as homemaking. We surveyed their answers for the years 1964-1969 and found the results charted in Table J-3:

TABLE J-3. CAREER PATTERNS OF NURSE FACULTY

1964 — 1969	*Diploma*		*AD*		*Baccalaureate*	
	Percent Faculty	*Percent of their Time Spent*	*Percent Faculty*	*Percent of their Time Spent*	*Percent Faculty*	*Percent of their Time Spent*
Nursing Service	50	36	41	33	32	34
Nursing Education	91	60	93	28	98	67
	25	100	28	100	36	100
Educational Administration	16	69	16	61	10	57
	7	100	5	100	2	100
Service Adminsitration	3	41	7	30	1	45
Non-Nursing	13	32	18	32	9	33
Student	28	37	30	33	35	37

From these responses, we determined that a larger percentage of baccalaureate faculty spent a greater percentage of their time in nursing education than did either diploma or associate degree faculty, while a larger percentage of diploma faculty spent a greater percentage of their time in nursing service than did either associate degree or baccalaureate faculty. In addition, a greater percentage of baccalaureate faculty spent 100 percent of their time in nursing education during these designated years than did either of the other two faculty types. As for educational and service administration, a smaller percentage of baccalaureate faculty were engaged in this activity than either diploma or associate degree faculty.

Not only did a greater percentage of baccalaureate faculty spend a greater percentage of their time in nursing education and less in nursing service and administration, but a greater percentage of this faculty type spent a higher percentage of time as students during the five-year period. Furthermore, a smaller percentage of baccalaureate faculty spent their time in non-nursing activities.

From this sample, we can extrapolate that baccalaureate nursing faculty patterns more closely resemble other collegiate faculty patterns in the distribution of time spent and proportion of time devoted as members of educational institutions. However, as faculty members, these nurses do not necessarily spend all of their time in the classroom; a substantial number of the faculty view themselves as primarily nursing educators, but they emphasize that term includes clinical instruction, administrative duties, and sometimes, research.

Another objective of our faculty questionnaire was to determine the amount of research and publishing being done by the three types of faculty. To this end, we asked those surveyed about any research activities and/or publications engaged in during the last five years. The results are shown in Table J-4:

TABLE J-4. RESEARCH AND PUBLICATIONS OF NURSE FACULTY

1964 – 1969	*Diploma*	*AD*	*Baccalaureate*
Percent faculty in research	3.0	6.5	19.0
Average number of research activities per faculty member	1.6	1.0	1.4
Percent faculty publishing	1.3	7.7	24.0
Average number of publications per faculty member	1.7	1.5	2.5

From these responses, it is clear a greater percentage of baccalaureate faculty was engaged in research activities and publishing, and certainly those who published, published more articles per person than did the other two types of faculty. Our questionnaire was more general than specific in inquiring about research, so the range of the responses included a variety of research activities ranging from "revising the curriculum" or "surveying what our graduates do after receiving their RN" to "research on open-heart surgery patients" and "research and development of self-instructional materials in maternal and child nursing". Very few of the faculty respondents were very specific about their research and much of it was unpublished and inaccessible to the staff so that these figures really tell us more about how the faculty view themselves in relation to research activity rather than determining how many faculty have been engaged in meaningful research in nursing, or the general quality of their efforts.

In almost all cases, those faculty who mentioned their publications were very specific about titles, journals, and dates; therefore, the figures relating to the percentage of faculty having published in the past five years reflect the actual situation quite accurately. These figures indicate that a greater percentage of baccalaureate faculty is publishing — and publishing more often — than either associate degree or diploma faculty members. And with the *caveat* concerning quality, the same conclusion can be drawn concerning research.

In order to determine the extent of professional organizational participation, or at least the percentage of faculty who see themselves as "professional", we asked the subjects to list their organizational memberships. The results appear in Table J-5:

TABLE J-5. ORGANIZATIONAL MEMBERSHIP AMONG NURSING FACULTY

Professional Organization	*Diploma*	*AD*	*Baccalaureate*
Percent faculty in ANA	74	87	87
Percent faculty in NLN	46	35	56
Percent in other professional nursing organizations	15	20	30
Percent faculty in non-nursing professional organizations	4	66	24
Percent faculty in no professional organizations	0	8	8

Some explanation is due at this point. Many faculty listed a state nursing association membership under "other professional nursing organizations"; however, because membership in the ANA automatically assures membership in the state nursing organization and vice versa, when we came across either one or the other or both listed, we counted it as one—membership in the ANA. In "other professional nursing organizations", we did not count honorary or social organizations, but did count other professional health organizations in this category.

From this data, it appears that the nursing faculty in all programs support some professional organization and if the ANA is considered *the* professional organization, then it is well supported by all three faculty types. In more than 50 percent of the cases, faculty members supported either the ANA or the NLN and many supported both.

An interesting figure is the percentage of associate degree faculty who see themselves as belonging to other non-nursing professional organizations. But from our sample, it appears that a greater percentage of the baccalaureate faculty belong to the professional nursing organizations than either of the other two faculties.

Our final questions involved trying to determine what problems the faculty members feel are the most serious facing nursing education today, and particularly, at their own institution. The results were alluded to earlier in this writing and they are shown in Table J-6. Incidentally, there was no effort to divide these responses according to type of nursing program.

TABLE J-6. PROBLEMS AND SOLUTIONS FOR NURSING EDUCATION

In Your Opinion, What is the Greatest Problem Facing Nursing Education Today?		What One Change Would Most Improve Nursing Education at Your Institution?	
Lack of qualified faculty	22 percent	Improve level of faculty	13 percent
Too many different and confusing kinds of programs preparing RN's	17 percent		
Lack of qualified students	5 percent	Improve level of students	2 percent
Costs	1 percent	Reduce costs	2 percent
Facilities: Need more and better	1 percent	Improve facilities	6 percent
Gap between nursing education and nursing service	4 percent		
Miscellaneous	44 percent	Miscellaneous	54 percent
Did not answer	7 percent	No Answer	23 percent

Regarding the responses to the greatest problem facing nursing education today, aside from the miscellaneous category, the greatest homogeneity occurred in the category "lack of qualified faculty", with 22 percent of the faculty concurring. A close second was the 17 percent feeling that "too many different and confusing kinds of programs preparing RN's" exist. In many cases, respondents did not limit their answer to one response but listed two or three, in which case we tallied the first response. But this indicates to us that there are at least two or three major concurrent problems facing nursing education, in the opinion of these faculty members, and that because of this, it was difficult to limit an answer to one problem. If we had tallied how many times "lack of qualified faculty" appeared as one of several answers, the percentage likely would have been significantly higher.

The following examples give an idea of the type of answers (indicated by 44 percent of the faculty members) which the staff included under "miscellaneous": "Student attrition"; "Our unwillingness to face reality"; "Evaluating clinical performance with validity, reliability, objectivity, uniformity, and practicality"; "Clinical services with antiquated nursing service practices"; "Faculty time to keep current with research findings, literature, etc., as well as clinical practice".

When asked what *one* change would most improve nursing education at their institution, 13 percent of the faculty mentioned more and better qualified faculty. The potency is somewhat reduced here, probably because so many individual problems cropped up — notice that miscellaneous (54 percent) figure is greater than in the other question — due to local crises. It was impossible to suggest any homogeneity out of the miscellaneous category because of the unique problems among the varying institutions. Since problems from institution to institution varied so greatly, the 13 percent homogeneity concerning lack of qualified faculty is quite meaningful.

FOOTNOTE

1. Tate, B., Research Associate, National League for Nursing. Personal Communication to the NCSNNE. 1969.

APPENDIX K

SUMMARY PROJECTIONS OF MANPOWER NEEDS AND ENROLLMENT PATTERNS

Manpower in nursing is a subject worthy of an entire study. It is also a subject which we felt we could not study independently, but rather, because it is so interwoven with all the specific foci of our study, we would be continually touching upon it during our investigations. For these reasons the staff relied on previous studies of nursing manpower for the bulk of information relating to projections of need, demand, and supply. We did, however, put together a straight line projection which was useful in guiding us through the initial stages of the study. The methodology and results of this projection are contained in Tables K-1, K-2, and K-3.

In reviewing the manpower studies conducted during the past eight years, the staff was amazed at the variety of methods employed in arriving at projections of need, demand, and supply for nursing manpower. An outline summary of these studies is presented in Table K-4 while a graphic report of their projections is shown in Figure K-1. Needless to say, the information derived from these studies, including their methodology and results, was of great help to the staff in formulating the recommendations. In the following paragraphs we will detail and analyze some of the more popular and widely used methods of forecasting manpower requirements.

TABLE K-1. MANPOWER PROJECTION

	ADMISSIONS						GRADUATIONS				
Year	High School Graduates (Girls)	Total Admissions R.N.	Percent High School Grads Admit	Diploma	AD	Baccalaureate	Total	Diploma (percent attrition)	AD (percent attrition)	Baccalaureate (percent attrition)	Nurses in Practice
'56–57	750,000	45,255	6.0	37,571	578	7,106					
'57–58	784,000	44,221	5.6	36,402	953	6,866			425		
'58–59	849,000	46,263	5.4	37,722	1,266	7,275		25,907 (31.0)	462 (26.5)		
'59–60	966,000	49,166	5.1	40,013	1,598	7,555	30,113	25,188 (30.8)	789 (51.5)	4,136 (41.8)	
'60–61	1,013,000	49,487	4.9	38,702	2,085	8,700	30,267	25,311 (32.9)	917 (37.7)	4,039 (41.2)	
'61-62	984,000	49,805	5.1	38,257	2,504	9,044	31,186	25,727 (35.7)	1,159 (42.6)	4,300 (40.9)	
'62–63	991,000	49,521	5.0	36,434	3,490	9,597	32,398	26,438 (31.7)	1,479 (44.4)	4,481 (40.7)	
'63–64	1,167,000	52,667	4.5	37,936	4,461	10,270	35,259	28,238 (26.2)	1,962 (40.9)	5,059 (41.9)	
'64–65	1,337,000	57,604	4.3	39,609	6,160	11,835	34,686	26,795 (26.5)	2,510 (43.8)	5,381 (40.5)	
'65–66	1,330,000	60,701	4.6	38,904	8,638	13,159	35,125	26,278 (30.7)	3,349 (43.7)	5,498 (42.7)	

TABLE K-1. MANPOWER PROJECTION

'66–67	1,344,000	58,700	4.4	33,283	11,347	14,070	38,237	27,452 (30.7)	4,654 (46.1)	6,131 (40.3)	
'67–68	1,378,000	61,389	4.5	31,628	14,870	14,891	41,555	28,197 (27.5)	6,213 (45.2)	7,145 (39.6)	
'68–69	1,434,000*	63,169[a] / 65,964[b]	Est. / 4.6	30,258[c] / 31,597[d]	16,929[c] / 17,678[d]	15,982[c] / 16,689[d]	39,323	23,232[e] (30.2)	8,327[e] (44.0)	7,764[e] (41.0)	Jan. '69 / 680,000
'69–70	1,492,000	65,001[a] / 68,632[b]	Est. / 4.6	28,730[c] / 30,335[d]	19,110[c] / 20,178[d]	17,160[c] / 18,169[d]	40,067	22,076[e] (30.2)	9,690[e] (44.0)	8,301[e] (41.0)	Jan '70 / 697,743
'70–71	1,549,000	66,886[a] / 71,254[b]	Est. / 4.6	27,089[c] / 28,858[d]	21,403[c] / 22,801[d]	18,394[c] / 19,595[d]	41,375	21,588[e] (30.2)	11,001[e] (44.0)	8,786[e] (41.0)	Jan. '71 / 715,676
'71–72	1,599,000	68,826[a] / 73,554[b]	Est. / 4.6	25,328[c] / 27,068[d]	23,814[c] / 25,450[d]	19,684[c] / 21,036[d]	42,628	20,613[e] (30.2)	12,377[e] (44.0)	9,638[e] (41.0)	Jan. '72 / 734,339
'72–73	1,639,000	70,822[a] / 75,394[b]	Est. / 4.6	23,442[c] / 24,955[d]	26,346[c] / 28,047[d]	21,034[c] / 22,392[d]	43,728	19,526[e] (30.2)	13,794[e] (44.0)	10,408[e] (41.0)	Jan. '73 / 753,658
'73–74	1,682,000	72,875[a] / 77,372[b]	Est. / 4.6	21,425[c] / 22,747[d]	29,004[c] / 30,794[d]	22,446[c] / 23,831[d]	44,722	18,286[e] (30.2)	15,230[e] (44.0)	11,206[e] (41.0)	Jan. '74 / 773,464
'74–75	1,719,000	74,988[a] / 79,074[b]	Est. / 4.6	19,272[c] / 20,322[d]	31,795[c] / 33,527[d]	23,921[c] / 25,225[d]	45,645	16,890[e] (30.2)	16,743[e] (44.0)	12,012[e] (41.0)	Jan. '75 / 793,640
											Jan. '76 / 814,106

* Data on the number of high school graduates (girls) for the years 1968–69 to 1974–75 obtained from a 1967 projection by the U.S. Office of Education and contained in *Facts About Nursing*, 1968 Edition, p. 87.

(a) Average annual change in total admissions for the years 1960–61 to 1967–68 = +2.9 percent per year. This average annual increase was applied to the actual admissions total in 1967–68 and to each subsequent year resulting in the totals listed in front of (a).

(b) Percent of high school graduates (girls) entering nursing programs for the years 1960–61 to 1967–68 averaged 4.6 percent per year. This percent was applied to the U.S. Office of Education projection of the number of graduates beginning with the year 1968–69 and to each subsequent year resulting in the totals listed in front of (b).

TABLE K-1. MANPOWER PROJECTION

(c) Average annual change in the share of total admissions for each program for the years 1960—61 to 1967—68 = Diploma, —3.7 percent per year; AD, +2.6 percent per year; Baccalaureate, +1.1 percent per year. These percents were applied to total admission (a) beginning in 1968—69 and to each subsequent year resulting in the totals listed in front of (c) for each program.

(d) Average annual change in the share of total admissions for each program for the year 1960—61 to 1967—68 = Diploma, —3.7 percent per year; AD, +2.6 percent per year; Baccalaureate, +1.1 percent per year. These percents were applied to total admissions (b) beginning in 1968—69 and to each subsequent year resulting in the totals listed in front of (d) for each program.

(e) Average attrition rate per year for the period 1960-61 to 1967-68 = Diploma (30.2 percent); AD (44.0 percent); Baccalaureate (41.0 percent). Attrition rates applied to the average of (c) and (d). (Example— 1968-69 Diploma Admissions were projected to be 30,258 + 31,597 = 61.855 ÷ 2 = 30,928 X 30.2 percent = 21,588 estimated graduations three years later in 1970-71.)

(f) We started with the figure of 680,000 nurses in active practice as of January 1, 1969, which was obtained from the Division of Nursing, Public Health Service. Then we added our estimate of the number of graduates in 1969 (39,323) and subtracted from this total a net attrition of 3 percent.

Example: January, 1969 —   680,000 RN's in practice

                                  +   39,323 Graduations, 1969

                                          719,323

                                   −   21,580 Net Attrition*

        January, 1970 —   697,743

*Net Attrition = Losses through the year due to resignation, retirement, or death, less gains resulting from the return of formerly inactive nurses plus the addition of foreign trained nurses licensed through endorsement.

TABLE K-2. ADMISSION DATA

a. Annual Changes in Admissions

Year	Diploma (percent)	AD (percent)	Baccalaureate (percent)	Total (percent)
'60– '61	- 3.3	+ 30.5	+ 15.2	+ 0.6
'61– '62	- 1.1	+ 20.1	+ 4.0	+ 0.6
'62– '63	- 4.8	+ 39.4	+ 6.1	- 0.6
'63– '64	+ 4.1	+ 27.8	+ 7.0	+ 6.4
'64– '65	+ 4.4	+ 38.1	+ 15.2	+ 9.4
'65– '66	- 1.8	+ 40.2	+ 11.2	+ 5.4
'66– '67	- 14.4	+ 31.4	+ 6.9	- 3.3
'67– '68	- 5.0	+ 31.0	+ 5.8	+ 4.6
	$\frac{-21.9}{8} = -2.7$ percent per year	$\frac{+258.5}{8} = +32.3$ percent per year	$\frac{+71.4}{8} = +8.9$ percent per year	$\frac{+23.1}{8} = +2.9$ percent per year

b. Share of Total Admissions

Year	Diploma (percent)	AD (percent)	Baccalaureate (percent)
'59– '60	81.4	3.2	15.4
'60– '61	78.2 (-3.2)	4.2 (+1.0)	17.6 (+2.2)
'61– '62	76.8 (-1.4)	5.0 (+ .8)	18.2 (+ .6)
'62– '63	73.6 (-3.2)	7.0 (+2.0)	19.4 (+1.2)
'63– '64	72.0 (-1.6)	8.5 (+1.5)	19.5 (+ .1)
'64– '65	68.8 (-3.2)	10.7 (+2.2)	20.5 (-1.0)
'65– '66	64.1 (-4.7)	14.2 (+3.5)	21.7 (+1.2)
'66– '67	56.7 (-7.4)	19.3 (+5.1)	24.0 (+2.3)
'67– '68	51.6 (-5.1)	24.2 (+4.9)	24.2 (+ .2)
	$\frac{-29.8}{8} = -3.7$ percent per year	$\frac{+21.0}{8} = +2.6$ percent per year	$\frac{+8.8}{8} = +1.1$ percent per year

TABLE K-3. ANNUAL CHANGES IN GRADUATIONS

Year	Diploma (percent)	AD (percent)	Baccalaureate (percent)	Total (percent)
'60– '61	+ 0.5	+ 16.2	- 2.3	+ 0.5
'61– '62	+ 1.8	+ 26.4	+ 6.5	+ 3.0
'62– '63	+ 2.8	+ 27.6	+ 4.2	+ 3.9
'63– '64	+ 6.8	+ 32.7	+12.9	+ 8.8
'64– '65	- 5.1	+ 27.9	+ 6.4	- 1.6
'65– '66	- 1.9	+ 33.4	+ 2.2	+ 1.2
'66– '67	+ 4.5	+ 39.0	+11.5	+ 8.9
'67– '68	+ 2.7	+ 33.5	+16.5	+ 8.7

$$\frac{+\,12.1}{8} = +\,1.5 \text{ percent per year}$$ $$\frac{+\,236.7}{8} = +\,29.6 \text{ percent per year}$$ $$\frac{+57.9}{8} = +\,7.2 \text{ percent per year}$$ $$\frac{+\,33.4}{8} = +\,4.2 \text{ percent per year}$$

Measurement of manpower requirements in nursing is essential in determining the adequacy of the existing manpower supply. These requirements are generally measured in terms of *need* or *demand*. In using *need* as a measurement, the most frequently employed concept is professional judgments of standards considered to produce optimum nursing care. An example of this type of measurement is found in the Surgeon General's Report, "Towards Quality in Nursing Care" (1963) where the most adequate hospital nursing care was judged to result when 50 percent of the care was provided by RN's, 30 percent by LPN's, and 20 percent by aides. This method of measuring manpower requirements is useful in that it attempts to project the most desirable current system of nursing care into the future; however, it relies on both the particular philosophies or beliefs of the professionals comprising the group, and the extension of a *status quo* utilization pattern.

When *demand* is used, the best available measure is total budgeted positions. The resultant figure includes all positions for nursing, whether filled or vacant, and supposedly indicates the number of nurses employers are willing and able to pay for. Caution has to be exercised when using the concept of "budgeted vacancies" for budgets are frequently padded with salaries for unplanned positions in order to provide for unanticipated emergencies. An additional limitation of this measure can be seen when projections are analyzed for future requirements. We find, in effect, that the total budgeted positions are specifically related to a current population base. At the national level, the future demand for nurses is the ratio of total active nurses, plus the unfilled positions, per 100,000 population. An example of this is shown in Table K-5. This is certainly the most familiar measure of manpower

TABLE K-4. SUMMARY OF MANPOWER NEED PROJECTIONS OF PREVIOUS STUDIES

Study	Projection of Need, Demand or Requirement	Projection of Supply in 1975	Basis for Projection (s)	Summary Highlights
Surgeon General's Report (1962)	1970 — (a) 850,000 (b) 680,000	(c) 650-680,000	(a) & (b) Based on professional judgments of the number needed to assume safe, therapeutically effective, and efficient nursing care.	Principal problems relating to manpower for which solutions must be found: Not enough capable young people are being recruited to meet the demand.
			(a) Determined not to be feasible for 1970. Criteria — that highest patient satisfaction is obtained when direct patient care is provided in the ratio 50 percent RN — 30 percent LPN — and 20 percent nursing aides.	Too few college-bound students are entering the nursing field. Continuing lag in the social and economic status of nurses discourages people from entering the field and remaining active in it.
			(b) & (c) Feasible goal — based on assumption that there will be between 41,000 (extension of present trend) and 53,000 graduates a year by 1969, that the present rate of return of inactive nurses continues, and that there is continued utilization of nurses trained in other countries — then the number of professional nurses in practice in 1970 can be estimated at between 650,000 — 680,000.	Available nursing personnel are not being fully utilized for effective patient care, including supervision and teaching as well as clinical care. Many basic questions need to be answered: What kinds of nurses and how many are needed to alleviate present shortages of personnel as well as to meet future requirements?

TABLE K-4. SUMMARY OF MANPOWER NEED PROJECTIONS OF PREVIOUS STUDIES

Source	Projection	Assumptions	Comments
Health Manpower Source Book Section 2 Revised (1966)	1975 — (a) 850,000 (b) 724,300 (c) 688,100	(a) Extended the requirement for 850,000 RN's, determined by the Surgeon General to be unfeasible in 1970, to 1975. (b) Based on a 2 percent annual increase in graduations (this was the average annual increase over the last 10 years) and a 4 percent annual attrition rate. (c) Based on the assumption that the 1963-64 graduation figure of 35,000 will remain constant over the next ten years and that the attrition rate will be 4 percent annually.	In order for the projection of 850,000 RN's by 1975 to be realized, admission to nursing schools must rise from 69,000 (3.7 percent of 17 year-old girls) in '64-'65 to 109,000 (5.5 percent) in '72-'73. Then using 67 percent of admissions, a percent which for many years has been the overall completion rate for students entering nursing school directly from high school, and assuming the attrition rate goes no higher than 4 percent, then by 1974 annual graduations will increase to 72,000 and the estimate of 850,000 RN's in active practice in 1975 becomes feasible.

How can the profession of nursing be made more attractive to potential recruits?

How can the best use be made of our limited number of nurses?

The manpower projections in this report do not seem to consider such important factors as: future productivity of nurses, technological change, substitution and availability of other inputs, and potential impact of the recommendations of this report on the manpower projections.

TABLE K-4. SUMMARY OF MANPOWER NEED PROJECTIONS OF PREVIOUS STUDIES

National Commission on Automation, Technology and Economic Progress (1966)	1975 — 830,000	No Projection

One of the most significant determinants of any manpower projection is the basic assumptions describing the expected nature and composition of the economy in the target year. The assumptions underlying the projection in this study are as follows:

(1) Civilian labor force of 91.4 million

(2) Peacetime conditions will prevail.

(3) Unemployment rate of 3 percent

(4) National Security expenditures (excluding space) will not be significantly different than they were in 1964.

(5) Economic, social and consumption patterns will continue to change at about the same rate as they have in the recent past.

(6) Scientific and technological advances of recent years will continue and research and development expenditures will continue to grow, although at a slower rate than during the decade of 1955-1965.

Technology is not expected to significantly affect growth in employment requirements for nurses, but should affect their job characteristics. Technology is just as apt to free nurses from many routine tasks enabling them to devote more time to patient care, as it is to create new areas of work.

New medicines, drugs, and treatments should increase the employment requirements for nurses. Many more people would be expected to seek medical help as a result of the availability of the medicine and treatments thereby creating a greater demand for nursing care. However, the effects of such developments will be offset to some extent by reductions in the periods of time patients are ill.

The projections did not take into account limitations in the future supply of nurses. They represent the nation's requirements for nurses in 1975 under stated assumptions, they are not predictions of what employment will actually be in 1975. Also, no attempt has been made to include the estimate of the number of nurses needed for replacement.

TABLE K-4. SUMMARY OF MANPOWER NEED PROJECTIONS OF PREVIOUS STUDIES

In developing specific industry projections one of the most significant factors affecting employment in each industry was the prospective level of demand for the product or service of the industry.

Occupational patterns were developed for the current year, projected to 1975, and then applied against the overall industry projection framework. The preliminary occupational projections resulting from the application of occupational patterns to industry totals were then analyzed and compared with the occupational projections developed independently. In general, the final projections presented in this report are based on judgment as to the effect of demand factors on specific occupations.

National Commission on Health Manpower (1967)	1975 — (a) 895,000 (b) 790,000

(a) Weighted heavily toward the increased use of short-term general hospitals where over half of the active RN's are employed.

During 1965-75, it is estimated that hospital patient days will rise approximately 42 percent due to growth of population, changes in its age and distribution, and Medicare.

The report qualifies its projection of nursing manpower requirements by saying "Sharp increases in nurses' salaries may discourage hospitals from adding nurses as liberally as they have heretofore, and the nurse-patient ratio may not increase quite as fast."

The supply estimate does not include those RN's on inactive status or not employed in nursing. Continued improvement in wages and working condi-

Appendix K 349

TABLE K-4. SUMMARY OF MANPOWER NEED PROJECTIONS OF PREVIOUS STUDIES

If the ratio of RN's to patients is assumed to rise by 10 percent in the next decade, as it did in the last, a 42 percent growth in hospital patient days should be accompanied by a 56 percent increase in hospital nurses. If the same rate of increase applies to other health institutions, total institutional requirements for nurses will grow by approximately 210,000 between 1965-75. Although demands from other sources are not expected to grow as quickly, they may still be sufficient to generate demands for 80,000 additional nurses.

(b) Based on an annual increase of 2 percent in graduations and an annual attrition rate of 3 percent.

tions would very likely result in the supply matching the projected demand by 1975. This would result because improved economic conditions would not only draw nurses back into practice, but would also slow the withdrawal of others from leaving the field.

Study	Projection		
Health Manpower 1966–1975 U.S. Dept. of Labor (1967)	1975 – 860,000 (240,000 growth) (150,000 replacement)	To meet the projected needs of 390,000 additional nurses by 1975, nursing schools will have to graduate an average of 43,000 per year over the 1966–1975 period.	The projection is an estimate of the effective demand for nurses in 1975, developed under a specific set of assumptions rather than perceptions of specific needs based on provision of specific standards or goals of medical care. The assumptions describe the nature and composition of the economy in 1975.

This study recognized that many factors affect the demand for nurses. The two most important being the number of persons requiring health care and the amount of funds spent on health care, from public and private sources.

The study uses alternative assumptions regarding population and expenditures

TABLE K-4. SUMMARY OF MANPOWER NEED PROJECTIONS OF PREVIOUS STUDIES

	These assumptions are: (1) GNP of about $1,058 trillion (2) Resolution of Vietnam by 1970. (3) Economic, social and consumption patterns will continue to change at about the same rate as they have in the past. (4) Rate of scientific and technological advances of recent years will continue. An analysis was then made of the number of patients who will need nursing care, expenditures for health care, technological developments, need for elimination of current shortages, and employer utilization patterns.	to discover how these different sets of assumptions would affect the manpower projections. The use of different assumptions about the population in 1975 has little affect on the estimates of 1975 requirements for health manpower. On the other hand, different assumptions about the level of health care expenditures over the 1965-75 period would have a great impact on the need for health manpower. Estimates of the need for nursing personnel utilize a continuation of patterns of employer utilization, rather than estimates of utilization that professional perceptions indicate would be needed to provide some desired level (or goal) of nursing care. Estimates of health manpower required based on professional perceptions of needs are generally higher than the levels indicated by projections of effective demand.	
Nurse Training Act — Program Review Report (1967)	1975 — 1,000,000	No Projection	Used the criteria of the Surgeon General's Report which were based upon professional judgment for 'safe, therapeutically effective, and efficient care' rather than projected vacancies and assumed the continuation of current patterns of organization for health care.	The Committee stated that 40 percent of the one million nurses needed by 1975 should be prepared at the baccalaureate and graduate degree levels to form a nucleus for planning, coordinating, and giving expert practice. The remaining 60 percent should be prepared to assume nursing responsibilities that are less complex in nature.

TABLE K-4. SUMMARY OF MANPOWER NEED PROJECTIONS OF PREVIOUS STUDIES

National Planning Association Center for Priority Analysis (1968)	1975 — (a) 840,000 (b) 1,091,000	No Projection	(a) Continued expansion of total expenditures for health and medical care at the existing rate level — a maintenance of effort level. (b) Expansion of effort to pursue realistically the health goal of narrowing "the gap between the potentialities of modern health technologies and the availability of medical care for most Americans." The center estimates that to attain this goal would result in health expenditures for medical care, from public and private sources, rising to 8.7 percent of GNP, or between $85-90 billion, in 1975.	National Planning Association in the first goals analysis study used the GNP and its allocation among various goals in a base year and then projected the increase in costs after 10 years. The present study translates these dollar costs into manpower terms, thereby providing a useful basis for considering manpower training and educational policies. The manpower projections for the goals refer to aspiration goals. All told, their projected requirements are larger than the labor force anticipated in the 1970's. However, these estimates can serve as a take-off point for further research to

The progress of the Nurse Training Act after three years seems to indicate that the nation will have made substantial increases in total numbers of nurses by 1970.

However, the number prepared at the baccalaureate and graduate levels will fall far short of the goal. The Committee recognized that meeting the 1975 goal for this group will continue to be a major challenge, however with sufficient Federal assistance its goals for quality care are attainable.

TABLE K-4. SUMMARY OF MANPOWER NEED PROJECTIONS OF PREVIOUS STUDIES

develop projections of expenditures and manpower needs for alternative combinations of priorities that would be feasible within the limits set by the available or the expected resources.

The estimates of shortage frequently refer to the future requirements in individual occupations that derive from a concept of social need. The aspiration goals used as the basis for manpower estimates in this study represent one definition of social need, a definition reflecting the trend of opinion in the U. S. in the mid-1960's. By contrast, shortages in the sense of unfilled positions existing at any moment in time, are likely to be considerably smaller than the comparable estimates related to a standard of need.

As shortages threaten to emerge for an occupation, they frequently set off pressures for salary increases and other improvements, which typically increase the number of people choosing to enter or remain in these occupations. The potentials of technology are also apt to be applied at a more rapid pace in an attempt to economize in the use of scarce and costly human skills. The current experimentation with computer-

TABLE K-4. SUMMARY OF MANPOWER NEED PROJECTIONS OF PREVIOUS STUDIES

oriented systems for recording medical histories and treatment as an aid in diagnosis is an example of these applications. Also expectations of shortages in occupations that are important to the nation's purposes serve to encourage government to introduce and expand programs enlarging opportunities for education and training in these fields.

Study	Projection	Basis	Comments
U.S. Public Health Service, Bureau of Health Professions Education and Manpower Training, Division of Nursing (1969)	(a) 1,000,000 (b) 750,000 – 881,000	(a) Based on professional judgments measured in terms of criteria considered to produce optimal levels of nursing care for patients. The criteria employed were those established by the 1962 Surgeon General's Consultant Group on Nursing for each field of nursing employment excepting psychiatric and mental health nursing where the criteria were updated in 1966 by the National Institute for Mental Health. Bases for projections of quantitative personnel needs for 1975 were applied to appropriate projection factors in each field. Needs for each field were aggregated in terms of individual nurses, not full time equivalents.	The study recognizes that the qualitative and quantitative needs for registered nurses in 1975 is practically impossible to achieve. In 1969 there were approximately 680,000 registered nurses in active practice. To achieve the indicated goal of 1,000,000 by 1975, more than half a million would have to be added to the work force over the next six years to provide for growth and replacement. The number of graduations annually from RN programs now stands at about 40,000. This means that graduations would have to increase along with the number of RN's returning to active practice and then attrition from practice decline appreciably in order for the goal to be realized. In order to attain the goal of at least a baccalaureate degree for 40 percent of the RN's it would be necessary to

TABLE K-4. SUMMARY OF MANPOWER NEED PROJECTIONS OF PREVIOUS STUDIES

(b) Fifteen different projections of supply were made by changing such factors as the admission, completion, and attrition rates. These projections fall within the range indicated and averaged 809,867.

quadruple the present number of graduates from baccalaureate and higher degree programs. Currently some 14 percent of the active RN's have the baccalaureate or higher degree.

The study accurately points out the advantage and limitation of using professional judgment to project needs and supply. It states "A major advantage of this method is that it attempts to free itself from the status quo. It is based on a conceptualization of a desirable system in which nursing care would be provided at some future time including determination of the appropriate amount and mix of care. A major limitation of the method is the fact that many of the criteria used, the judgments about the future status of nursing care, and the predictions about the demand for nursing care in the future represent the values and philosophies of the particular group of experts involved. Moreover, these projections would have to be reexamined from time to time in order to assess their continued relevance and meaningfulness."

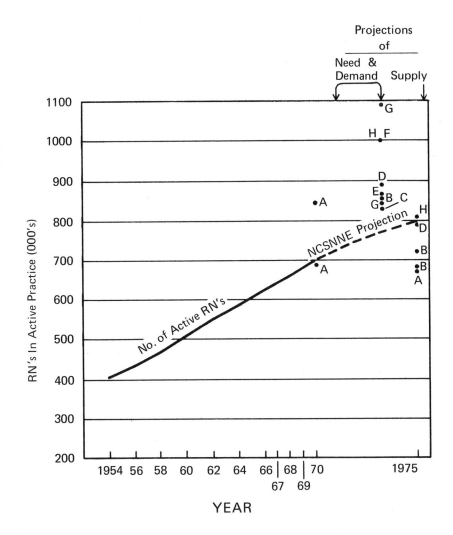

Figure K-1. Projections of Needs, Demands and Supply

KEY:

A = Surgeon General's Report (1962)
B = Health Manpower Source Book, Section 2, Revised (1966)
C = National Commission on Automation, Technology and Economic Progress (1966)
D = National Commission on Health Manpower (1967)
E = Health Manpower 1966–1975, U.S. Dept. of Labor (1967)
F = Nurse Training Act—Program Review Report (1967)
G = National Planning Association, Center for Priority Analysis (1968)
H = U.S. Public Health Service, Bureau of Health Professions Education and Manpower
    Training, Division of Nursing (1969)

TABLE K-5. NURSE TO POPULATION RATIOS IN SELECTED STATES 1966

State	*Nurse - Population Ratio*
National Average	313
Connecticut	536
Massachusetts	532
New York	408
Pennsylvania	395
Illinois	330
Nebraska	329
Kansas	303
Michigan	277
Indiana	259
Kentucky	198
Mississippi	157
Arkansas	133

Source: Facts About Nursing, 1968. p. 13.

requirements, but it assumes that only population growth will affect the demand. It ignores such factors as changes in patterns of utilization, increases in productivity, economic conditions, and changed demands for health care.

We discovered that each method used to measure manpower requirements had its virtues — and limitations. As long as one is aware of these characteristics, it seems that any of the measures can be employed successfully. What is illuminating, however, is that despite their differences in methodology, every study predicted a shortage of nurses in the future.

The concept of shortage leads us into the third dimension of manpower — and that is supply. The nurse-population ratio has gone steadily upward which would indicate that the supply of nurses has been responsive to the demand. If this is the case, what is all the clamor about? The point is that projections based on *demand* are somewhat more conservative than those based on *need*. Thus, using the nurse-population ratio as a guide, the *demand* is largely being met, but the supply, based on *need*, is still not being fulfilled.

Various interpretations of the concept of "shortage" and the many factors affecting manpower contingencies have resulted in conflicting opinions and judgments regarding the adequacy of the nurse supply. Better utilization and organization of the existing supply is felt by many to be the primary answer to the shortage problem. Technology and capital investment are also believed to be solutions for increasing the effectiveness of the existing supply. As the National Advisory Commission on Health Manpower stated, "Given the large number of non-practicing nurses, increasing the output of new nurses is not the best means of attacking the nurse shortage. The most important actions are those which will make nursing a more attractive profession and thus entice trained nurses back to duty, as well as lower the attrition rates of students and new graduates." In regard to admissions and graduations, Figures K-2, K-3, and K-4 give a picture of past, present and future admissions as well as information on nursing programs. The projections in Figure K-2 are those of the NCSNNE staff. Additional tables on admissions and graduations are those previously compiled by the staff and shown in Tables K-1, K-2, and K-3.

A statement from the Program Review Report of the Nursing Training Act appropriately summarizes our findings. "In the final analysis, the nature of nursing practice and the way in which nursing care services are organized will determine the number of nurses needed and the kinds of educational programs required to prepare them." Thus there seems no argument that the increasing demand for nursing service will result in a need for more nursing personnel and a supply must be developed to meet these goals.

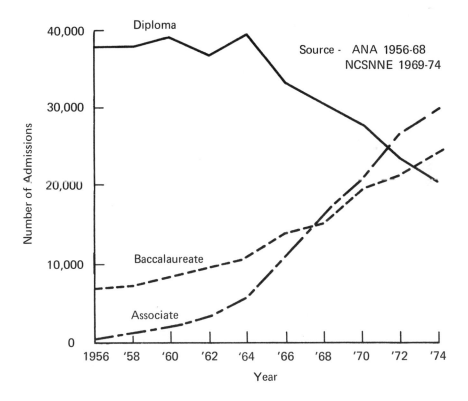

Figure K-2. Trends in Admission to Diploma, Associate and Baccalaureate Degree Programs.

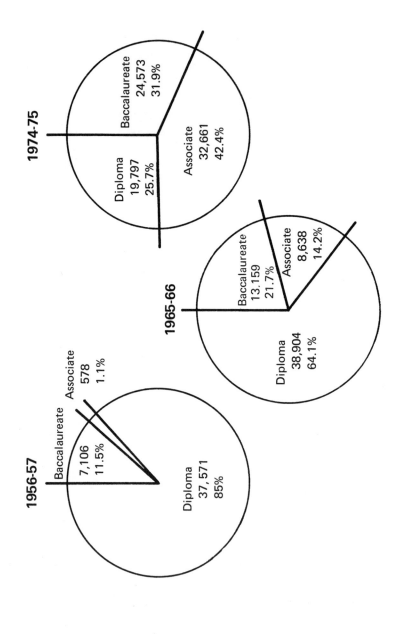

Figure K-3. Share of Admissions to Diploma, Associate and Baccalaureate Degree Programs

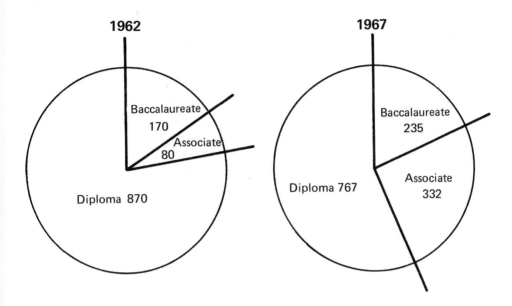

Source: *Facts about Nursing,* 1968, p. 106 and NLN State Approved
Schools of *Nursing,* 1969, p. 108.

Figure K-4. Number of Schools and Initial Programs in Nursing

APPENDIX L

NURSING MANPOWER: AN ANALYSIS OF FACTORS RELATED TO SUPPLY OF AND DEMAND FOR NURSES

One of the common generalizations made about nursing in the United States is that there is an extreme shortage of nurses. This generalization affects almost every policy decision made about nursing, and has tended to place heavy burdens on every effort to professionalize the occupation.

A shortage of nurses dictates that every preparatory program be maintained and expanded — with subsequent problems of quality and efficiency. A shortage of nurses suggests that as many aides, attendants, and assistants as possible be used to extend the arm of the qualified nurse — with attendant problems of quality and efficiency.

Throughout much of the literature on nursing manpower there weaves the theme of shortage, accompanied by the two traditional solutions to the problem: expand the number of nursing students; increase the number of aides.

The problem and its proposed answers have an almost seductive simplicity. For after all, is there not a crisis in terms of a nursing shortage? Surely, the papers, the health experts, and many of the nurses themselves say it is so.

But an over-hasty reliance on some of these sources may cause an over-hasty acceptance of their conclusions. Without denying for a moment that there are acute problems in providing needed nursing care, it is useful to examine the relationship between the predicted needs for nurses and the actual number of persons who are available for practice.

Since 1957, a series of manpower projection studies have almost uniformly predicted a sharply rising need for nurses coupled with a pessimistic doubt that the suggested numbers could ever be attained. Figure L-1 however, indicates that the actual number of active nurses has generally risen to equal and exceed the projected requirements year after year. (For more detail, see Appendix K)

There are observers who have seriously questioned many of the assumptions that have been made in developing these projections. Some have suggested that projected figures necessarily fail to take into account technological changes that can make practice more effective and efficient — thereby reducing, somewhat, the *per capita* need for nursing. Others, like Anderson,[1] simply suggest that the "social professions" always are uneconomic in their assessment of needs and generally over-estimate their requirements. However one may view such criticisms, there is evidence to suggest that our projected supply needs have been exceeded (whether they were "generous" or not) and yet we have a nursing shortage.

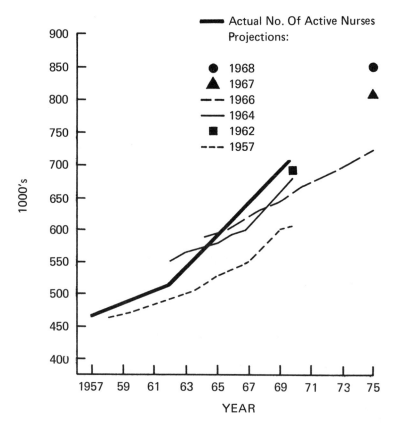

Figure L-1. Actual Number of Nurses in Relationship to Projected Numbers.

The paradox of this situation is revealed in Figure L-2. The supply of nurses in practice has grown faster than the population curve and we now have more nurses *per capita* (and per hospital bed) than we had in 1954. Certainly the demand for increased nursing care has been dynamic. As shown in Figure L-3, the relative change in a number of factors related to the need for nurses has been largely upward. Relatedly, however, the supply factors displayed in Figure L-4, with one exception, follow an ascending pattern. Only the percentage of high school graduates choosing nursing as a career has tended to decline. This particular variant represents a distinct warning that nursing is losing its relative attractiveness as an occupational choice.

If we accept the paradox that there are reported shortages in the face of increasing supply among nurses, we can attempt to analyze the problem using different viewpoints from the traditional cause-effect approach.

One can, for example, look at the analysis by Hoekelman which argues that: "By any of the criteria which define a shortage of personnel in any occupation, one cannot claim a shortage of registered nurses in this country."[2]

He then cites five conditions which support his claim: 1) unfilled positions in preparatory programs; 2) high drop-out rate during training; 3) relatively low rate of employment; 4) high rate of turnover; 5) moderate rather than a rapid growth of income.

In general, our compilation of data consistently substantiated his claims. While some nursing schools had waiting lists of applicants, most could accommodate more students and many reported a problem in the lack of qualified applicants.[3] Similarly, while there were institutional and regional variations, nationally almost one out of three nursing students dropped out of the preparatory program prior to completion.[4]

The rate of employment is a particularly problematic point to consider. As shown in Figure L-5, there were by several estimates, some 1,200,000 nurses living in the United States in 1968. These included all those who qualified for the R.N. after any type of preparation. Approximately one out of every four nurses, however, failed to maintain a license for practice. Another group, also approximating one of four, maintained a license, but did not practice. Of the remaining nurses, only 445,000 worked full-time — only somewhat more than one of every four. Making generous allowance for old age, health, and assorted conditions, one must recognize that the "shrinkage" in nursing is a remarkably important fact.*

So also with turnover. As indicated in Figure L-6, nursing shows a particularly high rate of turnover in comparison with public school education — an occupation fairly similar in terms of sex linkage, socio-economic background, and general salary conditions.

---

* For example, the two highest estimates of active nurses needed for 1975 are 850,000 and 1,000,000 respectively. The "total" figure of 1,200,000 nurses in 1968 could meet these figures easily if higher rates of activity obtained within the occupation (see Figure L-5).

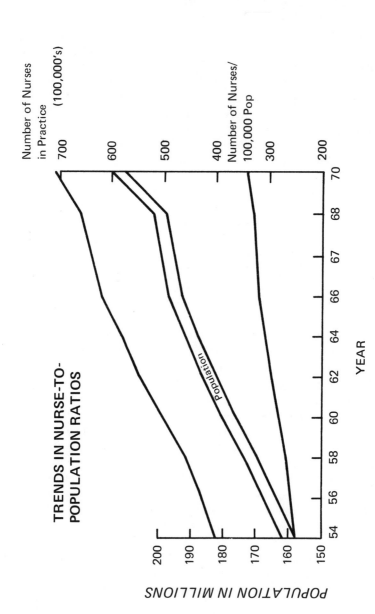

Source: Facts about Nursing, 1968; pg. 10

Figure L-2.   Trends in Nurse-to-Population Ratios.

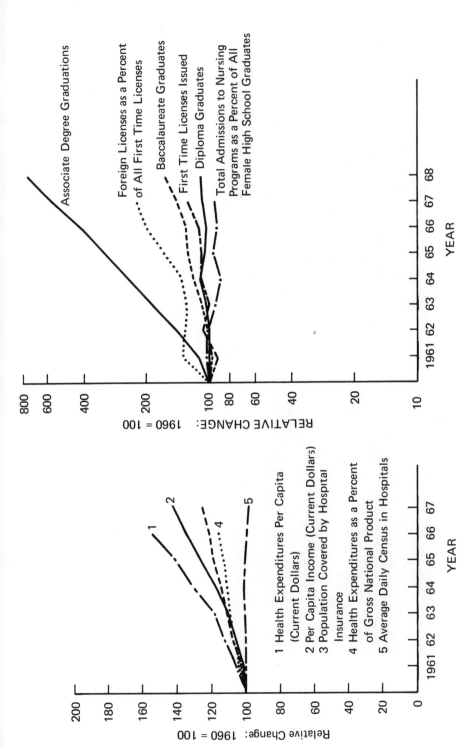

Figure L-4. Relative Change in Factors Related to Supply of Nurses

Figure L-3. Relative Change in Factors Related to Demand for Nurses.

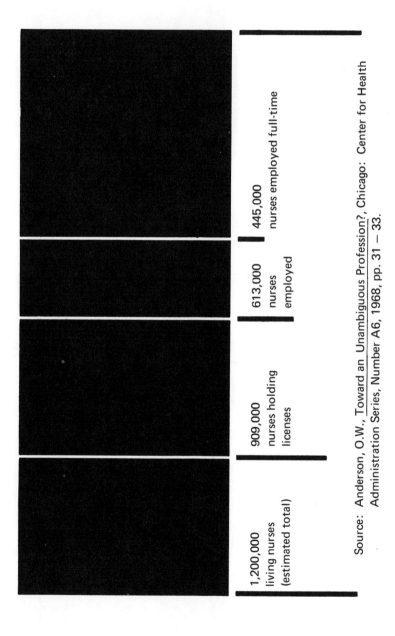

1,200,000
living nurses
(estimated total)

909,000
nurses holding
licenses

613,000
nurses
employed

445,000
nurses employed full-time

Source: Anderson, O.W., Toward an Unambiguous Profession?, Chicago: Center for Health Administration Series, Number A6, 1968, pp. 31 – 33.

Figure L-5. Recent Data on Employment Status of Nurses.

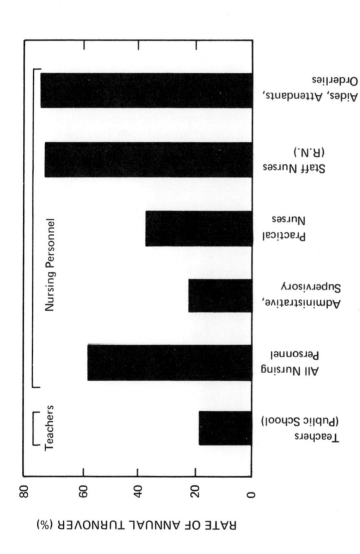

RATE OF ANNUAL TURNOVER (%)

Source: Technology and Manpower in the Health Service Industry, 1965 – 75, Manpower Research Bulletin No. 14. Washington, D.C., U.S. Dept. of Labor. 1967, p. 22.

Figure L-6. Rate of Turnover in Nursing Compared With Teaching.

368

Appendix LAppendix L

Average Weekly Salary Range	Number of Hospitals	Percentages	Estimated Number of Community Hospitals
less than $115	160	10.64	673
$115 – $125	211	14.05	822
$126 – $140	459	30.56	1788
$141 – $150	286	19.04	1114
more than $150	386	25.70	1503
Total	1502	100.00	5350

Source: American Hospital Association, Annual Reports, 1969. Chicago: 1970, p. 86.

Figure L-7. Estimate of Nurses' Salaries in Community Hospitals.

Finally, in terms of economic conditions, nursing has enjoyed recent advances in salary. As indicated in Figure L-7, however, seventy-five per cent of the community hospitals are still paying their nurse practitioners less than $7,500 per year. By way of a single personal comparison, beginning teachers in this writer's school district will have a starting salary of slightly above $7,200 this year. Even some of the recent gains in nurses' starting salaries have not produced corresponding increases in the salaries of experienced practitioners so that the net effect may be to diminish the career attractiveness of salary schedules.

In terms of our own assessment of the nursing shortage, we found it advantageous to view the continuation of career activity in terms of a concept of social behavior based on rewards (or reinforcement in more precise psychological terms). Rather than accepting shortage as a condition, this concept views it as a result. This suggests, in turn, that the shortage of nurses can be explained in terms like this: the social behavior of nursing is rewarded by a variety of benefits; if the sum total of these benefits is truly reinforcing to the individual (and relatively more reinforcing than alternative occupations) then we would expect to find career enhancement and increased duration of individual activity within the career pattern; if the sum total of these benefits has limited reinforcement for the individuals (and alternative occupations offer greater rewards) then we would expect to find withdrawal, turnover, and frustration symptoms within the occupation and its career pattern. In this light, nursing obviously suffers from a lack of sufficiently rewarding conditions. The result is personnel shrinkage and shortage.

If this analysis is viable, then, our traditional approaches to the nursing shortage are not aimed at the root causes of the problem. We are attempting to treat the symptoms by palliation rather than cure. And the patient is not only suffering, but may be losing the possibility of recovery.

Social reinforcers may be viewed as being either extrinsic or intrinsic to the crucial desires of the individual. Extrinsic reinforcers, such as pay and benefits, can provide for the necessary survival and security needs of the individual as developed by Maslow.[5] This approach suggests that until the basic needs of the individual for a living wage and reasonable economic security are provided, then, it is relatively useless to appeal to other motives as a springboard to action. That there are evident economic concerns over nursing compensation is generally recognized. The emphasis of nursing organizations on economic security, the increasing militancy of bargaining, and finally, the growth of unionism has dramatically scored the need to provide more reasonable levels of compensation.

Common reasoning also suggests that if we need more nurses to remain in direct patient care, then nurse practitioners need to see comparable compensation to the common alternatives of administration or education. Largely because there is a free (or relatively more free) interplay of supply and demand on college teaching salaries, we find qualified nurse academicians sometimes commanding higher salaries than equally prepared academicians in disciplines where the professorial pool is more filled. (See Appendix M)

Important as the extrinsic satisfactions are to the provision of security to the individual, Maslow emphasizes that each individual has a level of satiety for such reward, and that when this is reasonably attained, other needs must be met. Herzberg[6] is perhaps even more emphatic in his consideration of motivational factors because he suggests that certain kinds of rewards merely prevent dissatisfaction and that another grouping of reinforcements is necessary to provide satisfaction.

However we may wish to consider these concepts, it remains that there is a group of intrinsic satisfiers in nursing that could be extremely important to the long-range solution of manpower problems. If we examine the evidence of Hughes[7] and many others, we must recognize that the common reason given by students and practitioners for entering nursing is that of "wishing to help people." This would seem to suggest that the individuals themselves have identified as behavioral reinforcements the direct patient care functions, and, very likely, the development of the ability to enhance the quality of such personal service.

It is this very basic desire that is the critical issue underlying most of the controversy about nurse utilization. Figure L-8 is merely one randomly selected illustration of the point. Note that the staff nurse spends approximately 40 per cent of her time in direct patient care, but over half of that time is consumed in the passing of medications. She spends less time in direct patient care than the practical nurse, the orderly, other types of staff personnel, and even the student nurse. These time distributions have been confirmed by the studies of Christman and Jelinek,[8] by the investigation of Duff and Hollingshead,[9] and by numerous utilization surveys.

The problems with this situation are two-fold. First, we find that the use of nurses in health care facilities is contrary to the intrinsic motivations that brought them into nursing, that is, they are not being used primarily to care for people.

percent of time by type of staff

	Head Nurse	RN	LPN/ LVN	Nursing Aide	Orderly	Ward Clerk	Student Nurse	All types of staff
Direct patient care:								
Medications	7	23	6				10	9
Treatment and tests		9	12	7	11		7	8
Vital signs			9	8	5		6	6
Personal care		9	24	32	28		27	20
Supportive care								
Feeding								
Rounds	8							
Transport patient								
Indirect patient care:								
Charting	21	16	10			24	11	11
Other clerical	16	7				39		7
Patient servicing			6	12	10			6
Reports and conferences	16	10	6				10	7
Exchange of information								
Employee activities:								
Unit servicing				7	8			
Personal	10	10	12	16	18	12	9	13
Other general						10		

Source: Jacobs, S.E. "Older Patients Get More Care." *Hospitals.* 43:24:71, December 16, 1969.

Figure L-8. Hospital Utilization of Nursing Services.

Secondly, we find a great deal of evidence that the individuals actually functioning in the care role for patients are not those who have received the most preparation for the task, and likely are not capable of providing the same quality of care as is the registered nurse. The approach of "nursing through others" seems calculated to both limit the satisfaction of the nurse and limit, to some extent, the quality of care received by the patient.

A further dimension is involved in the matter of enhancing the quality of patient care. If most nurses wish to enter the field to "help" people, then, it follows that satisfaction should derive in great part from the development of greater knowledge and capacity to provide that care. Despite recent emphasis on the development of research into nursing practice, and the training of individuals to conduct such inquiry, it is essentially true that nursing today stands much as medicine did in 1909 when Abraham Flexner insisted that it either had to develop a greater scientific base for clinical practice or continue to provide less than adequate treatment.[10]   Thus nursing, for reasons of both intrinsic reward to its own practitioners and better care for its clients, must determine and apply greater knowledge to its practice.

In short, the traditional view of a nursing shortage as a cause for action has conditioned us to think in terms of increased recruitment and increased use of auxiliary personnel. The first answer has very likely had some adverse effect upon the extrinsic motivation for continuing in nursing; the second has had an adverse effect on what we have defined as intrinsic motivational factors.

With regard to the first point, Yett, who has made perhaps the most detailed economic studies of nursing manpower to date, states unequivocally:

> "Ultimately, any attempt to really solve the nursing shortage problem will require policies addressed to its demand, as well as its supply side. Sooner or later, it must be recognized that the shortage will persist as long as basic nursing salaries remain so low . . . . "[11]

And, again, the same author speaking in a different context points out the inherent dangers of our conventional approach to manpower shortage in these terms:

> "Without a program to translate the nation's needs into effective *demand*, the proposal to greatly *increase* the supply of nurses could cause large relative salary declines. Under such circumstances, nursing will become an even less attractive career than at present . . . "[12]

Recognizing the basic nature of this extrinsic reinforcement, we must still plead for understanding of the need for the intrinsic rewards that, too, must be present if there is to be an unambiguous profession of nursing. There must be career patterns established that not only provide for continuation of practice, but for its equal recognition as a leadership position along with posts in education and administration. There must be acceptance that the proper end of nursing as a profession is the extension of individual care. It is for this that persons enter the field; it is to this objective that education, administration, and practice must be directed. Finally, there must be understanding of the fact that change is life and that failure to change is entropy and death. If we are not actively engaged in pushing ahead the frontiers of knowledge concerning the practice of nursing, then we are already beginning to stagnate and fall back. In this search, nursing need not act alone. It can use the discoveries of medicine, the several health sciences, and the related academic disciplines. It is absolutely essential, however, that nursing be deeply engaged. If it leaves the field of discovery to others, without a commitment of its own, then the probability is slight that the intrinsic satisfactions of improved nursing practice can ever be sufficiently attained.

FOOTNOTES

1. Anderson, Odin W. *Toward An Unambiguous Profession? A Review of Nursing.* Chicago: Center for Health Administration Series. Number AC. 1968.
2. Hoekelman, Robert A. "Florence's Fable." *Newsletter of the Ambulatory Pediatric Association.* Vol. 5, No. 2 (February, 1970). p. 23.
3. Data obtained from a survey of nursing schools conducted in 1968 by the staff of the NCSNNE.
4. American Nurses' Association. *Facts About Nursing.* 1967. New York: American Nurses' Association. p. 106.
5. Maslow, Abraham. *Motivation and Personality.* New York: Harper and Brothers. 1954.
6. Herzberg, Frederick, Bernard Mausner, and Barbara Snyderman. *The Motivation To Work.* New York: John Wiley and Sons. 1959.
7. Hughes, Everett, *et. al. Twenty Thousand Nurses Tell Their Story.* Philadelphia: J. B. Lippincott Company. 1958.
8. Christman, L. P. and Jelinek, R. C. "Old Patterns Waste Half the Nursing Hours." *Modern Hospital.* Vol. 108, No. 1 (January, 1967). p. 79.
9. Duff, R. S. and Hollingshead, A. B. *Sickness and Society.* New York: Harper and Row. 1968.
10. Flexner, Abraham. *Medical Education in the United States and Canada.* Boston: D. B. Updike. The Merrymount Press. 1960. p. 26.
11. Yett, Donald E. "The Nursing Shortage and the Nurse Training Act of 1964." *Industrial and Labor Relations Review.* XIX. (January, 1966). p. 200.
12. U.S. Department of Health, Education and Welfare. *Nurse Training Act of 1964: Program Review Report.* Public Health Service Publication No. 1740. Washington, D.C.: U.S. Government Printing Office. 1967. p. 3

APPENDIX M

A BRIEF REVIEW OF TRENDS IN NURSING SALARIES

One of the biggest disappointments encountered during the course of the study was the lack of data on salaries paid to R.N.'s. For this reason the material contained in this Appendix is necessarily abbreviated.

Nevertheless some interesting observations and judgments can be made from the material that is available. Within nursing, the employment standards from the state nurses' associations (Table M-1), indicate that nurses employed in nursing education programs on the average receive the highest starting salaries. Those in nursing service administration rank second, and are followed by general duty nurses. Naturally, there are some exceptions to this ranking, but, in general, this seems to be the overall pattern.

In spite of their high ranking within nursing, the salaries of nurse educators do not compare well when measured against other educational personnel. In Table M-2, the school nurse stands near the bottom of the list in salary means among public school professional personnel. In the collegiate setting, the nurse educator fares better when her salary is compared with those of her counterparts in the other academic disciplines as shown in Table M-3.

In the hospital, where the largest number of nurses are employed, the Director of Nursing Service ranks second among those personnel in middle management positions. Regardless of the size of the hospital, the Director of Nursing receives a salary that is surpassed only by that of the Assistant

TABLE M-1. STATE NURSES' ASSOCIATION EMPLOYMENT STANDARDS (STARTING MONTHLY CASH SALARY)

Date of Standard	State	EDUCATION			GENERAL DUTY			NURSING SERVICE ADMINISTRATION			
		Teacher(a)	Ass't Director of Nursing Education	Director of Nursing Education	General Duty	Assistant Head Nurse	Head Nurse	Supervisor	Assistant Director	Associate Director(b)	Director(c)
1967	Alabama	750			542	600	625	708	750	833	1000
1967	Alaska				*475 to 522		*500 to 547				
1967	Arizona	*900 to 1321		1458	*600 to 725	*675 to 750	*750 to 800	*850 to 950		*900 to 950	*1000 to 1250
1967	Arkansas	*567 to 800	*675 to 850	* 800 to 2000	550 to 575		*600 to 650	650	700	750	850
1968	California	*1100 to 1274	*1338 to 1626		*710 to 782	*821 to 862	*905 to 950	*998 to 1048	*1100 to 1155	*1213 to 1274	*1213 to 1626
1968	Colorado	*772 to 985	1034	1479	*545*to 635	666	772	985	1034	1138	1479
1968	Connecticut	*792 to 875	1042	1667	*625 to 687	750	792	*812 to 875	1041	1250	1667
1967	Delaware	*583 to 750	—	*833 to 1000	542			450		500	650
1967	District of Columbia	*875 to 1333	*1042 to 1333		583		*729 to 779	*912 to 1017			

TABLE M-1. STATE NURSES' ASSOCIATION EMPLOYMENT STANDARDS (STARTING MONTHLY CASH SALARY)

Year	State	*550 to 650	*675 to 700	*725 to 750	*750 to 800	*800 to 1050	*1050 to 1250	*1050 to 1450		
1966	Florida	*550 to 650	*675 to 700	*725 to 750	*750 to 800	*800 to 1050	*1050 to 1250	*1050 to 1450		
1968	Georgia	*542 to 625	623	716	823	905	947	*1000 to 1500	*1083 to 1500	*1250 to 1667
	Hawaii	542	569							
1965	Idaho	425	445	465	490	500	610			
1968	Illinois	600	640	725	830	925	1110	1111	1220	1333
1967	Indiana	542	569	654	719	827	993	*625 to 750	*750 to 875	*792 to 958
1965	Iowa	400	445	475	510	575	650	*475 to 650	*550 to 700	
1966	Kansas	*600 to 625	*650 to 675	700	800	*650 to 800	*800 to 1000	1000		
1967	Kentucky	*542 to 570	*570 to 625	*600 to 625	*600 to 625	*650 to 675				
1966	Louisiana	*480 to 580	*500 to 525	*525 to 650	*630 to 750	*690 to 840	*594 to 1104	*806 to 1217	*861 to 1321	
1966	Maine	*542 to 567	*555 to 615	*611 to 671	*634 to 694	608	708	900		
1967	Maryland	*542 to 608	650	700	775	850	775	1017	1108	1142
	Massachusetts									
1967	Michigan	550	616	825	911	1031	1333			

TABLE M-1. STATE NURSES' ASSOCIATION EMPLOYMENT STANDARDS (STARTING MONTHLY CASH SALARY)

Year	State										
1966	Minnesota	*889 to 1000						*660 to 880			
1966	Mississippi	*583 to 683	833	1000	542	562	592	850	925	950	1000
1967	Missouri	752	779	1283	596	626	715	779		871	1100
1968	Montana	*650 to 1000			*541 to 617	*571 to 646	*600 to 675	650		775	975
1968	Nebraska	*880 to 970	1100	1340	*550 to 580	*615 to 649	*670 to 800	*825 to 970		*935 to 1100	*1165 to 1340
	Nevada										
1967	New Hampshire	*583 to 792	917	1000	542	585	650	737		*750 to 917	*833 to 1042
	New Jersey				535	561	591				
1967	New Mexico	*667 to 917	917	*1083 to 1333	542		593	653	685	754	979
1967	New York	*917 to 1083	1250	2250	*625 to 667	708	750	1083	1250	1667	2250
1967	North Carolina	*633 to 1250	*708 to 1000	*1042 to 1917	545	592	617	675	750	875	1000
	North Dakota						625	*667 to 833		*708 to 917	*750 to 1083
1967	Ohio	867	948	1083	*542 to 569	*596 to 623	650	761	867	948	1083
1966	Oklahoma				567						

TABLE M-1. STATE NURSES' ASSOCIATION EMPLOYMENT STANDARDS (STARTING MONTHLY CASH SALARY)

Year	State										
	Oregon										
	Pennsylvania										
1967	Rhode Island	*667 to 833	957	1018	*542 to 569	603	639	*875 to 1013	*917 to 1061	*972 to 1125	*1083 to 1452
1967	South Carolina	*633 to 750			450			400			600
1968	South Dakota				450						
	Tennessee				542						
1967	Texas	708	750	*833 to 1167	542	569	596	650		758	896
1965	Utah				400		430	450		560	
	Vermont				364	390	416	442			
1967	Virginia	600	667	833	540	570	605	680	750	825	910
1966	Washington	*852 to 1087	1141	1641	*600 to 700	735	852	1087	1141	1257	1641
1967	West Virginia				542	582	625	705	815	915	975
1967	Wisconsin	*675 to 825			575	605	640	705			
	Wyoming										

* Varies according to a specific schedule based on educational qualifications, experience, responsibility and/or size of institution

a) Standards exclude positions in hospitals with schools of nursing, where such positions often include the dual function of education and nursing service

b) Includes assistant director of nursing service if there is no associate director of nursing service

c) Excludes directors with responsibility for both nursing service and nursing education

TABLE M-2. MEAN SALARIES FOR SELECTED PUBLIC SCHOOL PROFESSIONAL
PERSONNEL 1966–1967

Superintendents	$ 12,975
Junior High School Principals	11,226
Senior High School Principals	10,507
Elementary School Principals	9,957
Counselors	8,630
Secondary School Teachers	7,109
Librarians	7,006
School Nurses*	6,664
Elementary School Teachers	6,622

*Does not include public health nurses who work in public schools in some cases.

Source: National Education Association, Research Division.
*23rd Biennial Salary Survey of Public School Professional Personnel. 1966-67.*Research
Report 1967 - R11.

National Education Association, Research Division. *Estimates of School Statistics.*
1968-69. Research Report 1968 - R16

Administrator. However, the staff nurse does not fare nearly so well when her
salary is compared. The smaller the hospital the higher the staff nurse ranks in
salary. But even here she is no better than half way up or down the list of those
functioning in middle management. When we examine the larger hospitals, the staff
nurses are completely at the bottom of the list. The data on these categories is
found in Table M-4.

Table M-5 displays the salaries of women college graduates seven years after
graduation. The salaries are listed according to undergraduate major and by
occupation. In either listing nurses, or nursing, rank approximately in the middle.

The data in this Appendix only reaffirm what is generally known and
accepted. That is, salaries for nurses have not been competitive. What the data does
not show is the increasing dissatisfaction of nurses with their economic status.
Recent walkouts, strikes, and threats of such actions have to a great degree been
directed against economic conditions within the profession. The resort to collective
bargaining is only an example of the nurses active interest in their economic
welfare. It may seem obvious that a profession should be concerned with its
economic rewards, but in nursing this has not been the case until the last few years.

Hospital administrators have perhaps been reluctant to raise the wages of
nurses for fear that it would set off competitive bidding among hospitals and other
occupations and result in an altered distribution of nurses and a higher wage bill for
each hospital. They have frequently tried to substitute lesser trained nursing

TABLE M-3. COMPARISON OF EDUCATOR SALARIES

Program	Median of Minimum Salaries Established for RN's in Full-Time Teaching Positions (1968) (a)				Median Annual Salaries of Full-Time Nurse Faculty Members in Nursing Teaching Positions in Nursing Educational Programs (1968) (a)				Median Salaries for Full-Time Teaching in Junior Colleges and Colleges and Universities (1968) (b)			
	No Degree	Bacc.	Masters	Doctorate	No Degree	Bacc.	Masters	Doctorate	No Degree	Bacc.	Masters	Doctorate
LPN SCHOOLS	$6,666 (N = 365)	$7,150 (N -383)	$7,848 (N =279)		$7,500	$8,640	$10,470					
HOSPITAL SCHOOLS	$6,960 (N = 263)	$7,696 (N = 309)	$8,520 (N = 291)		$7,500	$8,400	$9,650					
AD SCHOOLS		$7,000 (N = 92)	$8,000 (N = 107)			$8,000	$10,250					
COLLEGIATE SCHOOLS						$7,000	$9,200	$13,875				
COLLEGIATE FACULTY:												
INSTRUCTORS	$6,800 (N = 69)	$7,494 (N = 108)					$8,000*					$7,496
ASST. PROF.		$8,500 (N = 134)	$9,324 (N = 39)				$9,420*					$ 9,472
ASSOC. PROF.		$10,300 (N = 106)	$11,808 (N = 46)				$11,810*					$11,393
PROFESSOR		$12,500 (N = 72)	$13,500 (N = 66)				$16,000*					$14,713

(a) American Nurses' Association. *Survey of Salaries of Teaching and Administrative Personnel in Nursing Educational Programs.* September 1968.
(b) National Education Association. *Salaries in Higher Education 1967-68.* Note: Excluded faculty from medical, dental, and nursing schools.
N = Number of programs used in determining median.
* = Median salary included administration along with teaching.

TABLE M-4. HOSPITAL PERSONNEL SALARIES

Hospitals With 50 or Fewer Beds

Job Titles	*1965 Salary Average*	*Job Titles*	*1967 Salary Average*
Assistant Administrator	$6,627	Assistant Administrator	$8,428
DIRECTOR, NURSING SERVICE	5,776	DIRECTOR, NURSING SERVICE	7,106
Chief Technologist (Lab.)	5,510	Chief Technologist (Lab.)	6,695
Operating Room Supervisor	4,943	Operating Room Supervisor	6,460
Chief X-Ray Technician	4,597	Chief X-Ray Technician	5,674
STAFF NURSES	4,277	STAFF NURSES	5,589
Food Service Director	3,683	Food Service Director	4,597
Central Service Supervisor	3,462	Central Service Supervisor	4,333
Chief Admitting Officer	3,433	Chief Admitting Officer	4,160
Chief of Housekeeping	3,095	Chief of Housekeeping	3,879

Hospitals With 51 to 150 Beds

Assistant Administrator	$7,247	Assistant Administrator	$8,868
DIRECTOR, NURSING SERVICE	6,540	DIRECTOR, NURSING SERVICE	8,240
Chief Technologist (Lab.)	6,375	Chief Technologist (Lab.)	7,679
Chief X-Ray Technician	5,719	Chief X-Ray Technician	6,773
Operating Room Supervisor	5,314	Operating Room Supervisor	6,675
Food Service Director	5,074	Food Service Director	6,118
STAFF NURSES	4,642	STAFF NURSES	5,876
Central Service Supervisor	4,027	Central Service Supervisor	5,133
Chief of Housekeeping	3,784	Chief of Housekeeping	4,631
Chief Admitting Officer	3,334	Chief Admitting Officer	4,150

Hospitals With 151 to 300 Beds

Assistant Administrator	$11,633	Assistant Administrator	$14,229
DIRECTOR, NURSING SERVICE	8,953	DIRECTOR, NURSING SERVICE	11,109
Public Relations Director	7,635	Chief Technologist (Lab.)	9,106
Chief Technologist (Lab.)	7,399	Food Service Director	8,895
Food Service Director	7,264	Public Relations Director	8,852
Operating Room Supervisor	6,573	Operating Room Supervisor	8,132
Chief X-Ray Technician	6,293	Chief X-Ray Technician	7,811
Central Service Supervisor	5,866	Central Service Supervisor	7,475
Chief of Housekeeping	5,688	Chief of Housekeeping	7,187
Chief Admitting Officer	5,282	Chief Admitting Officer	6,447
STAFF NURSES	4,948	STAFF NURSES	6,246

Hospitals With More Than 300 Beds

Assistant Administrator	$12,503	Assistant Administrator	$15,204
DIRECTOR, NURSING SERVICE	10,327	DIRECTOR, NURSING SERVICE	12,378
Food Service Director	8,511	Food Service Director	10,240
Public Relations Director	7,635	Public Relations Director	9,148
Chief Technologist (Lab.)	7,622	Chief Technologist (Lab.)	8,867
Chief of Housekeeping	7,242	Operating Room Supervisor	8,657
Operating Room Supervisor	7,101	Chief of Housekeeping	8,460

TABLE M-4. HOSPITAL PERSONNEL SALARIES

Job Titles	Hospitals With More Than 300 Beds 1965 Salary Average	Job Titles	1967 Salary Average
Chief X-Ray Technician	$7,076	Chief X-Ray Technician	$8,072
Chief Admitting Officer	6,608	Chief Admitting Officer	7,795
Central Service Supervisor	6,346	Central Service Supervisor	7,531
STAFF NURSES	5,220	STAFF NURSES	6,461

Source: "Soaring Salaries Explored in Statistical Survey." *Modern Hospital.* 110:2:35. February, 1968.

personnel for the professionally trained nurse. There is increasing evidence this practice of "economic substitutability" has not in fact been economical at all, resulting in high turnover rates, lessening of quality standards, and other undesirable outcomes.

Competitive salaries for nurses will almost certainly help attract more students into the educational programs, slow the withdrawal of active nurses from the profession, and entice those nurses who are inactive back into service.

TABLE M-5. AVERAGE ANNUAL SALARY IN 1964 OF WOMEN WHO GRADUATED IN 1957 WITH BACHELOR'S DEGREES BY OCCUPATION AND UNDERGRADUATE MAJOR

Undergraduate Major	Salary	Occupation	Salary
Mathematics	$7,517	Chemists, Mathematicians	
Chemistry	6,535	Statisticians	$8,039
Psychology	6,393	Managers, Officials	7,466
Speech, Dramatic Arts	6,236	School Workers (Misc.)*	6,744
Social Sciences	6,232	Professional Workers (Misc.) **	6,490
Health Fields	6,190	Editors, Copywriters,	
History	6,188	Reporters	6,274
Sociology, Social Work	6,096	Social, Welfare, Recreation	
NURSING	6,094	Workers	6,137
Biological Sciences	6,027	Dietitians and Home	
Education	5,877	Economists	6,110
Physical Education	5,861	NURSES	6,078
English	5,840	Kindergarten Teachers	6,060
Home Economics	5,791	Senior High School Teachers	5,852
Languages, Foreign	5,788	Elementary School Teachers	5,843
Art	5,754	Technicians (Biological)	5,843
Business and Commerce	5,568	Junior High School Teachers	5,837
Music	5,566	Librarians	5,658
		Clerical Workers (Misc.)	4,813
		Secretaries, Stenographers	4,527

 * Includes counselors, principals and other non-teaching professionals
 ** Includes research workers and therapists as well as other professional workers not listed

Source: U.S. Department of Labor, Women's Bureau. *College Women Seven Years After Graduation.* Bulletin 292. Washington, D.C.: Government Printing Office. 1966. p. 54.

APPENDIX N

A BRIEF ANALYSIS OF RESEARCH PROJECTS IN THE DIVISION OF NURSING

T he practice of nursing has long been "known" to influence the delivery of total health service and contribute to the process by which a state of health is maintained or restored. Only during the past 30 years, however, has research capability and financial support been available to put these "knowns" under the scrutiny of scientific investigation.

Until the advent of government supported grants for extra-mural research through the Public Health Service in 1955, investigations were limited to those undertaken within the Public Health Service organization itself, the newly organized American Nurses Foundation, and those financed by private foundations that were beginning to move into the health research field. Since that date, the bulk of the support has come from PHS grants, and an analysis of the projects supported from 1955-1966, as shown in Table N-1, indicates that range and scope of investigation being conducted in nursing.

TABLE N-1. SCOPE OF RESEARCH IN NURSING ,1955-1968

Sample of Projects, indicated by titles, awarded
grants from Division of Nursing, U. S. Public Health Service

Nursing Roles and Functions

Role of the Nurse in Outpatient Departments
Specific Nursing Activities and Patient's Welfare
Nurse-Patient Relationship with Older Patients
Minimal Nursing Service Staffing Experiment
The Potential Role of the Professional Nurse
Factors Influencing Continuity of Nursing Service
Attitudes Toward the Patient and Patient Care
A Study of An Exterior Role for Professional Nurses
Identification of Researchable Nursing Care Problems
Optimal Organization and Facility for a Nursing Unit
Specific Nursing Behaviors Related to Patient Improvement
The Effectiveness of a Clinical Nurse Specialist Role
New Dimensions for Improvement of Clinical Nursing:
    Development of Criteria to Measure the Effectiveness of
    Clinical Nursing Practice
Crucial Variables in Nurse-Patient Interaction
Nurse Specialist's Effect on Recovery in Tuberculosis
Intensive Nursing Care in Acute Myocardial Infarction
The Role of a Nurse in Medical Education
Role Differentials and Nursing Ideology
Interpersonal Influences and the Nursing Function
Ritualism in Nursing and Its Effect on Patient Care
Ambiguities in the Nurse-Doctor Relationship
Factors Affecting Quality of Nursing Care
Community Nursing Services for Psychiatric Patients
A Longitudinal Study of Nursing Careers
Effects of Nursing Intervention on Illness Careers
A Study of Content Differentiation Between Technical and
    Professional Nursing

Nursing Education

Performance Variables in Collegiate Nursing Education
Curriculum Study of Hospital Schools of Nursing
Development of Programmed Units in Nursing
Defining Clinical Content of Graduate Nursing Programs
Investigation of Nursing Content — Baccalaureate Nursing
    Programs

TABLE N-1. SCOPE OF RESEARCH IN NURSING, 1955-1968

Satisfying and Stressful Situations in Basic Programs in
    Nursing Education
Outcomes of Degree and Diploma Nursing Education
Characteristics of Collegiate Nursing Students
Curriculum Research for Graduate Education in Nursing
Study of Costs of Nursing Education
Relationship of Nursing Education to Performance
Evaluation of an Experimental Nursing Curriculum
Nursing Student Selection and Job Satisfaction
Causes of Student Withdrawal from Nurse Training
Prediction of Success in Nursing Education
Vocational Motivation for a Career Teaching Nursing
Identifying the Core Content of an Advanced Nursing
    Curriculum
Improvement of Curricula in Schools of Nursing Through
    Selection and Application of Core Concepts of Nursing
The Use of an Academic Assistance Program to Curtail
    Failures in a Nursing Program
The Returns on Investment in Training for Nurses and
    Physicians
Development of Self-Instructional Materials in Pediatric
    Nursing
Facilitation of Student Learning Through Meaningful Use
    of Community Resources
Computer-Assisted Instruction of Basic Nursing Using
    Inquiry Method
Utilizing Team Teaching Concepts to Improve the Quality
    of Instruction in Teaching Medical and Surgical Nursing
An Independent Diploma Program Assesses its Effectiveness
    and its Future in Nursing Education
The Articulation of Clinical and Non-Clinical Learning
    in a 4-year Nursing Program
A Plan to Study and Initiate Curriculum Changes in the
    Present Diploma Program that will Prepare a Nurse with
    the Same Level of Competency in a Shorter Period of
    Time
Reorganization of Curriculum Content to Permit the
    Qualified Licensed Practical Nurse Who Meets Established
    Criteria to Acquire Advanced Standing in a Diploma Program
The Design, Implementation, and Evaluation of a Curriculum
    Leading to the Bachelor of Science in Nursing Degree
A Program for Upgrading the Culturally Disadvantaged
    Underachieving Nursing Student
Evaluation of Clinical Practice in a Diploma School of
    Nursing
Faculty Project for Strengthening Research Competence
An Evaluation and Study of Faculty Research Potential
Utilization of Sabbaticals for Research Training in Nursing
    Education

TABLE N-1. SCOPE OF RESEARCH IN NURSING, 1955-1968

Manpower and Professional Development

The Professionalization Process in Nursing
Factors Determining Selection or Rejection of Nursing as
      a Career
Men Who Enter Nursing: A Sociological Study
Decision to Re-Activate Nursing Career
A Method for Determining Intra-Hospital Nursing Needs
Student Program in Nursing for Adult Men and Women
An Economic Analysis of the Hospital Nursing Shortage
Employer Expectations vs. Staff Nurse Performance
Evaluation of Persons for Leadership Positions in
      Nursing in General Hospitals
Conferences — Communicating Nursing Research Results
      Improving Nursing Practice Through Research

In January of 1969, the Division of Nursing published a list of the then current nursing research grants.[1] With a budget appropriation of $3,325,000 for fiscal 1969, the Division of Nursing was supporting the work of 53 investigators involved in 58 projects. These projects were underway in 38 agencies and institutions in 21 states.

Nineteen of the 58 projects were in the general area of research development; 14 were specifically directed to increasing faculty research competency and to support faculty research. Five others were concerned with development of instruments or assessment of methods of communicating research findings.

There was one project in the area of nursing education — a curriculum study grant of a California university.

Heightened interest in definition and evaluation of new and expanded roles for the nurse practitioner is evidenced by the funding of seven projects in this area, the majority directed to assessment of the clinical specialist role.

Five grants supported inquiry in the general area of nursing careers. Both initial career choice; (e.g. "Men Who Enter Nursing: A Sociological Study,") and subsequent employment patterns, ("Anticipatory Socialization and Chosen Work Locale") are scrutinized.

There were 13 projects investigating effects of clinical nursing action in both the distributive and episodic areas of practice. The remaining 12 projects were essentially sociological in character, assessing the extent of interaction among nurses, between nurses and other health personnel and between nurses and patients, and their effect, direct and indirect, on patient welfare.

This review brings to light several features of research in nursing that must be adjusted in the years ahead. The first is the extremely modest level of funding. The paucity of this total figure of slightly more than $3¼ million in 1969 can be seen by comparison with the approximately $350 million in federal funds designated for medical research alone, not to mention additional grants for teaching and training as well as funds from private sources for a variety of purposes. Inevitably the development of a scientific body of practice in nursing will be slowed by such inadequate support.

A second feature is the concentration of research in nursing on educational and professional matters rather than clinical practice and its underlying roots in biological, physical and social sciences. More attention has been given to clinically founded studies in recent grants, and to some extent the emphasis of the past is understandable. The numbers of nurse researchers were few, their training primarily in the fields of education and administration, and the scope and character of researchable problems in nursing in the process of definition.

If the goals of health service for the American public are to be realized it is essential that research in nursing practice and its underlying scientific base move forward at an accelerated rate. Not only are nurses the largest single body of health professionals, but nursing problems represent one large constant in health care and probably constitute the major component of all health service. As research in nursing does advance, the range and type of studies to be performed by nurses will be clarified and the techniques, data, and findings developed in this field will have increasing usefulness to researchers in other disciplines. The consequence will be measurable in benefits of better health delivered with increasing efficiency and effectiveness.

FOOTNOTE

1. U.S. Department of Health, Education, and Welfare. Public Health Service, Division of Nursing. *Current Nursing Research Grants.* PHS Publication No. 1762. Rev. January 1969.

APPENDIX O
SUMMARY OF RECENT FEDERAL LEGISLATION AND FUNDING PROGRAMS FOR NURSING

In 1950, the federal government's total expenditures for nursing and nursing education amounted to $250,000 while in fiscal 1968, the total expenditures by the Department of Health, Education, and Welfare alone for nursing were approximately $130 million. Of this total, approximately $48 million was spent for the training of practical nurses while the balance of about $81 million was devoted to the preparation of R.N.'s. Refer to Figure O-1.

The turning point for increased federal assistance for nursing and nursing education resulted from the report of the Surgeon General's Consultant Group on Nursing that was submitted in 1963.[1] This group was charged with advising the Surgeon General of the needs for nursing personnel throughout the country and also with identifying the appropriate role of the Federal Government in assuring that adequate nursing services were available to the nation. A major result of this report was the passage in 1964 of the Nurse Training Act.[2]

The intent of the Nurse Training Act was to serve not as a panacea for the problems identified by the Surgeon General's Report, but rather to serve as the impetus whereby the quality and quantity of individuals in nursing would be steadily increased. To achieve these ends the Act provided for a balanced program of aid to nursing education. Facilities and programs were to be expanded and improved through the use of construction grants, teaching improvement grants, and payments to diploma schools. Programs of loans for nursing students and

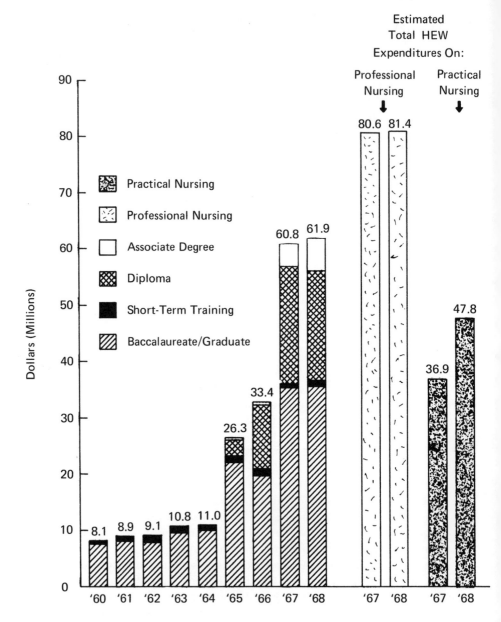

Figure O-1. Division of Nursing (HEW) Expenditures on Professional Nursing.

Figure O-1. Division of Nursing (HEW) Expenditures on Professional Nursing.

traineeships for graduate students were provided to attract more candidates into the profession and at the same time to make provision for the necessary numbers of teachers and leaders that would be needed in the future. Refer to Table O-1.

A provision of the Nurse Training Act required the Secretary of Health, Education, and Welfare to appoint a committee to review the progress of the programs authorized under the Act and submit a report to Congress by January 1, 1968 with recommendations regarding the deletion, continuation, expansion, or modification of any program. This was done and the result of this action was that in August 1968 the Health Manpower Act[3] was signed into law.

The basic function of the Health Manpower Act, in regard to nursing, was to extend the life of the Nurse Training Act to June 30, 1971. Certain modifications in existing programs under the Nurse Training Act and some additional programs were contained in this new legislation. A major change resulted in the program of diploma school formula grants being deleted and replaced by a program of institutional grants for all schools of nursing. This was the first time that any legislation provided institutional grants for nursing although this type of grant had been available to other health professions under previous legislation. Refer to Table O-2 for a tabulation of federal funds for nursing.

The Health Manpower Act also provided for a program of special project grants which extended the coverage under the Nurse Training Act to include such programs as: planning, developing, or establishing new nursing programs; modifying existing programs; assisting schools with special need for financial aid to meet accreditation requirements; assisting schools in serious financial straits to meet costs of operation; and research in education. In addition, the authority to accredit nursing programs was given to state agencies, certain regional bodies, and the Joint Commission on the Accreditation of Hospitals.

Like its predecessor the Nurse Training Act, the Health Manpower Act also requires a congressional report on the progress of its programs. This report is to be submitted by July 1, 1970.

It is unquestionable that nursing has made considerable progress under these programs of federal assistance. In the opening paragraph of this appendix it was indicated the extent to which federal assistance to nursing has grown over the past twenty years.

The trend is reflected in the 1971 authorizations. To keep this in proper perspective, however, we should illustrate examples of financial assistance to other health professions and compare these to nursing. The fiscal '71 budget from the federal government requests $113.6 million in institutional grants for medical, dental and related occupations—none for nursing. This is cited to indicate that, although nursing has received increasing federal assistance over the years, the nation's largest health profession still does not receive aid proportionate to the other health professions.

TABLE O-1. FUNDS AUTHORIZED AND AWARDED UNDER THE NURSE TRAINING ACT OF 1964

| | Fiscal Years | | | | | | | | | | TOTALS | |
| | 1965 | | 1966 | | 1967 | | 1968 | | 1969 | | | |
	AUTH. (000's)	AWD. (000's)	AUTH. (000's)	AWD. (000's)	AUTH. (000's)	AWD. (000's)	AUTH. (000's)	AWD. (000's)	AUTH. (000's)	AWD. (000's)	AUTH. (000's)	AWD. (000's)
Construction Grants	—	—	15,000	7,411	25,000	27,427	25,000	19,382	25,000	18,643	90,000	72,863
Project Grants	2,000	1,990	3,000	1,928	4,000	3,518	4,000	3,999	4,000	4,000	17,000	15,435
Payments to Diploma Schools	4,000	788	7,000	2,146	10,000	3,069	10,000	3,000	10,000	3,000	41,000	12,003
Traineeships	8,000	7,879	9,000	8,784	10,000	9,790	11,000	9,864	12,000	10,468	50,000	46,785
Student Loans*	3,100	3,090	8,900	8,871	16,800	12,677	25,300	16,390	30,900	16,008	85,000	57,036
Opportunity Grants	—	—	—	—	—	—	5,000	4,120	6,500	6,552	11,500	10,672
											294,500	214,794

* Includes Revolving Fund Obligations

Source: Division of Nursing, Bureau of Health Professions Education and Manpower Training, HEW.

TABLE O-2. FEDERAL FUNDS FOR NURSING

	FISCAL YEAR 1970			FISCAL YEAR 1971	
	Authorization[1]	Administration Request	Conference Agreement	Authorization[1]	Administration Request
(1) Construction Grants to Schools of Nursing	$25,000,000	$ 8,000,000	$ 8,000,000	$35,000,000	$ 8,000,000
(2) Scholarships	No specific authorization[2]	12,000,000	7,178,000	No Specific authorization[2]	17,000,000
(3) Loans	20,000,000	9,610,000[3]	16,360,000	21,000,000	9,610,000
(4) Special Project Grants for Improvement in Nurse Training	35,000,000	7,000,000	} 8,400,000	40,000,000	11,000,000
(5) Institutional Grants		NONE	} NONE		NONE
(6) Traineeships for Professional Nurses	15,000,000	10,470,000	10,470,000	19,000,000	10,470,000
(7) Special Fellowships in Nurse Research	No ceiling	650,000	650,000	No ceiling	650,000
(8) Research Training	No ceiling	700,000	700,000	No ceiling	700,000
(9) Research Grants	No ceiling	2,625,000	2,625,000	No ceiling	2,455,000
(10) Direct Operations[4]	No ceiling	4,265,000	4,265,000	No ceiling	4,702,000

[1] Legislative authority is provided under the Health Manpower Act of 1968, PL 90-490 (1-6); Public Health Service Act (7-10).

[2] While no specific amount is authorized in this budget, the allocation formula in the legislation-based on enrollment-would require approximately $30 million in 1970 and 1971.

[3] The President's Budget requests $9,610,000. However, the program level of operation would amount to $12,281,000 because of the addition of revolving funds.

[4] These funds provide for activities of the Division of Nursing other than those listed above, and include such areas as consultation and some contact money.

Source: American Journal of Nursing, April 1970.

FOOTNOTES

1.   U.S. Public Health Service. *Toward Quality in Nursing.* Report of the Surgeon General's Consultant Group on Nursing. (Pub. No. 992) Washington, D.C.: U.S. Government Printing Office. 1963. p. 55.
2.   "Nurse Training Act of 1964". Public Law 88-581, 88th Congress H.R. 11241. September 4, 1964. Washington, D.C.: U.S. Government Printing Office. 1964.
3.   "Health Manpower Act of 1968." Publication No. 90-490. 90th Congress. S. 3095. August 16, 1968. Washington, D.C.: U.S. Government Printing Office. 1968.

APPENDIX P

CAREER ENHANCEMENT PROGRAMS FOR THE LICENSED PRACTICAL/VOCATIONAL NURSE

D uring Phase I of the study, one of the preliminary acts of the Commission was to decide the delimitation of the investigation. In September, 1967 and again in early 1968, the Commission decided that, because of limitations in time and resources, the staff had to work toward the objectives of the study in terms of the licensed registered nurse (see Appendix A). This meant that the staff was not to make an in-depth study of all the "nursing assistant" groups. It was felt, however, that there were most likely to be valid generalizations concerning such problems as: the economics of nursing compensation, career inducements (or lack of them), career ladders; and that one area, relative to both the Commission's objectives and the concerns of the LPN, was the opportunity for continued personal development and upper professional mobility. Thus, the Commission and staff sought from the beginning to view the LPN as one disadvantaged sector of nursing and to think in terms of finding ways to move this section into the mainstream of professional nursing opportunities. With this in mind, the staff collected any information it was able to uncover, in the course of the general investigation, concerning career opportunities for the LPN/LVN. The following paragraphs comprise a brief summary of our findings.

One of the first programs which the staff identified for site visitation, was the program designed to provide means for practical nurses to become registered nurses, at the Helene Fuld School of Nursing of the Hospital for Joint Diseases and Medical

Center in New York City. This program was brought to our attention by both the nurse Commissioners and the nurse advisory panelists, and because of their recommendation, the staff included this program in its initial site visit plans (see Appendix H).

At approximately the same point in time, through the general search of the literature, one staff member found an article in *Nursing Outlook* which briefly described this same program.[1] A site visit was subsequently scheduled in April, 1969, and a member of the NCSNNE staff met with Miss Justine Hannon, Director of Nursing and Nursing Education, and various other staff members involved in the experimental program. This personal interview[2] and the article mentioned formed the basis for the following observations.

The Hospital for Joint Diseases and Medical Center has had an LPN program since 1945. In 1962, representatives of the New York State Department of Education visited the school, as is their custom, and raised the issue of the possibility of an LPN becoming an RN.

The hospital is located in East Harlem, and most of the nursing care was provided by LPN's from minority groups. In the interests of improved patient care and improved career and educational opportunities for their LPN's, and with the encouragement of the state education department, a curriculum was developed and a program established entitled "An Experimental Program in Professional Nursing Education", during the years 1962-1964. In 1964, 24 LPN's were admitted to the new program (1800 applications were received) and in 1966, 21 students graduated, of whom 20 passed the RN licensure examination and as of November, 1967, were practicing in New York City.

In order to be admitted into the program, the applicant must have graduated from an accredited secondary school (or possess a high school equivalency diploma) with the appropriate general academic courses. In addition, the applicant must: be a graduate of an approved school of practical nursing with a standing in the upper third of the class; be licensed to practice as a practical nurse; and have had a minimum of one year's employment as an LPN in an accredited health care institution. Finally, the applicant must take a series of tests, one being the NLN Pre-Nursing and Guidance Examination.

The main objective of the program is to enable the LPN to pass the New York State Registered Nurse Board examination in a minimum amount of time. Originally, the planners hoped for a 12-month course, and are still considering it, but as of the time of our interview, their feeling was that 15 months seemed more sound, educationally. According to the description of the program in *Nursing Outlook*, the 15-month course of study is divided into four semesters of 15 weeks each: the first semester consists of courses in integrated physical sciences, psychology, communications, and medical-surgical nursing theory and practice; the second includes integrated physical sciences, sociology, and medical-surgical nursing II, with content in public health, pharmacology, nutrition, and principles of mental hygiene throughout; the third offers courses in the humanities, trends in nursing, and maternal and child care, with emphasis placed on the family as a whole; the fourth consists of concepts of medical-surgical nursing and mental disorders, with increased depth in meeting the nursing needs of the acutely and the severely ill patient.

The students in this program have come from six states (generally near New York) and applications have come from more than 20 states. About one half of the students come from New York City and most have had more than the minimum one year of LPN work experience.

All of the faculty for this program have their Master's degree and have been especially recruited for the program, attracted mainly by its innovative nature.

The initial funding (developmental) came from the state and the operating costs have been accepted by the hospital board primarily for two reasons: the opportunity to recruit personnel who seem to be in short supply; acceptance of a responsibility to the local community.

By means of the AHA Newsletter for The Hospital School of Nursing, we were directed to several experimental programs to enable an LPN/LVN to become an RN. The Northwest Texas Hospital School of Nursing in Amarillo, Texas has a program for LPN's that lasts 20 months and is the first of its kind in the state of Texas to be approved by the Board of Nurse Examiners.[3]

In order to enter the program, an LVN must have had at least one year of professional experience. Additional factors to be considered are: the applicant's standing on the state board examination and in their LVN school, and the results of school-constructed tests. If the grades on the latter are satisfactory, the applicant then is granted one year's credit toward completion of the regular 30-month diploma program.

After entering the program, the student will take a first-year course in general education at an approved college and also some NLN tests. Upon satisfactory completion, the applicant will enter the regular senior class of nursing students of the diploma school.[4]

According to Mrs. Eunice King, Director, Department of Nursing, this experimental program had been in the planning stages for several years and the Board of Nurse Examiners approved it in February, 1970. The program is due to open in September, 1970 with approximately 12 students. Initially, the school received over 500 inquiries about the program.

In addition to supplying the community with a needed program, the school provides remedial work in mental health and hygiene, according to Mrs. King. Since many of the students are in need of financial help, the federal nursing scholarship program provides monetary assistance for most of the students.

The Providence Hospital School of Nursing in Southfield, Michigan, in their 14-month program to prepare LPN's to take state board examinations and become RN's, emphasizes the physical, biological and social sciences rather than courses in clinical nursing.[5]

The ASN (Advanced Standing Nurse) students complete the same requirements as the regular 20-month diploma students but vary their curriculum in that

Maternal and Child Nursing and Psychiatric Nursing are substituted for Fundamentals of Nursing and Introductory Medical-Surgical Nursing. The last eight weeks of the second term are spent following the regular diploma curriculum.

The program at Providence Hospital was begun as a pilot project in September, 1967 with the hospital's own funds, and in January, 1968, the Public Health Service awarded them a three-year grant to continue the project. By September, 1968, the school was prepared to accept 35 LPN's of which 27 graduated in December of that year. Like other similar programs, the one at Providence has received widespread interest, evidenced by a waiting list for the September, 1970 program.

September, 1970 will see yet another program opening -- South Chicago Community Hospital School of Nursing opens their pilot project which enables the LPN to become an RN in two rather than three academic years.[6] This project, the first of its kind in Illinois, will admit 10 LPN students who will take most of the same courses as other first year students but will emphasize Medical-Surgical, Maternal and Child Care, Leadership and Complex Nursing courses in the second year.

Up to this point, hospital schools of nursing which have programs to help the LPN ascend the career ladder in nursing have been discussed. At Maricopa Technical College, in Phoenix, there is an Associate Degree nursing program which has a pilot project to prepare LPN's to take the Arizona state board examination in registered nursing in approximately one calendar year.[7] These 20 LPN's are granted 23 semester hours of credit toward the Associate of Arts degree after they have been admitted into the program. As in the other programs discussed, these applicants must have graduated from an approved school of practical nursing, have a license to practice practical nursing in Arizona, have been employed for at least two years at an approved general hospital, possess a high school diploma and have an acceptable score on the College Qualification Test. The program received its first class in February, 1969 and successive classes in September, 1969 and projected for September, 1970.

An Associate Degree nursing program which has a policy of giving credit by examination to LPN's for admission to their AD program is Cuyahoga Community College in Cleveland. The LPN student can receive 12 hours of credit by examination but no more than five semester hours of this may be obtained in the nursing major. This policy was initiated in February, 1967.[8]

Skagit Valley College, Mt. Vernon, Washington, opened an advanced course in psychiatric nursing for LPN's in March, 1965, under the joint sponsorship of the Division of Mental Health Department of Vocational Education and the college. "All LPN's are eligible for this course which is designed to prepare them to work therapeutically with psychiatric patients, at the same time increasing their effectiveness in other areas of nursing."[9] This course carries 16 community college credits and consists of 30 hours per week for 12 weeks. As of December, 1967, at least 51 students who have worked in mental hospitals or psychiatric wards of general hospitals had completed the course. Unlike the other programs discussed, this program experienced a limited number of applications because of the lack of financial help plus the need of nursing services by the community institutions which employed them. The state mental hospitals have arranged to continue the salaries of those LPN's who enroll in the course but nursing coverage needs and budget limit the number of applicants.

In the United States today, hundreds of thousands of Licensed Practical/ Vocational Nurses represent one of the needed resources for recruitment into professional nursing. One community college nursing educator has written of practical nursing: "it is unfair and almost dishonest to enroll men and women with obvious ability and interest in nursing in a program that prepares them to occupy the lowest rung of the nursing ladder and prohibits their being used to their greatest potential."[10] For much the same reason, one associate degree program, "acting also on the premise that there were many capable members of the LPN category who might wish to develop full technical competence and receive recognition of this competence,"[11] initiated a program to upgrade LPN's to RN's.

The NCSNNE has recommended that nursing education be positioned in the mainstream of American educational patterns. It seems that many more programs to bring the LPN into the system are needed. Have the community colleges been used as well as they might in this endeavor? Why are some of these programs to upgrade the LPN 12 months in duration and others as long as 20 months? These are some questions that could be dealt with quite appropriately by the state master planning committees for nursing education whose establishment is recommended by the NCSNNE. The resolution of the dilemma of the LPN will not only work to the benefit of the individual nurse, but to the benefit of all those whose need is for adequate numbers of competent, professional nurses to assist in the extension of health care delivery.

FOOTNOTES

1. Feuer, Helen Denny. "Operation Salvage." *Nursing Outlook.* 15:11:54. November, 1967.
2. Interview. Hospital for Joint Diseases and Medical Center. New York, New York. 4/28/69.
3. *AHA Newsletter For the Hospital School of Nursing.* Vol. 2, No. 16. April 6, 1970.
4. Telephone Interview. Mrs. Eunice King, Director, School of Nursing. The Northwest Texas Hospital, Amarillo, Texas. June 24, 1970.
5. AHA., *op. cit.,* Vol. 1, No. 23. July 14, 1969.
6. *Ibid.,* Vol. 2, No. 17. April 20, 1970.
7. Mannion, Shirley E. "Upgrading LPN's to RN's." *Journal of Practical Nursing.* 19:9:31-32, 47. September, 1969.
8. Burnside, Helen. "Practical Nurses Become Associate Degree Graduates." *Nursing Outlook.* 17:4:47-48. April, 1969.
9. Irving, Susan. "Psychiatric Nursing Course For LPN's." *Nursing Outlook.* 15:12:44-45. December, 1967.
10. Harris, Virginia J. "This I Believe—About Practical Nursing Education." *Nursing Outlook.* 17:6:40-41. June, 1969.
11. Mannion, Shirley E., *op. cit.,* p. 31.

APPENDIX Q

A REPORT ON THE 1970 REGIONAL CONFERENCES ON IMPLEMENTATION

As the preparation of the final report and recommendations of this Commission neared completion in late 1969, the focus of attention shifted to appropriate methods of apprising the public and the professions of the details of the report and to effective means of securing the support of those concerned individuals and groups that were considered vital to the implementation of the recommendations.

As an initial step, two principal projects were undertaken. The first involved preparation of a summary report of the major recommendations for publication in the *American Journal of Nursing*, the final product being a 16 page document containing 15 recommendations. We hoped that this early widespread dissemination of major findings would provide the basis for discussion and formulation of questions well in advance of our second venture—a series of regional meetings to be conducted in the spring of 1970.

The planning for these meetings was initiated in September 1969 with a consideration of possible conference sites. In this investigation, priority was given to large metropolitan areas that would assure versatile travel schedules, adequate and conveniently located housing, and sites at which a School of Nursing could provide meeting facilities. Information relevant to these considerations was provided by our advisory panelists and by several of the regional education boards. Based on the above criteria, the final selection of sites included: Boston University,

Boston, Massachusetts; Catholic University, Washington, D. C.; Emory University, Atlanta, Georgia; Saint Louis University, St. Louis, Missouri; University of Minnesota, Minneapolis, Minnesota; University of Utah, Salt Lake City, Utah; and Stanford University, Palo Alto, California. The states included in each region were:*

Boston	*St. Louis*	*Palo Alto*
Connecticut	Arkansas	Alaska
Maine	Iowa	California
Massachusetts	Kansas	Hawaii
New Hampshire	Louisiana	Oregon
New York	Missouri	Washington
Rhode Island	Nebraska	
Vermont	Oklahoma	
	Texas	

Washington, D.C.	*Minneapolis*
Delaware	Illinois
District of Columbia	Indiana
Kentucky	Michigan
Maryland	Minnesota
New Jersey	Montana
Ohio	North Dakota
Pennsylvania	South Dakota
Virginia	Wisconsin
West Virginia	

Atlanta	*Salt Lake City*
Alabama	Arizona
Florida	Colorado
Georgia	Idaho
Mississippi	Nevada
North Carolina	New Mexico
South Carolina	Utah
Tennessee	Wyoming

*Because of the need to somehow balance numbers for the various meetings, arbitrary decisions were made concerning the states to be invited to specific locations. Usually this followed customary regional patterns, but in a few cases, exceptions had to be made. It should be emphasized that these regional meetings were not intended to set up lasting districts for implementation efforts.

Two day-long meetings were planned for each conference and compilation of invitation lists was begun in October.

Believing that the respective State Boards of Nurse Registration were best equipped to suggest to the staff the names of those individuals in each state who were in a position to influence public and professional opinion concerning health care and health education issues, each Board was requested to: examine the following list of positions; make appropriate additions or changes; and supply the names and addresses of the individuals holding each position.

INVITATION LIST FOR REGIONAL MEETINGS

Governor

President and executive secretary of state board of
    licensure for nurses

Chairmen of state legislature committees on health,
    licensing, and education legislation

President and executive secretary of the state nurses'
    association

President and executive secretary of the state league
    for nursing

President and executive secretary of the state medical
    association

Chairman of the medical association committee on
    nursing and/or liaison committee with nursing

President and executive secretary of state and regional
    hospital association

President and executive secretary of the state nursing
    home association

Chairmen and executive secretaries of the areawide
    planning agency(ies)

Program coordinator(s) of the regional medical program(s)

Chairman or president and executive secretary of the
    regional education board

Chief executive(s) of Blue Cross and Blue Shield Plan(s)

Executives of major insurance companies providing health
    insurance

(In addition, invitations were to be sent to all educational directors and deans and directors of nursing service in each state for the second day's meeting.)

The number of names submitted by each Board varied widely, ranging from a low of 13 to a high of 52 with a total of approximately 200 names received.

In addition to the State Boards, the national offices of the American Nurses' Association, The National League for Nursing, The American Medical Association, the American Hospital Association and the Division of Nursing of the Department of Health, Education and Welfare were contacted and invited to submit suggestions for inclusion on the invitation lists. Their suggestions numbered 115 names.

These two sources formed the basis for the invitation lists for the first day meeting in each city.

A second day of meetings in each location was planned for the Deans and Directors of all nursing education programs and for directors of nursing service of all the health care institutions in each region.

The 1969 edition of "State Approved Schools of Nursing — RN" compiled by the National League for Nursing Research and Development department was utilized in issuing invitations to the nurse educators except for the seven states in which the State Boards, in addition to the list we requested of them, provided a more current list of educational institutions.

Hospitals August 1, 1969, Part 2, provided a list of health care institutions and an invitation was directed to each 'Director of Nursing Service'.

The decision to arrange the two day's sessions with separate and distinct invitation lists is one that has provoked some comment and question and would, perhaps, benefit by further discussion.

The initial planning for implementation in a given state would demand prior consideration of such questions as: Which agency holds ultimate responsibility for education in the state, from whence does authority derive for conferring licensure, and what are the legal relationships between nursing and medical practice? Further, what is the informal, working relationship between such groups as comprehensive health planning, regional medical programs, home health care, and the university medical center? To what extent are nurses meaningfully involved in decision-making, and what are the informal communications channels utilized by concerned people to effect action in a given state? We believed that exploration and resolution of these questions would proceed with the greatest dispatch if representatives of state nursing organizations, medical societies, hospital associations, legislative bodies, and other involved agencies from each region met together on the same day.

It should be emphasized that there was no intent to separate nurses from 'others' and actually this could not have been accomplished even by design, for many of the organizational positions included in the first day lists are held by nurses and at every meeting more than 50% of the participants were, indeed, nurses. In addition, the rationale for the composition of the second day groups was to bring nurse educators and nursing service people together, since it had been our experience that these people have had little opportunity to meet and discuss concerns such as those related to our recommendations.

A survey of facilities indicated that very few schools of nursing in the country could accommodate a meeting of more than 300 persons and this factor was a very practical limitation on the number of people that we could handle at any single session, and this factor was the final point in our decision to hold two meetings at each location.

The expectation of the staff that all the available spaces would be filled, was, unhappily, not an accurate one. In Palo Alto, for example, the affirmative responses to the first day invitations numbered less than 15 just ten days before the scheduled date of the meeting; consequently, a decision was made to conduct just one session. It should be noted that curtailment of out-of-state travel by the governments of some of the western states and distances involved in travel from Alaska and Hawaii contributed somewhat to this situation. Ultimately, however, the only conference reserved to capacity was the second day meeting in Boston.

An invitation incorporating information concerning the Commission, the objectives of the proposed meetings and a preliminary program was prepared and issued in late February.

The following table indicates the numbers of invitations issued in each category:

1287	Schools in the 1969 NLN Blue Book
7137	Institutions listed in August 1, 1969 *Hospitals*
115	Suggestions from the National organizations
103	Participants in the Commissions 1969 regional meetings
1349	From State Board lists:

224 Minneapolis	191 Salt Lake City
96 Palo Alto	225 St. Louis
222 Washington	185 Atlanta
206 Boston	

100	Invitations issued in response to mail and telephone requests
10,091	Total number of invitations issued

While the lists were carefully compiled and the mailing performed by a specialized handling company, we did experience some difficulties in delivery because of the general mail strike, and we had no absolute assurance that all invitations were received — or received in time for acceptance.

An initial, heavy return of reply cards, averaging 150 per day for the first 10 days, seemed to support our belief that all available spaces would be reserved. Subsequently, a marked decrease in returns resulted in a final tally of 2484 (or 24.6% of the invitations extended) responses. Of these, 1676 (or 16.6% of those invited) accepted and 808 (or 8% of those invited) declined.

The actual number of registrants for the 13 meetings was 1439 or 14.3% of the total number of persons invited. The number of participants from each state is outlined in the following table. Numbers in parentheses represent individuals who attended a conference outside their own region due to conflicts in scheduling or prior commitments.

Minneapolis March 23 and 24, 1970

Illinois	7 (5)	37 (7)
Indiana	5	12
Michigan	6 (1)	16
Minnesota	16	56
Montana	4 (4)	3 (2)
North Dakota	5	7
South Dakota	12	5
Wisconsin	6	31
	61	167

Palo Alto March 26, 1970

Alaska	(1)
California	155 (1)
Hawaii	3
Oregon	11 (1)
Washington	10
	179

Washington, D.C. March 31 and April 1, 1970

Delaware	4	7
District of Columbia	12	20
Kentucky	2 (1)	5
Maryland	13	42
New Jersey	3 (1)	26
Ohio	1 (3)	21
Pennsylvania	7	86
Virginia	14	24
West Virginia	3	9
	65	243

Boston April 6 and 7, 1970

Connecticut	10	32
Maine	11	7
Massachusetts	24	97
New Hampshire	5	8
New York	23 (5)	62 (3)
Rhode Island	55	14
Vermont	6	5
	86	225

Salt Lake City   April 13 and 14, 1970

Arizona	4	4
Colorado	8 (2)	9
Idaho	3	5
Nevada	4	-
New Mexico	1	-
Utah	4	13
Wyoming	4	1
	31	35

St. Louis   April 14 and 15, 1970

Arkansas	-	2
Iowa	1	3
Kansas	3	10
Louisiana	2	7
Missouri	15	67
Nebraska	-	5
Oklahoma	8	6
Texas	2 (2)	11
	38	118

Atlanta   April 20 and 21, 1970

Alabama	13	16
Florida	6	17
Georgia	17	28
Mississippi	5	8
North Carolina	9	21
South Carolina	10	15
Tennessee	6	16
	68	123

At each meeting, one or more Commissioners were requested to provide for the participants a brief history of the Commission, the professional backgrounds and qualifications which the individual members brought to the deliberations, and an outline of the activities of the group over the course of the study. The program then proceeded to a presentation of the major recommendations of the Commission, viewed within the framework of these basic priorities:

1. The necessity for increased research into both nursing practice and education;
2. The requirement for changed educational patterns consistent with the need to conduct and apply research;
3. The need for increased financial support for nurses and for nursing to ensure adequate career opportunities that will attract and retain the number of individuals required for quality health care in the coming years.

The background and judgment involved in the formulation of the recommendations was outlined and graphic representations of much of the tabular material and data were provided.

The afternoon sessions in most cases, were devoted to smaller discussion groups with participants from each state assigned to the same group. Within existing space and staff limitations, an effort was made to group states having similar health care problems, education facilities, and geographic proximity so that there could be a sharing of information and resources.

Each group included a member of the Commission's study staff as a resource person and, at most of the meetings, members of the nursing advisory panel and the health professions advisory panel assisted in a resource capacity.

Each participant had been advised to read the summary report before the meeting, hence, discussion was most often focused on the clarification of details of certain recommendations, definition of terms, and elaboration of the thinking and judgment upon which a recommendation rested. At each meeting, participants were asked to write specific questions and comments for later review by the staff. Material from 13 meetings indicated that the major areas still in need of discussion were:

1.   Composition of state master planning committees for education and the source of committee authority to operate;
2.   Composition of the Joint Practice Commissions;
3.   The process by which schools acquire degree-granting powers and the relationship of this process to that of accreditation.

The most often asked question by far was: How, by whom, and when will implementation of the report be achieved?

Implementation will surely, and rightfully, be the responsibility and perogative of nursing. And while nurses will require the unstinting support of the other health professions and of the public, nursing is assured the support and assistance of the Commission and its staff.

Information to be used in designing a plan for effective delivery of that support was one prime objective of the regional meetings.

Cursory consideration of the often-posed question regarding implementation would seem to indicate that the objective was not attained. There is, however, encouraging evidence to the contrary. Requests for speakers, consultants, and materials have been steadily increasing since the meetings. Predictably, the nature of the requests have varied from state to state as the meeting participants returned home to identify the priorities for action, lines of communications, and resources available.

Widespread dissemination of information about the report was the second objective of the regional meetings. We hoped, by means of the meetings, to acquaint the leaders in the health care field in every state with sufficient data to enable each of them to serve in a resource capacity in his own region, association and practice agency, when the full length report appeared.

Evaluation of the regional meeting as a method of meeting that objective, of necessity, awaits action in the community. There is no question that a massive coordinated effort will be required if the recommendations, formulated on the basis of a long and searching look at the piece of the health care puzzle that is nursing, are to be explored, studied, weighed and implemented to allow nursing to maximize its vital contribution to the betterment of this nation's health care.

APPENDIX R

A COMPENDIUM OF FORMS

This appendix shows the arrangement and text of the major forms used by the NCSNNE during the study. Where a cover letter was used with the form, the content of that cover letter is shown preceding the form with which it was used. The cover letter is then identified by the same form number but a different sheet number in this compendium. The forms in this appendix are arranged in chronological order of their use. The following forms are included:

Form R-1.   Letter to executive directors of state nursing associations requesting copies of state or regional nursing studies (June, 1968)

Form R-2.   Interview materials for site visits (June, 1968)
        A.   Interview Guide
        B.   Interview Record
        C.   Interview Supplemental Information Request

Form R-3.   Nursing Education Questionnaires
                 A.   Deans or directors of nursing education programs
                                       (July, 1968)
                 B.   Directing officer or presidents of parent
                                       institutions (July, 1968)
                 C.   Former deans or directors of closed nursing
                                       programs (July, 1968)
                 D.   Administrators of institutions where nursing
                                       programs have closed (July, 1968)
                 E.   Presidents of colleges or universities which do not
                                       offer degree programs in nursing (October, 1968)
                 F.   Deans or directors of baccalaureate programs in
                                       nursing not formally accredited by the National
                                       League for Nursing (October, 1968)
Form R-4.   Letter of Invitation to participants of the March, 1969 regional
                 meetings (January, 1969)
Form R-5.   Faculty Questionnaire sent to faculty members in a sample of 278
                 preparatory nursing education programs (February, 1969)
Form R-6.   Nursing School Environment Inventory (March, 1969)
                 A.   Letter requesting participation and reply card
                 B.   Nursing School Environment Inventory
Form R-7.   Third draft of Probable Findings (June, 1969)
                 A.   Letter requesting participation in completing the
                                       questionnaire
                 B.   "National Commission for the Study of Nursing
                                       and Nursing Education," Reactionnaire: Probable
                                       Findings

FORM R-1   LETTER TO EXECUTIVE DIRECTORS OF STATE
NURSING ASSOCIATIONS

June 13, 1968

Dear Executive Director:

The study group of the National Commission for the Study of Nursing and Nursing Education has been in existence for approximately six months. This period of time has been devoted to preparing a plan of operation, talking with people in nursing and other health professions, attending national and regional meetings, and conducting an extensive literature search.

In regard to the literature search, we are aware that studies of nursing manpower, practice and education have been conducted in many states by State Nurse Associations and by various research groups. We are writing to ask your help in providing copies of any recently completed (the last two or three years) studies in your state or region, or by directing us to sources where we can obtain such copies.

As an additional favor we would like to have information regarding any studies currently underway with the idea that when these are completed we might obtain copies of the final reports.

Any information or assistance you can give us in this matter will be greatly appreciated.

Thank you.

Sincerely yours,

Richard E. Huse
Administrative and Research
Associate

REH:jd

Form R-1

FORM R-2 INTERVIEW MATERIALS

R-2A   Interview Guide
R-2B   Interview Record
R-2C   Interview Supplemental
        Information Request

INTERVIEW GUIDE

DESCRIPTION

A-1. What is the current objective of the project?

A-2. Has it changed since the project started? In what ways?

A-3. Please tell me about how and when the project got started.
  BE SURE TO IDENTIFY: Who had the idea
      Who became involved in getting the project started
      What were the *steps* taken to implement the idea

A-4. Please describe how personnel become assigned to this project?

A-5. Who participates in selecting personnel?

A-6. Who are the other personnel, not assigned to the project, with whom project personnel regularly work?

A-7. What are the responsibilities and relationships of these other people to the project and its personnel?

A-8. Has the project had any effect on the schedules and utilization of personnel or facilities?

CARE AND TREATMENT

A-8. Please tell me about the work of nursing personnel (cover each title, asking the same questions, where applicable. Ask for *EXAMPLES, EMPHASIZE* differences)
  a.   Physical Tasks?
  b.   Treatment Procedures?
  c.   Patient Interaction?
  d.   Patient evaluation and observations?
  e.   Training project personnel?
  f.   Participating in decisions? With whom? What kinds, e. g., discharge, providing for additional treatments, giving additional services, special examinations or tests.

A-9. Do some personnel specialize in certain functions? What are they?

A-10. How is what You are doing in this project different from what was being done previously?

A-11. How do you think it differs from what is generally being done?

A-12. What things are being done the same as before the project started?

Form R-2A

INTERVIEW GUIDE - Continued

PATIENTS

A-13. How does a patient become assigned to this (unit, dept. project)?

A-14. Are there plans regularly prepared to guide care of individual patients?

A-15. What things do plans include? (Request copies of typical plans, kept in confidence)

A-16. For which patients are plans prepared?

A-17. What is the criteria used which determines if a plan is needed?

A-18. Who is responsible for the plan preparation?

A-19. What are the steps involved in preparing a plan?

TRAINING

A-20. Did you develop special training for project personnel? Please tell me about it.

A-21. What training and background do you look for in obtaining personnel?

A-22. Do you expect this to change in the future? How?

A-23. If you have developed special training programs, may I have copies of course outlines, training manuals, or other materials.

EVALUATION

A-23. What do you consider to be the most successful part of the project?

A-24. What has been your biggest disappointment?

A-25. What has been your biggest problem in the development and carrying out of this project?

A-26. What are your plans for this project in the immediate future?

A-27. What do you consider to be the implications of this project for health care in the future?

A-28. Are there some types of people you find particularly successful? Unsuccessful?

A-29. How is patient care being evaluated?

A-30. How is the project being evaluated? (What data collected regularly by whom? analyzed and reported by whom, to whom)?

A-31. Do you plan any changes to your evaluation procedure? Why?

STUDENTS

B-1. Please tell me about your students? Where do they come from? What is their academic background?

B-2. What has been your recent experience with retention/graduation ratio? Is it changing?

Form R-2A (Sheet 2)

INTERVIEW GUIDE - Continued
STUDENTS (cont'd)

B-3. What are the areas in which you see the greatest source for optimism and strength for your student body in the future?

B-4. What are your areas of concern, or potential problems?

B-5. What are employers of students looking for? Where are your students first employed?

B-6. What are the academic performances of your students? (results of tests, boards, etc.)

FACULTY

B-7. Please tell me about your faculty. Where do they come from, what is their background?

B-8. Are there other qualifications which they have which you consider important?

B-9. What are some of the problems, if any, you have had in obtaining faculty?

B-10. Please tell me the rates of compensation for various levels. How does this compare with other schools?

B-11. What is your opinion of the status and standing of your faculty in comparison with others in your institution?

B-12. What do you consider the most important strengths of your faculty?

B-13. Are there important weaknesses you would like to tell us about?

PROGRAM

B-14. What are the objectives of your curriculum?

B-15. Please describe for me the content and articulation of your curriculum.

B-16. What is your degree of satisfaction with classrooms, laboratories, and teaching facilities?

B-17. Please tell me about your relationships with arts and sciences.

B-18. What efforts are made to individualize programs?

GENERAL

B-19. Please tell me what you consider to be your most important needs and requirements currently? How will these change in the future?

B-20. Are there other programs which you consider important, and worthy of study by us?

B-21. Please tell me about your physical plant and its facilities.

B-22. What are the things about your community and institution which are important to the success of your program?

Form R-2A (Sheet 3)

INTERVIEW GUIDE - Continued

MANPOWER

C-1. How have patient/personnel ratios been affected by the project? Have the types of patient care personnel changed?

C-2. Would wide application of this project change recruitment, retention, reentry, and other aspects of patient care personnel recruitment?

C-3. How has this project affected other local health care programs?

C-4. What measures have been used to maintain employee morale while introducing this project?

COSTS

C-5. What impact has the innovation of this project had on costs (to the patient, to the facility)?

C-6. How have salaries of patient care personnel been affected? Are they paid any differently than other personnel? Is this difference, if any, a permanent or temporary arrangement?

C-7. How will the project personnel be related to the structure and system for advancement? Are opportunities for advancement greater? Please describe the structure for salaries, and evaluation.

LEGAL

C-8. Have there been any legal issues (such as "scope of practice") raised during this project? If so, how have they been resolved?

INTERVIEWER

Comments on purpose of visit
Evaluation of interviews, including principal investigation, or director.
Evaluation and analysis of project
Follow-up requirements
Other notes, leads, commentary

Form R-2A (Sheet 4)

NATIONAL COMMISSION FOR THE STUDY OF NURSING
AND NURSING EDUCATION
208 Westfall Road
Rochester, New York 14620

<u>INTERVIEW RECORD</u>

AM

Interviewer _____ Date _____

PM

Institution _____

Address _____ City _____

Project or Program Title_____

Type(s) of Program or Project _____

Interviewee(s) _____ _____

Name	Title
_____	_____
_____	_____
_____	_____
_____	_____

Director, or Principal Investigator_____
    (If not interviewed)

Published Material (Collected, or to be sent) _____

_____

_____

Return to Interview Guide

Interviewer Comments and Summary

Form R-2B

INTERVIEW RECORD (Continued)

Question Number	Direct Reply	Conversational Commentary

Form R-2B (Sheet 2)

NATIONAL COMMISSION FOR THE STUDY OF
NURSING AND NURSING EDUCATION

INTERVIEW SUPPLEMENTAL INFORMATION REQUEST

Institution _____

Project or Program Studied _____

1.   Staff Involved_____ ____ _____ _____

                                (Title)   (no.)   (Duties)   (Ann. sal.)

2.   What is the source of project funding?_____

3.   What organization controls funds?_____

Educational Activities Data

STUDENTS

1.   Number_____
                          Please specify for each program

2.   Criteria for selection _____

FACULTY (Please specify for various programs, undergraduate, graduate, etc.)

1.   Number _____ _____ _____ _____

2.   Average Age   _____ _____ _____

3.   Average Years Teaching Experience _____ _____ _____

4.   Average Years Nursing Experience _____ _____ _____

Form R-2C

INTERVIEW SUPPLEMENTAL INFORMATION REQUEST - (Continued)

FACILITIES

1.   Please list *all* clinical facilities used, and the courses to which they apply:

        _____   _____

        _____   _____

        _____   _____

        _____   _____

2.   Please describe laboratory facilities, and if shared, indicate with which courses
      of study they are shared:

        _____   _____

        _____   _____

        _____   _____

        _____   _____

3.   How many classrooms for nursing alone? _____ How many shared? _____

      How would you rate their adequacy for your current programs?

        Superior _____ Very Good _____ Adequate _____

        Barely Adequate _____ Inadequate _____

      Please tell us why you arrived at this rating? _____

      _____

      _____

4.   Additional comments on educational activities _____

      _____

      _____

      _____

      _____

      _____

      _____

Form R-2C (Sheet 2)

INTERVIEW SUPPLEMENTAL INFORMATION REQUEST - (Continued)

Practice of Nursing

STAFF

1. What is the total number of people who have participated in the program since it started, and what disciplines?

(no.)	(Discipline)
_____	_____
_____	_____
_____	_____
_____	_____
_____	_____

FACILITIES

1. Please describe any special facilities and equipment provided for this project.

    _____

    _____

2. At this point, what changes in facilities could be made to improve the work of this project? _____

    _____

    _____

General

RECRUITMENT

1. Please list the most important sources of personnel recruited for this project.

    _____

    _____

2. Please compare the project staff with your regular staff for these factors:

	Regular Staff	Project
Average length of employment	_____	_____
Recruiting costs (per employee)	_____	_____
Average years of experience	_____	_____

Form R-2C (Sheet 3)

FORM R-3 NURSING EDUCATION QUESTIONNAIRES
(Including Cover Letters)

R-3A   Deans or Directors
R-3B   Directing Officers or Presidents
R-3C   Former Deans or Directors
R-3D   Administrators Where Programs Closed
R-3E   Presidents of Institutions Not Offering
            Nursing Degrees
R-3F   Deans or Directors of NLN Non-Accredited
            Baccalaureate Programs

National Commission for the Study of Nursing
and Nursing Education

NURSING EDUCATION QUESTIONNAIRE

1. Name of Dean or Director_____

2. Name and Address of Institution _____

    _____

    _____

3. T.ype of Program (Check one)   Associate Degree   ☐
                                    Baccalaureate Degree ☐
                                    Diploma   ☐

4. Administrative Control (Check one)   Hospital   ☐
                                          College or University   ☐
                                          Junior or Community College ☐
                                          Independent   ☐

5. Principal Source of Financial Support (Check one)

                                    Public ☐
                                    Private ☐

6. Enrollment as of February 15, 1968_____

7. Number of Graduates: Sept. 1, 1965 - Aug. 31, 1966_____

                            Sept. 1, 1966 - Aug. 31, 1967_____

                            Sept. 1, 1967 - Aug. 31, 1968 (Estimated)____

8. Within the last year has your institution revised the nursing curriculum or attempted instructional approaches which you consider innovative?

                    YES ☐   NO ☐

9. If the answer to question 8 was affirmative, please explain.

10. Within the last year has your institution made a decision either to enlarge the commitment to nursing education, to reduce it, or to discontinue operations?

                    YES ☐   NO ☐

Form R-3A

11.   If the answer to question 10 was affirmative, please explain.

12.   In your opinion, what are the two most serious problems facing nursing education today?

13.   At present what is the most serious problem confronting *your* institution?

14.   What one change would most improve nursing education in your institution?

July 9, 1968

Dear Administrator:

As you may know, our Commission is conducting research on nursing and nursing education with a view to making recommendations on the academic preparation necessary for future entrants into the profession.

The enclosed questionnaire is designed to explore the thinking of administrators on the major problems facing nursing schools. To identify these problems and their proposed solutions from another angle, we have also sent a related, but somewhat different, questionnaire to the director of nursing education at your institution.

You will notice that a few of our questions ask for your assessment of the quality of your nursing education establishment. Through this procedure we hope eventually to learn what particular elements contribute most to effective and viable nursing education. Rest assured that this information, as well as your other answers, will be treated in strictest confidence and that neither your nursing education division nor your institution will be identified in any material we may publish.

On the basis of the content of replies we may in the coming months ask to visit the nursing education program at your institution in order to study it in greater detail.

Thank you for your assistance.

Sincerely yours,

Jerome P. Lysaught
Director

JPL:jd

Form R-3B

National Commission for the Study of Nursing
and Nursing Education

NURSING EDUCATION QUESTIONNAIRE

1. Name of Directing Officer or President _____

2. Name and Address of Hospital or _____
        Institution   _____
                                         _____

3. In your opinion, what are the two most serious problems facing nursing
    education today?

4. At present what is the most serious problem confronting the school or
    department of nursing at your institution?

5. What one change would most improve nursing education at your institution?

Form R-3B (Sheet 2)

6. Compared with other schools of nursing how would you evaluate the quality of the school or department of nursing at your institution? In terms of: (For each item please check the appropriate column.)

	Upper Tenth	Upper Quarter	Upper Half	Lower Half	Lower Quarter	Lower Tenth
General Quality	____	____	____	____	____	____
Curriculum	____	____	____	____	____	____
Administration	____	____	____	____	____	____
Faculty	____	____	____	____	____	____
Student Body	____	____	____	____	____	____

7. Compared with other academic schools or departments (English, history, mathematics, etc.) in your institution or those elsewhere with which you are acquainted, how would you evaluate the quality of your school or department of nursing? In terms of: (For each item please check the appropriate column.)

	Upper Tenth	Upper Quarter	Upper Half	Lower Half	Lower Quarter	Lower Tenth
General Quality	____	____	____	____	____	____
Curriculum	____	____	____	____	____	____
Administration	____	____	____	____	____	____
Faculty	____	____	____	____	____	____
Student Body	____	____	____	____	____	____

8. Compared with other professional schools or departments (business administration, education, engineering, etc.) in your institution or those elsewhere with which you are acquainted, how would you evaluate the quality of your school or department of nursing? In terms of: (For each item please check the appropriate column.)

	Upper Tenth	Upper Quarter	Upper Half	Lower Half	Lower Quarter	Lower Tenth
General Quality	____	____	____	____	____	____
Curriculum	____	____	____	____	____	____
Administration	____	____	____	____	____	____
Faculty	____	____	____	____	____	____
Student Body	____	____	____	____	____	____

Form R-3B (Sheet 3)

July 9, 1968

Dear Educational Director:

   As you probably know, our Commission is conducting research on nursing and nursing education with a view to preparing a report for publication in about two years. As a first step in the area of education, we are making a survey of all professional preparatory institutions.

   We are aware that your school of nursing has closed. We have sent you the enclosed questionnaire because we feel that nursing educators whose schools have closed can, because of this experience, contribute information and ideas toward the solution of the major problems facing nursing schools. In an effort to get the viewpoint of college and hospital administrators on some of these problems, a related, but somewhat different, questionnaire has gone to the head of the institution at which you were formerly located.

   Information on completed questionnaires will be considered and treated as confidential and neither you, your former school of nursing, nor your institution will be identified in any material we may publish.

   Thank you for your assistance.

                                                  Sincerely yours,

                                                  Jerome P. Lysaught
                                                  Director

JPL:jd

Form R-3C

National Commission for the Study of Nursing
and Nursing Education

NURSING EDUCATION QUESTIONNAIRE

1. Name of Former Dean or Director _____

2. Name and Address of Former Institution _____

    _____

    _____

    _____

3. Date Nursing Education Establishment Closed _____

3a. How Long in operation _____

4. Type of Program (Check one)   Associate Degree ☐
                                   Baccalaureate Degree ☐
                                   Diploma ☐

5. Administrative Control (Check one)   Hospital ☐
                                         College or University ☐
                                         Junior or Community College ☐
                                         Independent ☐

6. Principal Source of Financial Support (Check one)

                                   Public ☐
                                   Private ☐

7. What one factor was most responsible for the closing of your school of nursing education?

8. Prior to your closing had your institution revised the nursing curriculum or attempted instructional approaches which you considered innovative?

                    YES ☐   NO ☐

Form R-3C (Sheet 2)

9. If the answer to question 8 was affirmative, please explain.

10. In your opinion, what are the two most serious problems facing nursing education today?

National Commission for the Study of Nursing
and Nursing Education

NURSING EDUCATION QUESTIONNAIRE

1. Name of Administrator _____

2. Name of Institution _____

    _____

    _____

    _____

3. Date Nursing School Closed _____

3a. How Long in Operation _____

4. In your opinion, what are the two most serious problems facing nursing education today?

5. What one factor was most responsible for the closing of the nursing school at your institution?

6. Compared with other schools of nursing how would you rate the quality of the school of nursing formerly at your institution? (For each item please check the appropriate column.)

	Upper Tenth	Upper Quarter	Upper Half	Lower Half	Lower Quarter	Lower Tenth
General Quality	____	____	____	____	____	____
Curriculum	____	____	____	____	____	____
Administration	____	____	____	____	____	____
Faculty	____	____	____	____	____	____
Student Body	____	____	____	____	____	____

Form R-3D

7. Compared with other *academic* schools or departments (English, history, mathematics, etc.) in your institution or those elsewhere with which you are acquainted, how would you rate the quality of the school of nursing formerly at your institution? (For each item please check the appropriate column.)

	Greatly Superior	Somewhat Superior	About the Same	Somewhat Inferior	Greatly Inferior
General Quality	_____	_____	_____	_____	_____
Curriculum	_____	_____	_____	_____	_____
Administration	_____	_____	_____	_____	_____
Faculty	_____	_____	_____	_____	_____
Student Body	_____	_____	_____	_____	_____

8. Compared with other *professional* schools or departments (business administration, education, engineering, etc.) in your institution or those elsewhere with which you are acquainted, how would you rate the quality of the school of nursing formerly at your institution? (For each item please check the appropriate column.)

	Greatly Superior	Somewhat Superior	About the Same	Somewhat Inferior	Greatly Inferior
General Quality	_____	_____	_____	_____	_____
Curriculum	_____	_____	_____	_____	_____
Administration	_____	_____	_____	_____	_____
Faculty	_____	_____	_____	_____	_____
Student Body	_____	_____	_____	_____	_____

Form R-3D (Sheet 2)

October 14, 1968

Dear President:

   As stated in greater detail in the enclosed press release, our Commission is conducting research on nursing and nursing education with a view to preparing a set of recommendations for the enhancement of this profession.

   One aspect of our study deals with the kinds of programs offered by schools of nursing at colleges and universities. In connection with this interest, we find we must explore the related point concerning those colleges and universities — particularly those with larger enrollments — which do not offer a degree program in nursing. We would greatly appreciate it if you would take the time to complete and return the attached questionnaire; it will be of significant help to us in analyzing the educational requirements for the future.

   Thank you for your assistance.

                                        Sincerely,

                                        Jerome P. Lysaught, Ed.D.
                                        Director

JPL:jd

Enclosures 2

Form R-3E

National Commission for the Study of Nursing
and Nursing Education

Name of Institution_____

Address   _____

                 _____

1.   Has a school or department of nursing ever been a part of your institution?

                        YES _____   NO _____

2.   If the answer to question 1. is "YES", why is the school of nursing no longer
      in operation?

3.   If a school or department of nursing was never a part of your institution,
      what is (are) the major reason(s) for the decision to omit it?

4.   Are you planning to introduce a school or department of nursing at your
      institution within the foreseeable future?

                        YES _____   NO _____

5.   If the answer to question 4. is "YES", what factors are responsible for your
      decision?

Form R-3E (Sheet 2)

October 18, 1968

Dear Dean or Director:

Thank you for completing and returning the questionnaire we mailed you in July. We hope that those few schools that have not yet completed and returned that questionnaire will do so before the scheduled November 1st processing date.

I am writing in the hope that you can provide us with some additional information which will help us form a more complete picture of nursing education in the United States. The enclosed survey is being addressed to those schools of nursing which offer a preparatory program, leading to the baccalaureate degree, which is not formally accredited by the National League for Nursing. We would like to know some of the background concerning the matter of accreditation and your institution's posture toward the matter.

As we stated in our letter of July 9th, information on completed questionnaires will be considered and treated as confidential and neither you, your school of nursing, nor your institution will be identified in any material we may publish.

Thank you for your assistance.

Sincerely yours,

Jerome P. Lysaught, Ed.D.
Director

JPL/jd

Enclosure 1

Form R-3F

National Commission for the Study of Nursing
and Nursing Education

Name of Dean or Director _____

Name and Address of Institution _____

_____

_____

1.   How many years has your school of nursing offered a preparatory program in nursing leading to the baccalaureate degree? Years _____

2.   Has your school of nursing ever applied for NLN accreditation?

YES _____   NO _____

2a.   If YES, has your school of nursing ever been accredited?

YES _____   NO _____

2b.   If your answer to 2 was NO, would you tell us why your institution has chosen not to seek accreditation.

3.   If your school of nursing has ever been accredited by the NLN and now lacks such accreditation, what was (were) the reason(s) for the loss of accreditation?

4.   If your school has applied for, but has never been granted, accreditation by the NLN, what is(are) the reason(s) for the failure of the NLN to accredit you?

Form R-3F (Sheet 2)

FORM R-4
LETTER OF INVITATION

January, 1969

This Commission was established in January 1968 to prepare a report on the function and education of nurses for future health service to the nation. The enclosed news release contains some further information on the Commission's formation and objectives.

In order to obtain grassroots feelings and suggestions, we are holding a series of conferences to obtain views and information from those people who will be directly concerned with our final report — including consumers, physicians, nurses, educators, health service administrators, and insurers.

Your experience and thoughts would be most valuable to us. I hope, therefore, that you will participate in a small group Conference in St. Louis, Missouri on March 3-4.

We would like you to meet at that time with other carefully chosen individuals whose special knowledge of the health concerns of the public and whose interest in the outcome of our study are of great significance.

Before the conference, we will send you a list of study questions and tentative findings prepared by our staff on the function and education of nurses in health service. These, along with the presentation of varying viewpoints by an invited panel, will furnish the discussion points for the conference.

Because our funds are quite limited, we hope that you or your organization will be able to provide for your conference expenses. If this is difficult, however, we will arrange to care for your expenses. Will you indicate your need on the enclosed card?

Form R-4

We earnestly solicit your attendance and your help. Recognizing the many problems to be found in nursing and its key role in the delivery of health care, many organizations and professional bodies are looking to this Commission for recommendations that can solve the current dilemmas and point the way to a brighter future. You can make a signal contribution to our efforts; we hope you will aid us in this endeavor.

Please return the enclosed reply card at your earliest convenience. As soon as we have word of your acceptance, we shall mail you a room reservation card for the Sheraton-Jefferson Hotel. Please send the card to the hotel promptly to ensure that your reservation is in order.

The meeting will begin promptly at 1:30 p.m. on March 3 at the Sheraton-Jefferson and will close at noon on March 4. Additional details and information will be mailed to you shortly after we receive your reply.

We look forward to seeing you in St. Louis.

Sincerely yours,

Jerome P. Lysaught   W. Allen Wallis
Study Director   President

Form R-4 (Sheet 2)

FORM R-5
FACULTY QUESTIONNAIRE
(Including Cover Letter)

FACULTY QUESTIONNAIRE

This faculty questionnaire is part of a larger study being conducted by the National Commission for the Study of Nursing and Nursing Education. The questionnaire has been designed to indicate the background, education, and career activities of faculty members in institutions preparing students for nursing.

A report based on the results of this investigation as well as on other research conducted by our Commission will be published by the Commission some time in 1970. It is hoped that the continuing cooperation of many persons will make this report a valuable contribution to nursing education in the United States.

PLEASE RETURN THIS COMPLETED QUESTIONNAIRE TO THE ADMINISTRATIVE HEAD OF YOUR NURSING EDUCATION UNIT

Institution _____

Address of Institution _____

_____

_____

                    Mr.

Name of Faculty Member Miss

                    Mrs. _____

Form R-5

If married, occupation of spouse_____

(Title and Type of Work)   (Employer)

Academic Preparation and Earned Degrees (Supply all information regarding preparation and earned degrees. List institutions separately in chronological order of attendance, beginning with undergraduate work.)

Institution   Location   Major   Date of Attendance   Degree

List Courses (given for college credit) you have taken during the period, September 1966 — June 1968. Omit this information if during this time you were enrolled full-time at a school of nursing or at a university.

Institution   Location   Course   Number of Credits

Form R-5 (Sheet 2)

Income for Last Three Years:

Contract Salary (before education). Please enter your salary in either the Academic
  Year or the Calendar Year Column, depending on whether your institution pays
  your salary by the academic or by the calendar year.

	No. of Months for Which	
Academic Year	Salary is Paid. (Academic year is usually nine months)	Calendar Year
1967-68 _____	_____	1967-68 _____
1966-67 _____	_____	1966-67 _____
1965-66 _____	_____	1965-66 _____

Amounts from other academic sources (teaching summer school, etc.). Please
  specify dates:

If you were employed as a faculty member in a school of nursing during the years
  1961 and 1962, please also enter your salary for that period below:

	No. of Months for Which	
Academic Year	Salary is Paid. (Academic year is usually nine months)	Calendar Year
1961-62 _____	_____	1961-62 _____

List all Courses You Normally Teach in an Academic Year:

Form R-5 (Sheet 3)

Career Since Receiving RN (Account for all years including periods of non-paid employment, i.e., homemaking. List present position first.)

<u>Dates</u>   <u>Employer</u>   <u>Location</u>   <u>Title</u> <u>and</u> <u>Type</u> <u>of</u> <u>Work</u>

Present Employment Status:

                                            Full-time   Full-time not

Rank _____ on Tenure _____ on Tenure _____ Part-time _____

If part-time, percent of normal load as defined by institution _____ %

Percent of your official duties assigned to:

        Teaching   _____ %

        Administration   _____ %

        Research   _____ %

        Nursing Practice or Service   _____ %

        Other (Specify).   _____ %

Form R-5 (Sheet 4)

Professional Organization Memberships:

College Activities Outside Nursing Education Department:

Research Activities (Last five years):

Publications (Last five years):

Other Professional Activities:

Form R-5 (Sheet 5)

In your opinion, what is the most serious problem facing nursing education today?

What one change would most improve nursing education at your institution?

_____
                                                                Signed

FORM R-6 NURSING SCHOOL ENVIRONMENT INVENTORY

March 11, 1969

Dear Director:

On at least two occasions over the last six months, we have sent you survey forms and questionnaires with a request that you help us in collecting data for our national study of nursing and nursing education. This important, but doubtless bothersome, chore results from your institution having been selected on a randomized sampling basis as one of 278 departments or schools of nursing representative of all those across the country. We know that these instruments require time and patience to complete, and we can only assure you that we are putting our best efforts into the analysis and synthesis of your replies to insure that our Commission has the best information available on which to base their recommendations.

We also recognize that our distribution of the earlier forms has caused you some particular problems. For example, our information concerning the number of full-time faculty members at your institution is obviously out-dated and several of you received an incorrect number of faculty questionnaires. Also, we recognize that many of the questions on salary and institutional problems appeared too personal and penetrating in the eyes of some faculty members. We must say, in this case, that we have been unable to find adequate and specific data on these several points and that the staff and the Commission feel the areas covered by the surveys are vital ones that must be explored. Proper classification of information, moreover, required identification of institutions so that different types of programs, different regional areas, and other variables might be categorized in our analyses. Naturally, all results are treated as confidential and no individual or institution will be identified in our reports or papers.

We greatly appreciate your aid and your responses. Hopefully, you will continue to advise us, and criticize those points that are unsettling. We, on our part, will strive to improve both our methods and our instruments. In these efforts, I know we are united in a common determination to enhance the future of nurses and nursing.

Form R-6A

We now must come to you, however, about another instrument developed in accordance with our over-all study plan. We have designed a questionnaire modeled after the "Medical School Environment Inventory" which has been used with excellent results by individuals concerned with improving medical education. Our form is called the "Nursing School Environment Inventory" and we would like to have it completed by your *full-time* faculty and graduating students. Its purpose is to distinguish different characteristics and climates among the sample institutions, and to develop some descriptive norms.

To insure your receiving the correct number of questionnaires, we ask that you send us the number of: a) your full-time nursing school or department faculty members; and b) the number of students in your graduating class. Please insert these figures in the appropriate places on the enclosed postcard and return it to us.

When we receive your card, we will mail you the necessary number of forms for distribution to your faculty and students. Return envelopes will be included with the questionnaire so that each faculty member and student can individually return the completed questionnaire form directly to us.

Thank you for your continuing assistance.

Sincerely,

Jerome P. Lysaught
Project Director

JPL/jd

Form R-6A (Sheet 2)

Name _____

Title _____

Institution _____

Address _____

_____

Number of Full-time Faculty Members _____

Number of Students in Graduating Class_____

Form R-6A (Sheet 3 - Reply Card)

April 9, 1969

Thank you for sending us the number of full-time faculty members and graduating students in your institution. We greatly appreciate your continuing willingness to participate in this national study of nursing.

We have enclosed a sufficient number of Nursing School Environment Inventories to enable you to distribute one copy to each full-time faculty member and each graduating student. Also enclosed are stamped, self-addressed envelopes for the use of these persons in mailing their completed questionnaires to us.

It is not necessary for anyone to give his name or to sign the questionnaire. However, if there are graduate students at your institution who will receive the questionnaire, please ask them to indicate this fact in parentheses after the word student on the front of the form.

Thank you for your assistance; the Commission and our staff value your contribution to this investigation.

Sincerely,

Jerome P. Lysaught
Director

JPL/jd
Enclosures 2

Form R-6B

Form R-6B

NAME _____

SCHOOL AND INSTITUTION _____

_____

ADDRESS _____

_____

NURSING SCHOOL
ENVIRONMENT INVENTORY

National Commission for the Study of Nursing and Nursing Education, Inc., 1969.
Adapted from Edwin B. Hutchins, "Medical School Environment Inventory,"
Association of American Medical Colleges, 1962, with the permission of the author.

Form R-6B (Sheet 1)

DIRECTIONS

The following statements refer to the general environment (facilities, faculty and student body) of your nursing school. The statements may or may not be totally characteristic of your school, but try to decide which statements are most characteristic and which are not.

Please use the following scale in rating each statement:

4 – TRUE

3 – MORE OFTEN TRUE THAN NOT

2 – MORE OFTEN FALSE THAN NOT

1 – FALSE

Record your answers by circling the appropriate number at the left of each item. Your statements should tell us what you believe your school environment is like rather than what you might personally prefer. You won't *know* the answer to many of these statements, because there may not be any really definite information on which to base your answer. *Your response will simply mean that in your opinion the statement is to some degree true or false about your nursing school.* Do not omit any item.

Form R-6B (Sheet 2)

4 – TRUE

3 – MORE OFTEN TRUE THAN NOT

2 – MORE OFTEN FALSE THAN NOT

1 – FALSE

Rating
(Circle one number
for each statement)

4 3 2 1   1. The goals and purposes of the work are clearly defined for the student.

4 3 2 1   2. This nursing school is outstanding for the emphasis it places on student scholarship and research.

4 3 2 1   3. In many of the basic sciences classes students have an assigned seat.

4 3 2 1   4. The faculty often seems more interested in the scientific aspects of a case than in the welfare of the patient.

4 3 2 1   5. Faculty members are very oriented toward practical application in their approach to education.

4 3 2 1   6. Faculty members frequently discuss topics which have no apparent relation to the total course.

4 3 2 1   7. Very few instructors try to give the student the kind of practical training she will need for the practice of nursing.

4 3 2 1   8. Most clinical faculty members are liberal in interpreting regulations and treat violations with understanding and tolerance.

4 3 2 1   9. Instructors frequently give unannounced quizzes or tests.

4 3 2 1   10. Departmental advisers seem unaware that a well-rounded program of study includes courses in the behavioral sciences.

4 3 2 1   11. The academic atmosphere here is not very helpful to the student who wants to get down to the business of practicing nursing.

4 3 2 1   12. Faculty members frequently go out of their way to establish friendly relations with students.

4 3 2 1   13. Assignments are usually clear and specific, making it easy for students to plan their studies effectively.

Form R-6B (Sheet 3)

4 – TRUE

3 – MORE OFTEN TRUE THAN NOT

2 – MORE OFTEN FALSE THAN NOT

1 – FALSE

Rating
(Circle one number
for each statement)

4 3 2 1   14. Instructors really get students interested in their subjects.

4 3 2 1   15. Faculty advisers are always available to help the student with the planning of her nursing career.

4 3 2 1   16. The faculty here stresses the study of the patient as a whole person.

4 3 2 1   17. There are many facilities and opportunities for individual creative activity.

4 3 2 1   18. Members of the nursing staff at the hospital conducting the students' clinical training participate enthusiastically in clinical patient conferences.

4 3 2 1   19. Most of the courses stress basic science or scholarship and really probe into the fundamentals of their subjects.

4 3 2 1   20. Faculty members typically exhibit great interest in and enthusiasm for their special fields of interest.

4 3 2 1   21. Faculty members here really push the students' capacities to the limit.

4 3 2 1   22. Students quickly learn what is acceptable and what is not acceptable in this school.

4 3 2 1   23. The faculty here lays great stress on ethical behavior.

4 3 2 1   24. Instructors generally feel that students should take comprehensive notes in lectures.

4 3 2 1   25. Examinations here generally provide a good opportunity for the student to display his knowledge and understanding of the course material.

4 3 2 1   26. Patient responsibility on the part of the student is closely supervised to guard against mistakes.

Form R-6B (Sheet 4)

4 – TRUE

3 – MORE OFTEN TRUE THAN NOT

2 – MORE OFTEN FALSE THAN NOT

1 – FALSE

Rating
(Circle one number
for each statement)

4 3 2 1   27. Faculty members rarely eat with students.

4 3 2 1   28. Many of the faculty seem bored with their teaching assignments.

4 3 2 1   29. The clinical faculty generally expects the student to know a great deal about his patients.

4 3 2 1   30. In many courses the broad social and historical setting of the material is not discussed.

4 3 2 1   31. The faculty rarely encourages a student to read in areas of the student's own interest.

4 3 2 1   32. Many courses stress the speculative or abstract rather than the concrete and tangible.

4 3 2 1   33. The faculty is very impatient with students who are content just to get by.

4 3 2 1   34. Frequent tests are given in most courses and oral quizzes are common in the clinical years.

4 3 2 1   35. Counseling and guidance services here are really personal, considerate, extensive.

4 3 2 1   36. It is hard to prepare for examinations because students seldom know what will be expected of them.

4 3 2 1   37. Very few of the professors here try to get students interested in the humanities or in the broad social context of nursing.

4 3 2 1   38. In many courses there are projects or assignments which encourage students to work in small groups.

4 3 2 1   39. Very little of the instruction here will be useful to students who go into practice.

Form R-6B (Sheet 5)

4 – TRUE

3 – MORE OFTEN TRUE THAN NOT

2 – MORE OFTEN FALSE THAN NOT

1 – FALSE

Rating
(Circle one number
for each statement)

4	3	2	1	40.	Students with superior academic ability are admired by other students.
4	3	2	1	41.	Student competition facilitates the acquisition of knowledge here.
4	3	2	1	42.	There is a lot of interest in the philosophy and methods of science.
4	3	2	1	43.	The students try to help each other.
4	3	2	1	44.	A lecture by an outstanding behavioral scientist would be poorly attended by the students here.
4	3	2	1	45.	It is hard to find any students in the library on weekends.
4	3	2	1	46.	The environment of the nursing school stimulates interest in things other than pure nursing.
4	3	2	1	47.	The problem of comprehensive patient care is given little attention here by the students.
4	3	2	1	48.	There is very little group spirit here.
4	3	2	1	49.	Students are concerned only with the physical aspects of nursing.
4	3	2	1	50.	Students compete actively among themselves.
4	3	2	1	51.	Student attendance at specially organized extracurricular programs related to nursing is good.
4	3	2	1	52.	Students frequently study or prepare for examinations together.
4	3	2	1	53.	A controversial speaker always stirs up a lot of student discussion.
4	3	2	1	54.	Students are more interested in nursing patients with rare and exotic diseases than those with more common illnesses.
4	3	2	1	55.	The student government is active and outspoken.

Form R-6B (Sheet 6)

4 – TRUE

3 – MORE OFTEN TRUE THAN NOT

2 – MORE OFTEN FALSE THAN NOT

1 – FALSE

Rating
(Circle one number
for each statement)

4 3 2 1   56. Most students here have strong intellectual commitments.

4 3 2 1   57. Hazing, teasing and practical joking are fairly common.

4 3 2 1   58. Courses which deal with psychological problems or personal values are resented.

4 3 2 1   59. The competition for special honors is very rough.

4 3 2 1   60. Student elections generate a lot of intense campaigning and strong feeling.

4 3 2 1   61. Students are so preoccupied with their nursing studies that they rarely concern themselves with anything else in social or informal discussion groups.

4 3 2 1   62. Personal hostilities are usually concealed or resolved as quickly as possible.

4 3 2 1   63. Student government or leadership does not participate in student affairs unless called upon by the administrative authorities on campus.

4 3 2 1   64. Students who are not ordinarily neat will take extra pains to have a professional bearing when in the presence of patients.

4 3 2 1   65. There is a recognized group of student leaders at this school.

4 3 2 1   66. Students who work hard for high grades are likely to be regarded as odd.

4 3 2 1   67. Students are concerned only with the work at hand and have few interests beyond this area.

4 3 2 1   68. Many students here are content just to get by.

4 3 2 1   69. It is usually quite easy to get a group decision here without much discussion.

Form R-6B (Sheet 7)

FORM R-7 THIRD DRAFT OF PROBABLE FINDINGS

R-7A   Letter Requesting Participation
R-7B   Reactionnaire

This Commission was established in January 1968 to prepare a report on the function and education of nurses for future health service to the nation. The enclosed news release contains some further information on the Commission's formation and objectives.

Recently, the Commission sponsored three regional conferences across the country to consider the problems of the nursing profession. Invitations were sent to persons who would be directly concerned with the recommendations of the Commission; nurses, physicians, health service administrators, insurers, consumers, and educators. These meetings appeared highly successful in bringing out the issues and creating a productive dialogue. We are writing you at this time because we think you can make a valuable contribution to the continuation of these processes.

During the meetings, those persons present had an opportunity to express views on questions and indicated findings prepared by our staff for the Commission, and also heard commentaries by a panel of consumers and a panel of health professionals. More importantly, however, we asked the participants to provide us with a formal record of their thinking by giving us written reactions and comments on specially designed response forms.

Form R-7A

We consider it essential at this stage to obtain the widest possible range of thinking in regard to the issues found in the study, and also to expose our approach to these issues to those who will be most affected by them. Consequently, we are sending your organization a revised version of the questions and findings used at the conferences. We would like to ask you to review them and then complete the response sheet. It should be emphasized that we are interested in your *organization's point of view* concerning our indicated findings rather than in the personal point of view of the individual who might complete the forms. Please return both the booklet of questions and findings with your comments and the completed answer sheet to us in the self-addressed envelope.

We anticipate that our staff will begin preparation of a final report early this fall and that the Commission will release its recommendations early next year. The report should receive wide publicity when it is issued.

We look forward to receiving your completed materials.

Sincerely,

Jerome P. Lysaught
Director

JPL/jd

Form R-7A (Sheet 2)

(Name of Organization)

NATIONAL COMMISSION FOR THE STUDY OF NURSING AND NURSING EDUCATION

This study has been divided into three parts: Study Area A — The Nursing Role, Study Area B — Nursing Education, and Study Area C — Nursing Careers. Questions, which we and our advisors believe are addressed to the important issues in each area, are followed by a listing of sources for data, and then by the findings we think are indicated by the data. This booklet contains a total of 119 findings.

We would like you to review the questions and findings and then, on the enclosed answer sheet, indicate the extent of your organization's agreement with each finding. If you have a comment or suggestion concerning a question or finding, please identify it by number and enter the comment at the bottom of the page on which the finding appears.

DIRECTIONS

On the answer sheet, print the name of your organization in the space after NAME. Do *not* supply any of the other information requested. Print the name of your organization on the line provided at the top of this page of the booklet.

As you read each probable finding in the booklet, blacken the appropriate space on the answer sheet as follows:

        A — Strongly Agree

        B — Agree

        C — No Opinion

        D — Disagree

        E — Strongly Disagree

DIRECTIONS FOR USING ANSWER SHEET

In marking your answers on the answer sheet, make sure that the number of the probable finding is the same as the number on the answer sheet. Please read and follow the directions at the top of the answer sheet. Be sure to use a No. 2½ or softer writing pencil. Avoid using ball point or ink.

Form R-7B

Study Area A: The Nursing Role

QUESTION 1

In the field of health care, certain major trends in caring for patients are discernible. For example, there is increasing emphasis on routine examinations, rehabilitation, health screening, and comprehensive care. How will these trends affect future roles of nursing personnel?

A. *Sources for Data:*

1. Visits to selected locations; 2. Literature: *Journal of Medical Education*, 4/68; *1965 New York Academy of Medicine Conference Proceedings; Journal of Public Health*, 9/68; *Bulletin New York Academy of Medicine*, 2/68; 3. Reports: *Health is a Community Affair; Technology and Manpower in the Health Service Industry 1965–75; National Advisory Commission on Health Manpower*, Vols. I & II; *ANA-AMA Conference Proceedings 1964, 1965.*

B. *Probable Findings:*

LEGEND

> A — Strongly Agree
> B — Agree
> C — No Opinion
> D — Disagree
> E — Strongly Disagree

1. The computer and related technological innovations will be used in the performance of almost all "routine" work, including parts of various measurements such as "vital signs;" recording, such as charting, EKGs; etc. As technological advances are incorporated into health care, nurses will increasingly concentrate on aspects of care which are unsuitable for automation. Examples are fostering attitudes conducive to recuperation in patients and overseeing complex rehabilitation regimens.

2. In almost all settings nurses will work as members of teams.

3. Consumer and social demands will require more comprehensive, less wasteful care.

4. Consumer needs will require additional emphasis on specialization in nursing. Some of the specialties might be health teaching and counselling, family health, health service coordination, etc.

5. Advances in communications will more quickly provide information about the patient's condition and access to knowledge dealing with applicable treatment. This speedup might allow more personal contact between health care personnel and patient.

6. Government (at all levels) will employ more and more health personnel. It will become more deeply involved in planning application of resources, and setting standards for the delivery of patient care.

Comments:

QUESTION 2

Future patterns of health care delivery and changing health care settings will require nursing personnel to function in some ways that differ from existing practice. What demands will arise for individual clinical performance in care and treatment; for participating with other health personnel; for coordination and administration of health services?

A. *Sources for Data:*

1. Visits to selected locations; 2. Literature: *The Nursing Profession* (Davis); Nursing, Medical, Hospital, and Health Journals; 3. Video-tapes from innovative locations; 4. Training materials; Nursing Care Plans, Hospital Research and Educational Trust; 5. Reports: *Health is a Community Affair; Program Review Report, Nurse Training Act 1964; ANA-AMA Joint Conferences* 1964, 1965.

B. *Probable Findings:*

LEGEND

> A — Strongly Agree
> B — Agree
> C — No Opinion
> D — Disagree
> E — Strongly Disagree

Nurses will:

7. Increase their capabilities for the care of the critically ill—cardiac, organ transplants, implants, "life-death" situations.

8. Devote more resources than previously to "total family" mental and physical health maintenance.

9. Increase emphasis on nurse leadership of health teams in other than critical illness situations.

10. Develop team and skill methods, as well as technology, to eliminate practice that is uneconomical.

11. Increase coordination of technology and personal observation; this improvement in coordination will enable nurses to more precisely assess a patient's state of health.

12. In future health care settings, develop capabilities and specializations different from current practice.

Comments:

Form R-7B (Sheet 3)

QUESTION 3

What physiological, psychological, and sociological capabilities and aptitudes will nursing personnel need if they are to successfully carry out future responsibilities and functions?

A. *Sources for Data*

1. Visits to selected locations; 2. Literature: *The Nursing Profession,* Davis; *American Journal of Nursing; Nursing Research; Nursing Outlook;* 3. Reports: *Quality of Nursing Care,* F. Reiter 1963; NLN, Assessing Nursing Service in Long Term Care Facilities; etc.

B. *Probable Findings*

LEGEND

   A — Strongly Agree
   B — Agree
   C — No Opinion
   D — Disagree

E — Strongly Disagree

Nurses will demonstrate:

13. Improved integration of physical care and psychological assurance.

14. Increased capability to deal with the psychological problems caused in patients and their families by impending death, dismemberment, and disfigurement.

15. Ability to use computers and other technological tools in the delivery of improved patient care.

16. Greater willingness to intercede on behalf of the patient if institutions and doctors fail to provide needed care.

17. Ability to provide care for groups of patients in the patients' environment, not just in health facilities, while maintaining adequate standards of safety and quality.

Comments:

Form R-7B (Sheet 4)

QUESTION 4

Will the skills and capabilities required of nurses also be displayed by other health care personnel? What skills and capabilities will nurses alone possess? Are there important nursing skills and capabilities attainable by women but not by men?

A. *Sources for Data:*

1. Visits to selected locations; 2. Literature: Doctoral Dissertation—Rodney F. White; 3. Reports: *Williamsburg Conference on Virginia's Nursing Problems,* 3/68; 4. *Conference on Manpower for Medical Laboratory,* 10/67; 5. Occupational studies prepared as basis of position descriptions used by Government and Military Services.

B. *Probable Findings:*

LEGEND

    A — Strongly Agree

    B — Agree

    C — No Opinion

    D — Disagree

    E — Strongly Disagree

18. Nurses will share some skills and capabilities with other health care personnel.

19. In some instances, nurses will acquire capabilities which other health personnel will not possess.

20. Men will be able to perform most patient care as well as women.

Comments:

From R-7B (Sheet 5)

QUESTION 5

Will future patient care needs be better met if nursing is delineated into "professional" and "technical" practice?

A. *Sources for Data:*

1. Visits to selected locations; 2. Literature: *Sickness and Society* and background material; 3. Reports: *Proceedings of the New York Academy of Medicine,* 1968 Health Conference; 4. Research: *Nurse-Physician Teamwork,* Dr. Barbara Bates, 1966; etc.

B. *Probable Findings:*

LEGEND

A — Strongly Agree

B — Agree

C — No Opinion

D — Disagree

E — Strongly Disagree

21. Patient care by the individual nurse in a single setting often calls for the possession of a range of skill and knowledge extending from the use of "technical" procedures to the evaluative and decision-making capabilities implied by "professional."

22. "Professional" and "technical" are inadequate designations. Rather, there will be a range of capability levels, defined by the degree of skill and knowledge necessary to accomplish required patient care.

Comments:

Form R-7B (Sheet 6)

QUESTION 6

Can we foresee patient care needs which present trends may not meet, and to which nursing should direct its attention and efforts?

A. *Sources for Data:*

1. Visits to selected locations; 2. Reports; *Conference on Decision Parameters in Screening Large Populations,* 1968; *Health is a Community Affair; Proceedings of the New York Academy of Medicine Health Conferences* 1965 and 1968; 3. Research: *Nursing Attendant's Role in Mental Health*—Fuhrer; and other behavioral studies.

B. *Probable Findings:*

LEGEND

A — Strongly Agree

B — Agree

C — No Opinion

D — Disagree

E — Strongly Disagree

23. Patients who require less than acute but more than simple ambulatory treatment may in the future receive inadequate health care. Nurses can help ensure that the health needs of this group are met.

24. Because of a failure to identify their special needs, certain population groups, such as the aged and those who live in rural areas, may receive inadequate health care. Nurses can help minimize such lapses in the health care system.

Comments:

Form R-7B (Sheet 7)

QUESTION 7

To what extent do innovations in patient care influence the perception and evaluation of health care quality?

A. *Sources for Data:*

1. Visits to selected locations; 2. Literature: *Sickness and Society*, and background material; 3. Reports: 1958 Report to ANF, *Patient Relationship and Healing*—Whiting; *Quality of Nursing Care*, F. Reiter; 4. Research: *Nursing Attendant's Role in Mental Health*—Fuhrer; other behavioral studies.

B. *Probable Findings:*

LEGEND

> A — Strongly Agree
> B — Agree
> C — No Opinion
> D — Disagree

E — Strongly Disagree

25. Patients' evaluation of care quality is in most cases only slightly influenced by the fact that the care received incorporated innovative practices. Most patients lack the opportunity to contrast care before and after the introduction of an innovation.

26. Innovations in patient care can have a strongly positive influence on the evaluation of care quality by health professionals. Among the innovations exerting an affirmative influence are those concerned with:

> A. Expanded or changed roles for personnel.
> B. Use of teams to provide patient care.
> C. Application of advanced or more sophisticated methods and techniques.

Comments:

QUESTION 8

What kinds of patient care innovations and what kinds of institutional settings are most likely to make major contributions to the quality of health care in the future?

A. *Sources for Data:*

1. Visits to selected locations; 2. Reports: *Health Manpower —Perspective 1967, Proceedings of the New York Academy of Medicine Health Conferences 1965 and 1968;* 3. Manuals: U. S. Army; Office of the Surgeon General, *Enlisted Medical Occupational Specialty Training;* and others.

B. *Probable Findings:*

LEGEND

> A — Strongly Agree
> B — Agree
> C — No Opinion
> D — Disagree
> E — Strongly Disagree

27. Innovations are possible in almost any setting.

28. Innovations most likely to make major contributions will arise in settings other than those found in the traditional health care field. For example, community health care clinics evolved through O.E.O.; the Kaiser plan was instituted through the efforts of labor unions; important rehabilitation advances have come from insurance industry efforts to rehabilitate disabled workers, thereby reducing the length of time benefits must be paid.

29. Public agencies' financial and research support will favor innovations which affect mass health care and involve non-profit and/or public organizations.

30. The acceptance of innovations sometimes depends upon factors only remotely connected with or even distinct from the innovation. For example, established health agencies may organize new services less to meet apparent needs than to prevent non-health organizations from entering the field.

Comments:

Form R-7B (Sheet 9)

QUESTION 9

What differences exist between institutional statements about nursing care and actual practice? If actual practice varies from stated procedures and goals, and results in patient care of lower quality than institutional statements would indicate, how can practice be brought into closer accord with these statements?

A. *Sources for Data:*

1. Visits to selected locations; 2. Manuals: *Standards for the Nurse,* Series GS610, U. S. Civil Service Commission 5/68; 3. Reports: "Management Evaluation of Nursing Services," AHA Conference Report 1968.

B. *Probable Findings:*

LEGEND

A — Strongly Agree

B — Agree

C — No Opinion

D — Disagree

E — Strongly Disagree

31. Institutional statements concerning nursing care are generalized and represent ideals toward which actual practice is expected to strive.

32. In the future, even though nursing care improves in quality, a gap will continue to exist between institutional statements about nursing care and actual practice, because statements will continue to express an ever higher goal in patient care.

33. Researchers are studying in detail the effect on the patient of the various elements of care subsumed under nursing. As knowledge of this kind increases, institutional statements such as job descriptions and procedural manuals will become more specific. Thus these statements about nursing may in the future vary less than currently from actual practice.

Comments:

Form R-7B (Sheet 10)

QUESTION 10

Do institutional requirements for nursing, such as administrative and "hotel" functions, inhibit the introduction of innovations designed to improve patient care? How can administrators ensure that an innovation which enhances patient care is incorporated quickly and efficiently into current practice?

A. *Sources for Data:*

1. Visits to selected locations; 2. Reports: *National Advisory Commission on Health Manpower*, Vol. I, 1967; Proceedings of the AHA meeting, 1968; 3. Position Paper: "Toward a New Politics and Economics of Health," Institute for Policy Studies, 1968.

B. *Probable Findings:*

LEGEND

        A — Strongly Agree

        B — Agree

        C — No Opinion

        D — Disagree

        E — Strongly Disagree

34. Currently, nursing personnel are expected by various institutions to perform many functions in addition to direct patient care. For the most part, these are administrative and "hotel" functions, but may include medical, laboratory, and pharmaceutical as well. These additional functions often receive priority over caring for patients because they have to be undertaken to "keep things going." Moreover, the institutional system rewards accomplishment in these areas more liberally than accomplishment in patient care.

35. If nurses and health institutions do not take the initiative in introducing changes to meet public expectations for improved patient care, public agencies will establish standards and enforce them.

36. Patient care innovations judged of value by health administrators will be quickly incorporated into nursing practice by greater use of on-the-job training. Institutions will also enroll nurses in formal nursing education programs to learn the skills required to apply innovations.

Comments:

Form R-7B (Sheet 11)

Study Area B: Nursing Education

QUESTION 1

What are the discernible trends in the institutional patterns for the preparation of nurses? Which educational institutions, or groupings of institutions, will be changing? What will be the nature of those changes?

A. *Sources for Data:*

1. Literature (Montag, Brown, Roberts, etc.); 2. ANA Position Paper and Published Reactions; 3. Educational Reports and Statements (ANA, NLN, AMA, AHA, AAJC, Joint Committees, etc.); 4. Nursing Advisory Panel; 5. Commissioners; 6. Visits to selected locations; 7. Reports *(National Advisory Commission on Health Manpower*, Vol. I & II, *Health Manpower Perspective 1967*, State Studies on Nursing Education); and 8. Special Analysis (Altman Report).

B. *Probable Findings:*

LEGEND

> A — Strongly Agree
> B — Agree
> C — No Opinion
> D — Disagree
> E — Strongly Disagree

37. The number of hospital schools of nursing will continue to be reduced for a combination of economic, social, and educational reasons.

38. The larger and stronger hospital schools will work out cooperative programs with institutions of higher education.

39. The greatest growth among institutions will be that of the community/junior college with more of them becoming engaged in the health field.

40. Many community/junior college programs presently lack satisfactory clinical training for their students.

41. Current and projected figures indicate that the combined output (graduates) of all institutions will be inadequate to meet the demand for nursing services.

42. Little in the way of "revolutionary" institutional change seems likely.

43. Many hospital schools of nursing will reduce the length of their program from three to two and one-half years or two years to meet the competition of community/junior colleges.

44. Hospitals and other health care facilities must assume responsibility for extended orientation and on-the-job training programs for first-time nurse employees.

Comments:

Form R-7B (Sheet 12)

QUESTION 2

What are the most pressing problems and needs currently of nursing preparatory institutions? What are short-term and long-term answers to these needs?

A. *Sources for Data:*

1. Commission Questionnaire to 1,250 institutions and heads of programs; 2. Literature (NLN, ANA, and AHA reports and publications); 3. Reports *(National Advisory Commission on Health Manpower,* Vol. I & II, *Surgeon General's Commission Report of 1963,* etc.); 4. *Nurse Training Act* Report; 5. Nursing Advisory Panel; 6. Commissioners; 7. Visits to selected locations; 8. Faculty Questionnaire developed by Commission staff.

B. *Probable Findings:*

LEGEND

         A — Strongly Agree

         B — Agree

         C — No Opinion

         D — Disagree

         E — Strongly Disagree

45. Probably the single most pressing need is for qualified faculty—with no quick or easy solution in sight.

46. Finances rate a close second. Nursing schools are distinguished by lack of endowment, high costs in comparison to many other institutions (arts and science, for example).

47. Other problems include: lack (and geographic maldistribution) of qualified student applicants; hospital schools unfilled; some other schools having to turn away qualified students.

Comments:

Form R-7B (Sheet 13)

QUESTION 3

What are the strengths, weaknesses and trends among nursing faculty?

A. *Sources for Data:*

1. *Facts About Nursing;* 2. General Literature (Montag, Brown, etc.); 3. *Report of the Health Manpower Commission;* 4. *Review of Nurse Training Act;* 5. Faculty Questionnaire developed by the Commission staff; 6. Nursing School Environment Inventory Questionnaire employed by Commission staff; 7. State studies on Nursing Education; 8. NIH Study Group Proceedings.

B. *Probable Findings:*

LEGEND

> A — Strongly Agree
>
> B — Agree
>
> C — No Opinion
>
> D — Disagree
>
> E — Strongly Disagree

Comments:

48. Over one out of five faculty members do not have a college degree.

49. Over three out of five have no better than baccalaureate preparation.

50. Graduate institutions that prepare nursing faculty are restricted in number and most frequently their programs are aimed at limited educational objectives, such as nursing education or administration.

51. The most dynamic growth in graduate programs is that in clinical specialization. These clinical programs are vying strongly for a small pool of competent faculty.

52. Most nurse faculty members lack research competence.

53. There is little experimentation in applying innovative changes in teaching methodology.

Form R-7B (Sheet 14)

QUESTION 4

What changes are taking place among the body of nursing students in terms of academic excellence, differing socio-economic-racial background, etc? How will these changes affect institutions educating nurses in the future?

A. *Sources for Data:*

1. Professional organizations (ANA, NLN, Student Nurses Association); 2. Commission questionnaire to students; 3. Questionnaires to preparatory institutions; 4. Nursing Advisory Panel; 5. State studies on nursing education and student recruitment; 6. On-site visits to *all* educational institutions being visited for any purpose.

B. *Probable Findings:*

LEGEND

> A — Strongly Agree
> B — Agree
> C — No Opinion
> D — Disagree
> E — Strongly Disagree

54. A wider range of socio-economic groups is being drawn into nursing with students from the upper middle class entering collegiate programs and disadvantaged students being more actively recruited at all levels.

55. In the future, nursing students will demonstrate slightly higher completion and retention rates, but the proportion of high school students entering nursing will decrease.

56. Student unrest and discontent with many of the traditional institutions and programs will become manifest.

57. There will be sharp differentiation in job placement among graduates of different preparatory programs.

Comments:

Form R-7B (Sheet 15)

QUESTION 5

What changes are taking place in, or are being recommended for, the nursing curriculum?

A. *Sources for Data:*

1. On-site visits to those educational institutions identified for us by the Nursing Advisory Panel, the Commissioners, and other consultants as schools representative of the best in both traditional and changing curricula; 2. Questionnaires specially developed for those institutions indicated by one or more of the groups in 1 above (but not a unanimous choice) to determine what changes are taking place; 3. The recommendations of the various state studies that have attempted to assess what should be changed in the curriculum; 4. Analyses of the literature and current recommendations of the professional bodies; 5. Papers presented at NLN Council of Baccalaureate and Higher Degree Programs, 1968.

B. *Probable Findings:*

LEGEND

> A — Strongly Agree
> B — Agree
> C — No Opinion
> D — Disagree
> E — Strongly Disagree

58. Few institutions are involved in large-scale curriculum changes. Moreover, in general, such innovations are relatively uncontrolled for purposes of measurement and evaluation.

59. One rather clear trend, however, is an increase in the number and quality of programs preparing students for the role of nurse clinician. These programs are more patient centered than some that seem designed to prepare their graduates for education or administration.

60. A few graduate schools are beginning to introduce research methods and basic statistics into the curriculum. Graduates of these programs will have received some preparation for research as well as the knowledge needed to measure and evaluate innovations which may be introduced at the institution which eventually employs them.

61. A few schools are developing programs that take into account differences in preparation and learning capacity among students.

Comments:

QUESTION 6

What are the trends in financing of nursing education?

A. *Sources for Data:*

1. U.S. Office of Education surveys of finance of higher education published under various titles; 2. Flitter and Rowe, *Study on Cost of Nursing Education;* 3. U.S. Public Health Service unpublished data on institutional finances; 4. Published data on expenditures in medical and dental education and other professional fields.

B. *Probable Findings:*

LEGEND

        A — Strongly Agree

        B — Agree

        C — No Opinion

        D — Disagree

        E — Strongly Disagree

62. As evidenced by the growth of nursing programs in junior colleges and colleges, the public is sufficiently aware of the need for nurses to allocate public funds to nursing education as the transition continues from hospital schools to educational institutions.

63. The public will continue to respond favorably to growing support for nursing education through broad based community taxation as opposed to the "user's tax" which is present in hospital diploma programs.

64. Diploma school educational resources represent a significant portion of current investment in nursing education. All planning for future education should take these resources into account.

65. The endowment and general foundation support of nursing education is low. These factors inhibit the entry of private colleges into this field and explain the withdrawal of several from nursing education.

66. Increased financial support to both institutions and to individuals (students, faculty members, researchers, etc.) is necessary if nursing education is to meet the demands placed upon it.

Comments:

QUESTION 7

What changes are taking place in other "health schools" that will affect the future of nursing education?

A. *Sources for Data:*

1. Reports and liaison with the Association of Allied Health Schools; 2. Reports and liaison with the Association of American Junior Colleges; 3. Other professional organizations and associations (e.g., Medical Technology and its Back to Work Educational Program); 4. Council on Medical Education of the AMA; 5. Association of American Medical Colleges; 6. Health Advisory Panel and Commissioners.

B. *Probable Findings:*

LEGEND

A — Strongly Agree

B — Agree

C — No Opinion

D — Disagree

E — Strongly Disagree

67. Some allied health schools will attempt to subsume the preparation of nurse practitioners.

68. Most attempts at the development of a core curriculum in the health sciences have been unsuccessful.

69. Community/junior colleges are becoming more independent and self-directed in their development of health curricula.

Comments:

QUESTION 8

What are the needs for advanced (either graduate or specialized) education in nursing?

A. *Sources for Data:*

1. Nursing Advisory Panel and Commissioners; 2. On-site visits to those educational institutions offering (or planning to offer) advanced programs in nursing; 3. Reports on state studies and recommendations in the *Report on Health Manpower* and other federal publications; 4. Review of current literature from the professional organizations; 5. Faculty questionnaire developed by Commission staff; 6. Health Professions Advisory Panel.

B. *Probable Findings:*

LEGEND

> A — Strongly Agree
> B — Agree

C — No Opinion

D — Disagree

E — Strongly Disagree

70. Advanced education is among the most critical needs in all nursing.

71. Qualified faculty to staff graduate programs (for example doctoral holders with research competence) are well-nigh unobtainable.

72. There is an imperative need for advanced clinical education.

73. Institutions offering advanced education in nursing lack adequate financial resources. Financial aid to these institutions and to their students is insufficient to meet requirements.

Comments:

Form R-7B (Sheet 19)

QUESTION 9

What are the needs for continuing and in-service education in nursing in order to provide for up-dating and up-grading?

A. *Sources for Data:*

1. On-site visits to both educational and service institutions—particularly the latter that are developing new procedures and requirements for nursing service that will become the focal point for in-service education; 2. Nursing Advisory Panel and Commissioners; 3. Current literature and reports on retention and retraining of nurses.

B. *Probable Findings:*

LEGEND

A — Strongly Agree

B — Agree

C — No Opinion

D — Disagree

E — Strongly Disagree

74. New aspects of health care and delivery are going to increase the variety and rapidity of in-service edu-cation.

75. Social change and technological advances will place increased emphasis on continuing education.

76. The need for increased numbers of qualified "faculty" for in-service education will likely be greater than the current number of faculty engaged in hospital schools of nursing. Shortages will be even more ex-aggerated.

77. Colleges and universities will expand and/or establish continuing education centers for professional nurses.

78. Employers do not expect the nurse to assume per-sonal responsibility for her own development of exper-tise.

79. Developments in educational technology and the availability of individualized instructional material will afford nurses new and less formal opportunities to up-date their knowledge and skills.

Comments:

Form R-7B (Sheet 20)

Study Area C: Nursing Careers

QUESTION 1

What general economic factors are influencing the development of the nurse's functions? What is the significance of these factors for manpower planning?

A. *Sources for Data:*

Toward Quality in Nursing; Nurse Training Act Review; Report of the Health Manpower Commission; Technology and Health Manpower; Facts About Nursing; 1967; Health Manpower 1966–1975; National Conference on Medical Costs Report; Medical Care Prices — A Report to the President from HEW; Hospital Effectiveness Report; Medicare and the Hospitals. Yett, "Yes, Virginia, There Is a Shortage of Nurses — But It's Not Quite So Simple as That." Journal articles. State studies of nurse manpower and staffing. Review of experimental staffing patterns in selected health institutions.

B. *Probable Findings:*

LEGEND

> A — Strongly Agree
>
> B — Agree
>
> C — No Opinion
>
> D — Disagree
>
> E — Strongly Disagree

80. It appears that two major economic factors are influencing nursing functions: a recurrent manpower shortage and a rising level of salaries.

81. These factors are causing health service agencies to substitute less well trained personnel for registered nurses and to place the registered nurses increasingly in leadership positions.

82. Manpower planning generally, and personnel practice in health agencies specifically, must recognize the need for several levels of nursing personnel broadly falling into two categories: 1) highly competent persons to provide leadership (generally identified as clinical specialists, teachers, researchers, or administrators), educated at the baccalaureate and higher levels; 2) the quantitatively larger number of persons to provide direct personal care, educated through associate degree, diploma, or other nurse training programs.

Comments:

QUESTION 2

What factors appear to be of central importance in understanding the problem of the supply of nurses?

A. *Sources for Data:*

Report of the Health Manpower Commission; Health Manpower 1966–1975; CASH studies of hospital management; Veteran's Administration Division of Management Systems Studies; *Nursing in Illinois;* site visits to institutions with excellent recruitment and retention programs.

B. *Probable Findings:*

LEGEND

> A — Strongly Agree
> B — Agree
> C — No Opinion
> D — Disagree
> E — Strongly Disagree

83. Effective utilization of nurses is essential in providing the volume of nursing care needed in the future. It is even possible that automation combined with sound management may reduce the proportion of nurses in relation to the volume of nursing service to be delivered.

84. The analysis of the nurse manpower situation by the Health Manpower Commission suggests that proportionately fewer nurses will be available in the future to provide a larger volume of health care. Consequent to such a probability is a critical need to advance the quality of nursing practice, and a need for sound management and training of substitute personnel. Both depend on the preparation of an adequate supply of leaders in nursing.

85. Successful recruitment and retention programs do not depend on one or two solutions alone, but rather on a complex of programs developed at national and regional levels, and within individual institutions.

86. The high rate of turnover in nursing and vast number of inactive nurses are not simply a product of the dominantly feminine composition of the profession and low wages resulting from the absence of normal market forces in the non-profit setting. Rather, they result, in large measure, from treating the nurse role as subservient, routine, and somewhat trivial.

Comments:

QUESTION 3

Are there enough spaces in colleges and universities to prepare the number of highly educated nurses needed in the future? Would the establishment of a post-baccalaureate program for nursing (similar to the MAT or MBA) attract liberal arts graduates into nursing?

A. *Sources for Data:*

National League for Nursing, *State Approved Schools of Professional Nursing;* state surveys and reports on nursing education resources; *Toward Quality in Nursing; Report of the Health Manpower Commission; Facts About Nursing; Manpower Resources in Hospitals; Health Manpower Perspective, 1967; Health Manpower 1966–75.* Letter survey of sample of deans in coeducational and women's colleges regarding choice of nursing for postgraduate study if an MAT type program were available.

B. *Probable Findings:*

LEGEND

A — Strongly Agree

B — Agree

C — No Opinion

D — Disagree

E — Strongly Disagree

87. In spite of vacancies in some baccalaureate programs in nursing, there is a need to expand the capacity of such programs to supply a sufficient number of persons trained at this level.

88. Women college graduates in the liberal arts, including mature women able to enter the labor force, now represent a vast, practically untapped, reservoir of potential recruits for nursing. Masters level programs in clinical nursing similar to the MAT in teaching or MBA in business would prove attractive to such persons.

89. The National League for Nursing would accredit such programs, and one such program has been approved.

Comments:

QUESTION 4

Do the manpower requirements for nursing personnel dictate that the diploma schools be retained and continue to provide graduates to fill nursing positions?

A. *Sources for Data:*

National League for Nursing, *State Approved Schools of Professional Nursing;* state studies of nurse manpower resources and educational resources; *Toward Quality in Nursing; Report of the Health Manpower Commission; Facts About Nursing; Manpower Resources in Hospitals; Health Manpower Perspective, 1967; Health Manpower 1966–1975;* ANA, "A Position Paper."

B. *Probable Findings:*

LEGEND

        A — Strongly Agree

        B — Agree

C — No Opinion

D — Disagree

E — Strongly Disagree

90. Despite the trend for diploma schools to close or merge with colleges, the diploma schools operated by hospitals will continue to play a significant part over the next five to ten years in educating the number of nurses required.

91. Even after diploma schools have ceased to play an important role in producing nurse manpower, the experience and educational resources of hospitals will prove to be valuable assets in providing a setting both for clinical instruction of nursing students and for in-service education.

Comments:

QUESTION 5

Does the need in American society for upward mobility require the organization of a career ladder for advancement within nursing? Should nursing education serve as a ladder to permit advancement from one level to another?

A. *Sources for Data:*

Center for the Conservation of Human Resources publications; journal articles and conference proceedings.

B. *Probable Findings:*

LEGEND

> A — Strongly Agree
> B — Agree
> C — No Opinion
> D — Disagree
> E — Strongly Disagree

92. In a full employment economy, opportunity for career advancement is essential to retain personnel.

93. Public policy implicit in current legislation and thinking on manpower calls for the opportunity for advancement from lowest to highest levels within a career. The presence of various capability levels within nursing provides an excellent setting for implementing public policy.

94. Career development within nursing provides for advancement primarily through entry into administration and teaching rather than through clinical practice or research relating to patient care.

95. Baccalaureate and higher degree programs have lacked adequate means for the recognition of lower levels of education and experience. This situation has caused excessively long periods of education for those who start on the bottom rung, and has discouraged upward mobility.

96. Development of a core curricuulm leading into various health careers could improve the possibilities for mobility.

97. Although nurses express no great desire to become physicians, the logic of the career ladder concept suggests that such an option should be available to them and to persons in other health disciplines.

Comments:

Form R-7B (Sheet 25)

QUESTION 6

Do the facts regarding career patterns of women, and nurses in particular, indicate that more men need to enter the field? Is the recruitment of men essential to provide a large enough pool of persons who can make the lifetime commitment necessary to attain the high levels of education and competence required by contemporary health service?

A. *Sources for Data:*

President's Commission on the Status of Women, *American Women;* Robson, *Sociological Factors Affecting Recruitment in Nursing;* Davis and others, *The Nursing Profession; Facts About Nursing;* Luther Christman, unpublished papers; Women's Bureau publications; interviews with nurse leaders and journal articles.

B. *Probable Findings:*

LEGEND

A — Strongly Agree
B — Agree
C — No Opinion
D — Disagree
E — Strongly Disagree

98. More men need to enter nursing, especially to enlarge the pool of persons who can make the long-term career commitments necessary to provide the number of leaders required in the field.

99. Men will enter nursing in increasing numbers as the salary and career advancement opportunities improve.

100. Nursing recruitment programs are not now designed to publicize career information about nursing for men and a male role in nursing, nor directed to military corpsmen, a likely target group.

Comments:

QUESTION 7

Should advanced levels of nursing practice be recognized in state licensing laws by setting requirements above the RN; or is the Academy of Nursing the proper agency to recognize these levels of practice?

Should licensing laws be so designed as to require persons who hold the RN to complete the bachelor's degree?

Should such laws require reexamination for renewal of licensure?

A. *Sources for Data:*

Lesnik and Anderson, *Nursing Practice and the Law;* Sarner, *The Nurse and the Law; Facts About Nursing;* issue of *Nursing Clinics of North America* on "The Nurse and the Law;" "Regan Report on Nursing Law;" Nathan Hershey, articles published in various journals and conference proceedings; personal interviews with leaders in nursing.

B. *Probable Findings:*

LEGEND

> A — Strongly Agree
>
> B — Agree

C — No Opinion

D — Disagree

E — Strongly Disagree

101. It is unlikely that opinion within major health professions or public opinion will support more special licensing. Therefore, the Academy of Nursing will develop as a major avenue for recognition of advanced levels of nursing practice.

102. Other professions, notably teaching, have brought about phased improvement of practitioners over a period of years through raising educational requirements. A similar pattern might have broad appeal in nursing.

103. Nurses need not show evidence of continuing study and self-improvement to renew their licenses to practice. Whether or not evidence of continuing study should be required for relicensure is an issue before all health professions. Such a requirement can be viewed as an important factor in improving the quality of nursing care.

Comments:

Form R-7B (Sheet 27)

QUESTION 8

Are there indications that medicine will recognize an increasingly scientific content and rising level of specialization in the role of the nurse?

A. *Sources for Data:*

   Sickness and Society; articles in medical publications; interviews with leaders in organized medicine; publications and conference proceedings of the AMA Committee on Nursing; reports of state nurse-physician liaison committees.

B. *Probable Findings:*

LEGEND

> A — Strongly Agree
> B — Agree
> C — No Opinion
> D — Disagree
> E — Strongly Disagree

104. Organized medicine is seeking to develop collaborative relationships with other autonomous health professions with respect to setting standards of education and accreditation, and in defining roles.

105. From the point of view of nursing, such a relationship might be desirable if it were founded on a colleagal association involving understanding of the nature of nursing functions, medical support for efforts to improve the quality of nursing care in hospitals, and recognition of the capacity of nurses to perform sophisticated roles, as in well-child care and care of the chronically ill.

106. Both within organized medicine and among individual practitioners there is understanding of nursing functions and some sentiment in favor of a significantly more sophisticated role for well educated nurses. This suggests that a colleagal association can be established if the case for it is properly made.

Comments:

QUESTION 9

What effect has accreditation had on nursing education and manpower?

The Health Manpower Training Act of 1968 modified previous legislation to provide that agencies other than the NLN may accredit nursing education programs for the purpose of qualifying for federal funds. What impact will this change have on the development of the nurse's role?

A. *Sources for Data:*

Interviews with nursing leaders and leaders in other health professions and institutions.

B. *Probable Findings:*

LEGEND

> A — Strongly Agree
> B — Agree
> C — No Opinion
> D — Disagree

E — Strongly Disagree

107. It is generally recognized that accreditation in nursing education has substantially improved the quality of programs, particularly in eliminating the performance of nursing service by students under the name of education.

108. Generalizations regarding the deleterious effect of accreditation on the supply of nurses cannot be supported, inasmuch as a whole complex of social factors, including the enlarged range of occupational choice and educational opportunity available to women, are the determinants of the supply.

109. The growing demand for health service, and the increasing sophistication and rising salaries of personnel are irreversible trends forcing the elevation of the nurse role. Consequently, standards for the accreditation of education programs will reflect the rising level of nursing practice no matter what agency is responsible for accreditation.

Comments:

Form R-7B (Sheet 29)

QUESTION 10

Is there an arena for resolving issues concerning preparation and utilization of health personnel that arise between consumers and providers of health service?

A. *Sources for Data:*

Interviews with leaders in the health field; observation of trends in comprehensive health care planning and consumer representation.

B. *Probable Findings:*

LEGEND

A — Strongly Agree

B — Agree

C — No Opinion

D — Disagree

E — Strongly Disagree

110. Consumers are in the process of building representation through health insurance plans, third party contractors, federal departments and agencies, comprehensive health planning agencies, and Congress. However, the arena for resolving issues of preparation and utilization of health personnel that arise between consumers and providers of health service is not fully formed.

111. Given a shortage of nurses, consumer demand for more health services tends to force the most highly trained nurses into leadership positions. In view of these circumstances, the consumer's influence on the preparation and utilization of nurses is now at most only indirect. However, the consumer may become a more direct force in delineating the nurse role as he becomes better organized and obtains a greater voice in planning and policy making.

Comments:

Form R-7B (Sheet 30)

QUESTION 11

What are the implications for the nurse role of current struggles (among community groups, levels of government) for control of various elements within the health field?

A. *Sources for Data:*

Interviews with leaders in the health field.

B. *Probable Findings:*

LEGEND

        A — Strongly Agree

        B — Agree

        C — No Opinion

D — Disagree

E — Strongly Disagree

112. If these struggles result in the organization of new kinds of services (such as hospital outreach clinics), they will very likely broaden and deepen the nurse role, because personnel will have to develop the levels of competence required to staff such services.

113. Recent Congressional programs have provided funds for programs that would tend to develop advanced levels of the nurse role. Foundations that are knowledgeable about nursing appear to recognize a need for specialization and for increasing the scientific content of nursing.

Comments:

QUESTION 12

What part do hospital administrators play in defining and influencing the role of the nurse; and, what arguments will convince them of the value of allowing nurses to function at more complex levels?

A. *Sources for Data:*

Interviews with American Hospital Association leaders and with selected hospital administrators. Journal articles on hospital organization.

B. *Probable Findings:*

LEGEND

> A — Strongly Agree
>
> B — Agree

C — No Opinion

D — Disagree

E — Strongly Disagree

114. Hospital administrators have had and will continue to have very considerable influence over the role of the nurse in view of their responsibility for designing the overall system for operation of the institution and for securing the personnel required.

115. Hospital administrators will recognize the value of a sophisticated role for the nurse when they can observe it, as in the case of highly qualified nursing personnel in coronary and intensive care units, as contributing to the effective and economic operation of the institution.

Comments:

QUESTION 13

What role can nursing play in the control of health care costs?

A. *Sources for Data:*

Research studies documenting the effect of nursing practice on improvements in health; review of patient data in the course of site visits.

B. *Probable Findings:*

LEGEND

> A — Strongly Agree
> B — Agree
> C — No Opinion
> D — Disagree
> E — Strongly Disagree

116. Excellence in nursing practice contributes to the prevention of illness, and reduces readmissions and the average length of stay of patients in hospitals. These factors contribute importantly to control of costs.

117. Nurses can contribute to cost control through improvement in the utilization of personnel. New developments in this respect have been the participation of nurses in management research designed to assess the levels of nursing competence required to treat patients with different conditions; a growing consciousness among nurses of the need for systematic allocation of assignments in the nursing team in accord with levels of competence.

118. It has been demonstrated that with proper experience and education nurses can assume expanded roles in such areas as the treatment of ordinary childhood illnesses and management of chronic illness and the aged. Assumption of such roles by nurses contributes to better utilization of personnel than if the highly trained talents of physicians are used to perform them, and therefore acts as a control on cost.

119. Nurses have contributed to cost saving by developing new and more efficient methods for performing treatments and procedures.

Comments:

Form R-7B (Sheet 33)